KU-713-916

Computed Tomography
of the Gastrointestinal Tract

Computed Tomography
of the Gastrointestinal Tract

Edited by

ALEC J. MEGIBOW, M.D.

Associate Professor of Radiology
New York University Medical Center;
Chief, Body CT and Gastrointestinal Radiology
University Hospital
New York, New York

EMIL J. BALTHAZAR, M.D.

Professor of Radiology
New York University Medical Center;
Director of Abdominal Imaging
Bellevue Hospital
New York, New York

*With **672** illustrations*

The C. V. Mosby Company

ST. LOUIS • TORONTO   1986

MOSBY

A TRADITION OF PUBLISHING EXCELLENCE

Editor: Carol Trumbold
Assistant editor: Anne Gunter
Project editor: Barbara Merritt
Editing and Production: Patricia Gayle May
Book design: John Rokusek

Copyright © 1986 by The C.V. Mosby Company

All rights reserved. No part of this publication may be reproduced, stored in a retrieval system, or transmitted, in any form or by any means, electronic, mechanical, photocopying, recording, or otherwise, without prior written permission from the publisher.

Printed in the United States of America

The C.V. Mosby Company
11830 Westline Industrial Drive, St. Louis, Missouri 63146

Library of Congress Cataloging-in-Publication Data

Computed tomography of the gastrointestinal tract.

  Includes bibliographies and index.
  1. Gastrointestinal system—Radiography.
2. Tomography. 3. Gastrointestinal system—Diseases—Diagnosis. I. Megibow, Alec J. II. Balthazar, Emil J.
[DNLM: 1. Gastrointestinal System—radiography.
2. Tomography, X-Ray Computed. WI 141 C738]
RC804.T65C66 1986   616.3'3'07572   86-8489
ISBN 0-8016-3376-1

AC/MV/MV 9 8 7 6 5 4 3 2 1   01/A/050

CONTRIBUTORS

MICHAEL E. BERNARDINO, M.D.

Professor of Radiology
Chief of Abdominal Imaging
Emory University School of Medicine
Atlanta, Georgia

JEAN DeTOEUF, M.D.

Department of Gastrointestinal Radiology
Hopital Erasme, Cliniques Universitaires
de Bruxelles, Université Libre de
Bruxelles, Belgium

LOUIS ENGELHOLM, M.D.

Director of Gastrointestinal Radiology
Department of Gastrointestinal Radiology
Hopital Erasme, Cliniques Universitaires
de Bruxelles, Université Libre de
Bruxelles, Belgium

DONALD H. HULNICK, M.D.

Assistant Professor of Radiology
New York University Medical Center
New York, New York

DAVID P. NAIDICH, M.D.

Associate Professor of Radiology
New York University Medical Center
New York, New York

FABIENNE RICKAERT, M.D.

Department of Anatomical Pathology
Hopital Erasme, Cliniques Universitaires
de Bruxelles, Université Libre de
Bruxelles, Belgium

HARVEY V. STEINBERG, M.D.

Assistant Professor of Radiology
Emory University School of Medicine
Atlanta, Georgia

MARC ZALCMAN, M.D.

Department of Anatomical Pathology
Hopital Erasme, Cliniques Universitaires
de Bruxelles, Université Libre de
Bruxelles, Belgium

ELIAS A. ZERHOUNI, M.D.

Associate Professor of Radiology
Director of CT and MRI Research
Johns Hopkins Hospital
Baltimore, Maryland

Indeed, if a little knowledge is dangerous,
where is the man who has so much as to be out of danger?

Thomas Huxley (1825-1895)

Collected Essays

PREFACE

The discovery and recent technological advances in computed tomography have substantially changed the practice of radiology, including that of abdominal imaging. While the clinical use of computed tomography in the diagnosis of diseases involving solid viscera (liver, pancreas, spleen) and retroperitoneal organs was established and accepted early, its use in the gastrointestinal tract lagged behind in development. This is explained mainly by the poor quality images obtained from second generation scanners and by a lack of unified technique and coordinated effort to evaluate primary gastrointestinal lesions. The ability of the newer generation scanners to accurately assess the thickness of the bowel wall and to determine the existence and degree of extramural involvement has added a totally new dimension to our diagnostic proficiency.

As gastrointestinal radiologists by training and experience, we became interested in the appearances of gastrointestinal pathology on computed tomography and since 1980 started to rapidly accumulate material. In the summer of 1983, Dr. Elias A. Zerhouni, then of the De Paul Hospital in Norfolk, Virginia, introduced us to his work with air distention of the colon and gas insufflation of the stomach. This technique provides a uniform, simple, and reliable methodology to examine the stomach and colon. Aside from an accurate, reproducible method for examining the wall of the alimentary tract, improved contrast resolution provides a better appreciation of subtle findings in the perivisceral fat.

We like to underline however, that in spite of the high-quality images obtained today, computed tomography should be considered complimentary to conventional contrast examinations. It opens a totally new horizon and gives access to important clinical data inaccessible to conventional barium studies. Although confusion and controversy still exist in regard to the place of computed tomography in evaluating primary gastrointestinal lesions, a continuously enlarging body of evidence attests to its undeniable importance. We have attempted to allow the reader to form his or her own conclusions by providing correlations between barium images and computed tomograms.

Our intention in writing this book is to present in a comprehensive volume an up-to-date evaluation of the role, significance, indications, and limitations of computed tomography of the gastrointestinal tract. The first chapter on technique outlines our schedules for oral contrast administration as well as maneuvers utilized to optimize air contrast techniques. In the following chapters the computed tomographic findings of a large variety of gastrointestinal lesions, including their complications, are described and illustrated. In addition, a close correlation with barium studies and a complete review of the literature is provided. A chapter on percutaneous abscess drainage has been included to give the reader precise technical information and data base for referral of patients for this important procedure. Finally an atlas of radiographic-gross pathologic and microscopic correlations is provided to aid the reader in understanding the pathologic basis of radiographic abnormalities seen by CT. Most of our illustrations were made from images obtained on GE 9800 and 8800 scanners and selected from pathology material seen in our institution. They reflect the experience at NYU Medical Center in our extensive use of computed tomography in the evaluation of the gastrointestinal tract.

We believe that this book can be used effectively by the student in radiology, by the clinical radiologist, and by the gastroenterologist, general practitioner and general surgeon interested in selecting the most helpful and cost effective radiologic examination for the patient. Finally, we like to gratefully acknowledge the enthusiastic cooperation of our contributors, all of whom are very experienced in the field of abdominal CT.

Alec J. Megibow
Emil J. Balthazar

ACKNOWLEDGMENTS

We take this opportunity to recognize the contribution made by our technical staff who patiently and efficiently obtained high-quality images many times under difficult circumstances: Jim Bain, Norman McKinley, Elba Cardona, Derrick Smith, Ken Hardt, Eddie Lopez, Rudy Rosa, Lisa Salvatorelli, George Clinton, Brad Haspel, Vinnie Breen, Ron Simmons, Kathy Hughes, Tomi Brandt, Deborah Harrigan, Michael Harbeson, Gloria Agramonte, Regina Adamousky, Melvienee Gilyard, Ladislav Kamenar, and Carolyn Tyson. We are particularly thankful to our CT supervisors, Daniel Rivera, Bellevue Hospital CT; Barbara Coakley, University Hospital CT; and Irene Cleary, Faculty Practice Office CT, for their enthusiasm and willingness to adopt our evolving methods of examining patients. We are indebted to Jennie Lopez and Jane Crafts for typing the manuscript and to Martha Helmers and Stanley Willard for their professional photography work. Special appreciation and thanks are given to Dr. Richard V. Gordon for his cooperation and help in selecting interesting case material from our affiliated Veterans Administration Hospital. Lastly, we would like to thank the editorial staff of The C.V. Mosby Company, and specifically Carol Trumbold, for their skillful contribution and helpful suggestions needed for completion of this work. Dr. Alec Megibow would like to thank his wife, Marilyn, and his children, David and Matilda, for their support and patience.

CONTENTS

Computed Tomography
of the Gastrointestinal Tract

Chapter One

TECHNIQUES OF GASTROINTESTINAL COMPUTED TOMOGRAPHY

CLASSICAL TECHNIQUES

Alec J. Megibow

Successful interpretation of all computerized tomographic examinations requires accurate identification of normal anatomic structures enabling the confident recognition of pathological processes and masses. This principle applies to any computer tomography (CT) examination of the abdomen, regardless of indication. The sensitivity of CT diagnosis of gastrointestinal pathology is directly proportional to bowel opacification and distention. When a portion of the alimentary tube is adequately distended, the intestinal wall may be accurately assessed.

In 1978 Kressel outlined the advantages CT has over traditional imaging modalities for evaluation of the gastrointestinal tract. These include: (1) sharp, transverse tomographic images show the relationship of organs to the alimentary tube; (2) vessels, ducts, nodes, masses, cysts, ascites, blood, and hemorrhages can be seen rather than presenting as nonspecific displacements; (3) mesenteric fat can be easily imaged; and (4) the bowel wall itself can be seen.[1] These same advantages apply today. However, improved equipment, particularly the use of higher reconstruction matrices and fast scan times, has significantly improved spatial resolution to the point where these advantages can be more routinely realized.

Because thickening of the intestinal wall is the basic radiopathologic finding signifying disease, it is of the utmost importance to ensure that the apparently thickened portion of the bowel is in fact distended. This chapter focuses on the various oral contrast agents available to the radiologist for computed body tomography and schedules that will result in uniform, homogeneous bowel opacification. We consider special problems of opacifying each level of the alimentary tube. Finally we attempt to categorize special indications requiring modified oral contrast administration.

Oral contrast agents

Routine use of oral contrast agents was realized to be a necessary adjunct to all body CT examinations early in clinical experience with this method.[2,3,4] The ideal contrast agent has the capacity to accurately identify a given loop of bowel, be palatable and nontoxic, not produce artifacts, and should distribute evenly through the gut. In the segments in which it is not present as a bolus, it is hoped enough contrast agent residue would be present to identify the loop.

Two positive contrast agents are available; solutions of water-soluble, iodinated compounds or suspensions of barium sulfate. Both agents must be significantly diluted to prevent the production of streak artifacts. Commercial barium preparations are available in weights ranging from 1.2% to 2.0%.* Iodinated, water-soluble solutions are used at 2% to 3% concentrations in water. Early experience with USP barium sulfate at low concentrations was unsuccessful because of difficulties in maintaining the barium in suspension; therefore commercial preparations for CT scanning contain suspending agents that avoid flocculation and ensure homogeneous distribution in the bowel. When barium suspensions were initially developed

---

*E-Z CAT, Redi-CAT, manufactured by E-Z-EM Company, Westbury, New York; Tomo-CAT, manufactured by Lafayette Company, Indianapolis, Indiana; Baro-CAT, manufactured by Mallinkrodt, Inc., St. Louis, Missouri.

for CT, it was hoped that they would coat the intestinal mucosa thus being able to identify a bowel loop after the bolus had traversed that segment of the intestine. This hope has yet to be realized.[5,6] Thus relatively large amounts must be consumed before the examination to ensure that the loops are filled when scanned.

In our practice we routinely use barium sulfate suspensions in *all* routine CT scanning procedures. We favor barium sulfate because it is palatable, unabsorbed by the intestine, and does not have the irritant properties of water-soluble solutions, which may increase peristalsis leading to motion-induced image degradation. Barium has an added advantage in patients undergoing systemic chemotherapy in whom the nausea may limit the amount of contrast tolerable. Ball et al. recently

have shown image-degrading precipitation of water-soluble contrast solutions in the stomach. The percipitate generates streak artifacts. Elimination requires buffering of the oral contrast agent.[6a]

There are specific instances when water-soluble contrast agents are indicated. These include scans performed for blunt abdominal trauma; scans of immediate preoperative or postoperative patients; scans performed for suspected gastrointestinal perforation; and as a bowel marker for any CT interventional procedure. The major factor underlying all of these indications is the possibility of an occult gastrointestinal perforation. Federle et al. have shown a higher incidence of bowel perforation occurring in patients with blunt trauma to the abdomen than has been clinically apparent.[7] CT

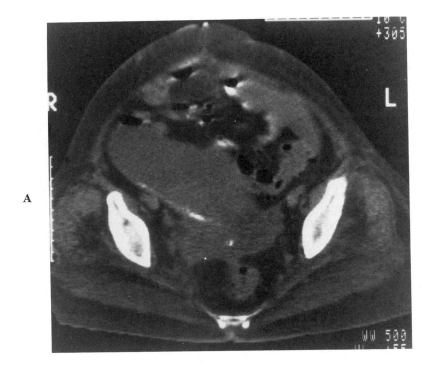

Fig. 1-1. Unsuspected ileal perforation with pelvic abscess. **A,** CT scans of the midpelvis in a patient who developed a fever 5 days following aortic aneurysm surgery. There is an amophous fluid collection. A small area of increased density represents extravasated oral contrast.

may visualize this abnormality in two ways. First, small amounts of free air may be seen particularly near the falciform ligament; secondly, oral contrast material may be seen in the peritoneal cavity.[8] Obviously in these cases water-soluble contrast agents are preferred because of the potential complications resulting from barium entering the peritoneal cavity[9] (Fig. 1-1). We have recently been requested to scan patients immediately before operative procedures, sometimes within 1 hour of induction of general anesthesia. Although these cases were not emergencies, increasing government restrictions on hospital stays are forcing a more telescoped work up. These patients are given water-soluble agents. Postoperative patients, particularly those having undergone resection of bowel or those with a fresh anastomosis, should also be given water-soluble contrast agents, especially when an abscess or leak is suspected.

Factors involved in contrast distribution

Uniform bowel opacification is critical to successful CT interpretation. Uniformity is based on intestinal transit time and the status of the luminal content of the bowel. Transit time is controlled by many endogenous and exogenous factors. These factors should be considered when administering oral contrast material.

Endogenous factors include interplay of diverse controls such as cortical hunger centers, autonomic nervous system, gastrointestinal hormones, prostaglandins, and thyroid hormones. Exogenous factors such as drug therapy, narcotic intake, or recent surgery diminish intestinal motility.[10]

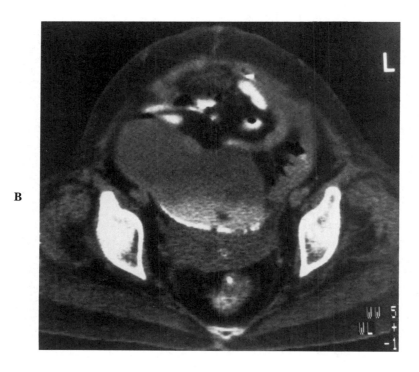

Fig. 1-1, cont'd. B, CT scan of same patient approximately 30 minutes later shows increasing amounts of oral contrast medium collecting in the fluid, indicating communication with the bowel. At surgery a loop of ileum was perforated, communicating with a large pelvic abscess. Water-soluble contrast material was used in this case because of a history of fever in postoperative patients.

In our experience complete opacification of the small bowel can be achieved within 45 minutes of ingestion of the contrast material in most *ambulatory* patients. Patients who are not ambulatory may require a longer prescan contrast administration time because of the imbalance of factors outlined earlier. Complete opacification can generally be achieved by consumption of 500 to 600 ml (15 to 18 ounces of oral contrast material). As stated previously, this amount should be consumed 30 to 45 minutes before the beginning of the examination. Optimally the contrast material should be consumed steadily, approximately one 6 ounce cup each 10 minutes over the waiting period. This ensures uniform distribution. Utilizing this schedule of contrast administration we routinely achieve opacified ileal loops and right colonic opacification in over 95% of patients. Colonic visualization beyond the proximal ascending colon is not routinely achieved by this method. Best results are obtained when patients are kept NPO. Outpatients are usually restricted from between 3 to 5 hours (the meal before) the examination. This is an added safety measure because an empty stomach is preferred when intravenous contrast agents are administered.

Visualization of the proximal bowel

Visualization of distal small bowel loops is easily achieved given sufficient time and volume of oral agent. Adequate opacification and distention of the stomach, duodenum, and proximal jejunum is more difficult. In the duodenum, the largest flux of water into the lumen of the intestine occurs. Receptors in the duodenum that are sensitive to pH, fats, and osmotic pressures slow gastric emptying and promote large amounts of pancreatic and mucous secretions—all of which serve to dilute the gastric contents and maintain an isosmotic solution when compared to blood.[11] The duodenum is also a site of vigorous peristalsis, making this segment of the intestine and the proximal jejunum difficult to opacify uniformly.[12] In order to overcome the dilutional effects of the duodenum, the patient must consume *additional* contrast material in order to have this portion of the gastrointestinal tract filled during the time of the scan. Thus immediately before the scan begins, as the patient lies on the scan couch, he or she is given one additional cup of oral contrast material. This distends the stomach, fills the duodenum and proximal jejunum, and overcompensates for the dilutional activity within the duodenum. Regardless of how much contrast material the patient has consumed prior to entering the scan room, this additional cup of contrast material is *essential* and must not be neglected in any CT examination regardless of the indication (Fig. 1-2). This step must also be performed when patients undergo CT scans of both the chest and the abdomen. If the chest is scanned first, the additional cup of contrast material should be administered when the diaphragm is reached and before proceeding to obtain sections in the abdomen.

Controversy has arisen concerning differences in transit time between water-soluble contrast agents and barium sulfate suspensions. Hyperosmotic solutions of water-soluble iodinated products tend to shift the gradient of water transport from the blood to the lumen because the unabsorbed molecules must be maintained in isotonic solutions. This accounts for the cathartic, "irritant" properties of these compounds. This irritant property is thought to stimulate peristaltic activity.[11] Whether the irritation actually occurs at the concentration utilized in CT scanning (2% to 4% solution) is questionable. A commercial barium preparation has added osmotically active agents to speed the passage of the bolus to the small bowel.* This suspension works best at slightly higher concentrations (2.0% weight:weight) than routine barium suspensions because the osmotically active additives draw water into the proximal intestinal lumen thus reducing visibility.

---

*Redi-CAT, manufactured by E-Z-EM Company, Westbury, New York.

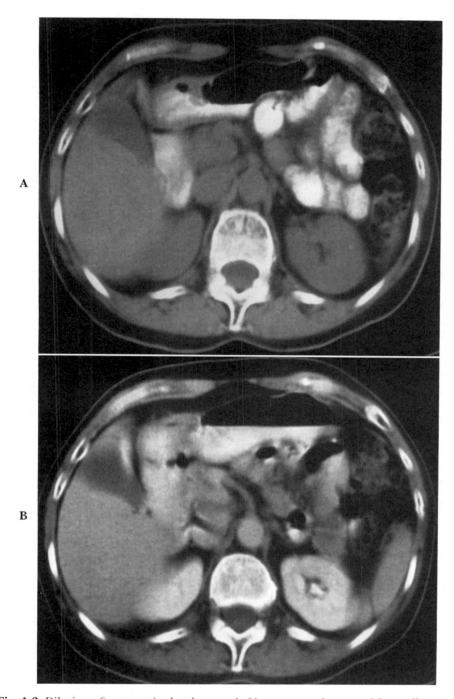

Fig. 1-2. Dilution of contrast in duodenum. **A,** Non-contrast images with excellent opacification of the duodenum and proximal jejunum. **B,** Scan at same level 10 minutes later, following administration of intravenous contrast material. Although some oral contrast material is still present, it is markedly diluted by influx of fluid into the duodenal lumen and proximal jejunum. If the upper abdomen is rescanned, additional oral contrast material should be administered to overcome this effect.

Glucagon

Glucagon was recommended as a routine adjunct to abdominal CT early in CT experience because 18 second scan times were routine and the streak artifacts generated from peristaltic activity produced severe image degredation, often resulting in nondiagnostic examinations.[13,14] As faster scan times became more routine, glucagon was no longer recommended.[15]

We routinely use intravenous glucagon in all CT examinations.* Even with 2 second scan times, bowel relaxation and hypotonia induced by glucagon provides scans of superior resolution to those performed without it. We administer 0.1 mg intravenously immediately following the administration of the final cup of contrast material. These doses have proved effective in inducing hypotonia for upper gastrointestinal examinations.[16,17] Glucagon can be administered with the intravenous contrast bolus. Hypotonia occurs within 1 minute and lasts from 9 to 17 minutes. The site and mechanism of action on the gastrointestinal tract is unknown. A 1 mg dose vial can provide enough glucagon for ten CT examinations. In New York City, this increases the cost of the CT examination by $1.80. Glucagon is particularly helpful in paralyzing the duodenum, which is useful in the examination of the pancreas. It must be remembered that glucagon causes contraction of the pyloric sphincter, therefore oral contrast material given to visualize the duodenum should be administered *prior to* the injection of glucagon. Contraindications to its use are insulinoma and pheochromocytoma. Although the drug is safe for most diabetic patients, we do not administer it to brittle patients on insulin therapy.

*Glucagon USP for injection manufactured by Eli Lilly Company, Indianapolis, Indiana.

SPECIALIZED TECHNIQUES FOR LEVELS OF THE GASTROINTESTINAL TRACT
Esophagus

The peristaltic activity of the normal esophagus results from sequential activation of muscles dependent on efferent nerve impulses from higher centers. The primary peristaltic wave sweeps from the cricopharyngeus muscle to the lower esophageal sphincter and can push a bolus of water through its length within 1 second. Coupled with momentum generated from hypopharyngeal muscle contraction water moves faster than the primary wave even in the horizontal position. Any material remaining within the esophagus will be swept through by secondary contractions. This results in our inability to opacify the normal esophagus for the length of time necessary for CT examinations. Because the esophagus is fixed in its mediastinal location, it is generally not difficult to recognize during thoracic CT examinations. Oral contrast material helps to differentiate the convex border of the esophagus from adjacent mediastinal adenopathy. Furthermore, if the esophagus appears thick-walled, a contrast agent should be available to distend this portion of the alimentary tube. In these cases we administer a pastelike suspension of barium sulfate.* This material clings to the esophageal wall and is not efficiently cleared by normal peristaltic activity. We use the contrast agent in the evaluation of intraluminal esophageal masses because it allows a more precise delineation of the borders of the lesion. Its most common use is to correlate an impression seen on a routine esophagram, ensuring that the area of the impression is in fact scanned during the esophageal CT (see Chapter Two for further details).

*Esopho-CAT manufactured by E-Z-EM Company, Westbury, New York.

Stomach

Gastric opacification is necessary not only to evaluate the stomach but also to accurately outline the extent of pathological processes in the upper abdomen. This is routinely achieved by ensuring that the patient consumes at least 6 ounces (180 ml) of oral contrast medium immediately before commencement of scanning as discussed previously. This additional contrast material should be administered regardless of how much the patient has previously consumed. In our practice, this is routinely administered after the patient has come to the scanner just before lying on the scan couch. Consumption in the sitting position provides more uniform distribution, prevents pooling of contrast material in the dependent gastric fundus, and leads to reliable gastric distention. This helps avoid false-positive diagnoses related to the inability to evaluate segments of normal wall thickening, particularly in the region of the esophagogastric junction and the pylorus. Apparent masses in the left adrenal gland, retroperitoneum, and pancreatic tail have been mistakenly diagnosed only to turn out to be a partially opacified gastric fundus.[18,19] We have seen several cases in which the splenic vessels can be seen to traverse the posterior aspect of the gastric fundus, showing portions of the stomach actually posterior to this vascular axis (Fig. 1-3). Inadequate opacification would surely result in mistaking this segment for a retroperitoneal, particularly adrenal, mass. When pathologic processes involving the stomach are suspected, alterations in patient positioning may be necessary to ensure that the portion of the stomach is maximally distended. Thus antral processes may be studied with the patient in a right-side-down decubitus position and fundal pathology may be studied with the patient in a left-side-down decubitus position. The prone position may help distend the fundus in thin patients in whom there is a suspicion of a left adrenal mass. Other agents have been used to visualize the stomach. These include water, mineral oil, and air.[20,21] These agents provide negative contrast, allowing identification of the viscus as well as evaluation of the wall. We describe our experience with air contrast techniques subsequently. At times one may want no gastric opacification. One may not wish to administer gastric contrast in scans directed at evaluation of liver metastases.[22] This eliminates streak artifacts generated from the air contrast level in the stomach. With present day equipment, algorithms eliminate the objectionable streaking and we therefore use oral contrast in every case.

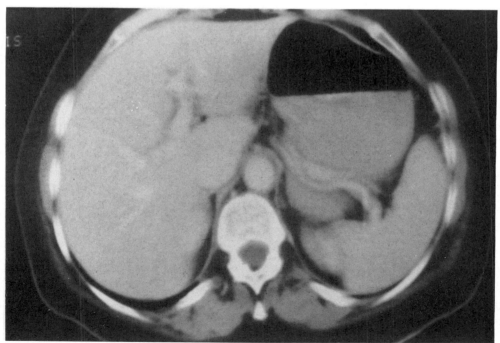

Fig. 1-3. Gastric fundus posterior to splenic vessels. A portion of the gastric fundus can be seen posterior to the splenic artery and vein. Poor filling of the stomach can lead to the false diagnosis of a left adrenal mass.

Duodenum

The duodenum is the most difficult segment of the abdominal gastrointestinal tract to reliably opacify. The motility in the duodenum is greater than the motility in any other segment of the small bowel and is particularly active when the stomach is stretched as with large volumes of oral contrast material.[11,12] Because of its close anatomic relationship to so many important structures, the segment becomes critical to visualize (Fig. 1-4). Routine administration of 0.1 mg of glucagon intravenously *following* a 6 ounce cup of oral contrast material generally produces sufficient hypotonia to reliably opacify the duodenal sweep. Haaga et al. have used the right-side-down decubitus position to routinely visualize the segment, particularly in cases in which pathologic processes in the pancreatic head were suspected.[23] Alternative air contrast techniques are discussed subsequently.

Small bowel

Filling of the small bowel is generally achievable by the schedules described previously. With the advent of faster scanners providing improved spatial resolution, unfilled bowel loops are less difficult to recognize. The problem patient is the cachectic individual who has no fat separating structures. Therefore particular effort must be directed at ensuring adequate contrast consumption.

If a "mass" is encountered and an unfilled bowel is thought to be the cause, a repeat cut obtained over the region may show the loop to be filled with contrast material. The physician monitoring the patient is responsible for this determination, and in optimal practice, a physician should view the scans before the patient is "off the table."

Another aid in recognition of a bowel loop is gained by attempting to track mesentery or mesenteric vessels associated with the loops. This is particularly useful in postoperative patients, especially those having undergone retroperitoneal surgery. Because of the recent postoperative status, they may not be able to drink sufficient amounts of contrast material and varying degrees of postoperative ileus may render optimal bowel opacification difficult. Furthermore, because unopacified fluid-filled bowel may simulate an abscess collection, it is important to look for the mesenteric attachments. The mesenteric axis appears as a central fat density surrounded by a fluid-filled loop. Occasionally a vessel may be seen within the mesenteric fat (Fig. 1-5). Another finding that may be of occasional use is to obtain a thin (less than or equal to 5 mm) cut over the region of question. The improved spatial resolution obtained when using a thin cut may show valvulae conniventes, thus identifying the "mass" as a loop of bowel.

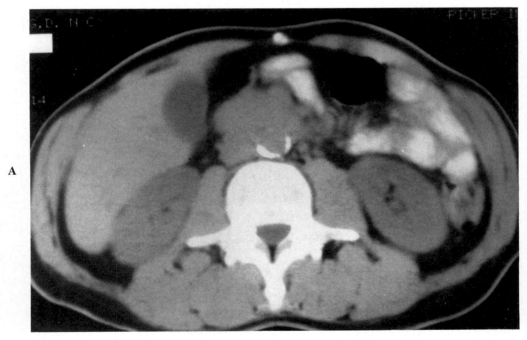

Fig. 1-4. Unopacified duodenum simulating peripancreatic nodes. **A,** CT scan in a patient with gastric carcinoma suggests the presence of peripancreatic lymphadenopathy appearing as lobulated densities deforming the contour of the pancreatic head.

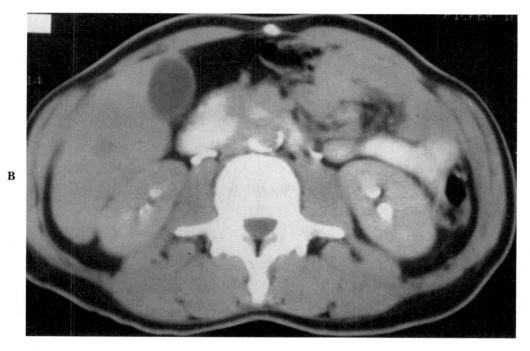

Fig. 1-4, cont'd. B, Repeat scan following ingestion of 6 ounces of additional oral contrast material. Enhanced scan clearly shows the "mass" accounted for by an unfilled duodenal sweep.

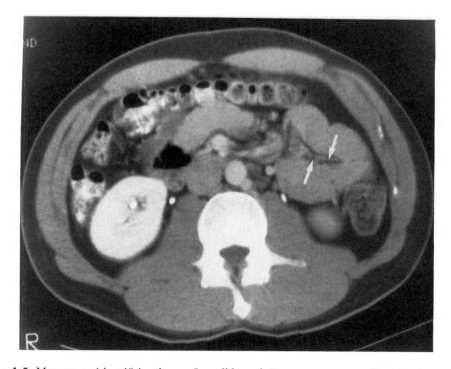

Fig. 1-5. Mesentery identifying loop of small bowel. Poor contrast opacification is present in the jejunum. Notice the fat and vessels in the central mesentary subtending this loop of bowel *(arrows)*.

Areas of difficulty in assessing the small bowel include the proximal jejunum at the ligament of Treitz, which is often mistaken for the pancreatic tail; posterior mid-ileal loops insinuated between the aorta, cava, and psoas muscles; and dilated ileal loops deep in the pelvis that fall into the cul-de-sac and pararectal recesses (Fig. 1-6). In patients who have undergone abdominoperineal resection, small bowel loops are "free" to fall into the presacral recesses of the lower pelvis. A high index of suspicion must be maintained before falsely mistaking an unopacified bowel loop for recurrent tumor (Fig. 1-7). Masses seen in these areas should always be considered as bowel loops and either rescanning after time or with thin cuts should be routinely performed to ensure that a suspected mass is in fact not in a loop of bowel. Occasionally we have been forced to recall a patient to the scanner, flooding the bowel with excess oral contrast material (700 to 800 ml), and rescanning to avoid a false-positive diagnosis (Fig. 1-8). As an individual's experience in CT interpretation accrues, the possibility of poor bowel opacification can be suspected by evaluating the entire scan for patient body habitus and status of opacification on other images. Often it becomes necessary to question the technician responsible for administering the contrast material as to the reliability of the patients consumption, possible vomiting, or omission of oral contrast administration. When scanning in a pressured "emergency" situation it is better to delay the scan for 45 minutes to allow sufficient bowel filling and minimize false-positive diagnosis.

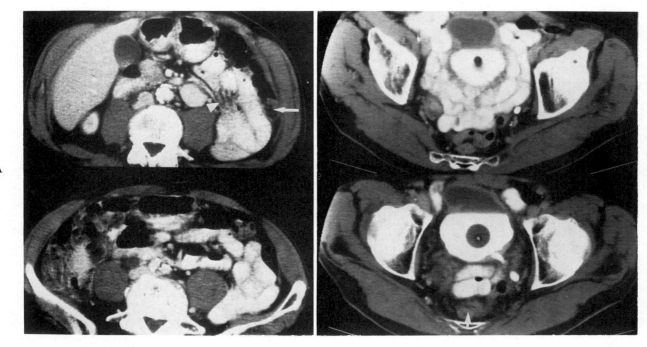

Fig. 1-6. "Posterior" location of small bowel. **A,** Two scans of a patient with scant peritoneal fat. Notice the jejunum tracking posterior to the left psoas muscle and descending colon *(arrow)*. Notice the mesenteric vessels following the bowel loops *(arrowhead)*. The need for uniform bowel opacification is obvious. **B,** Scans through the pelvis of the same patient as in **A.** Loops of ileum extend caudally to the retrovesical space immediately anterior to the rectum *(arrow)*. Other loops are draped over the anterolateral portion of the urinary bladder. These positions of small bowel are most likely to occur in thin patients; particular care should be taken to ensure that these patients consume full amounts of contrast material as outlined in the text.

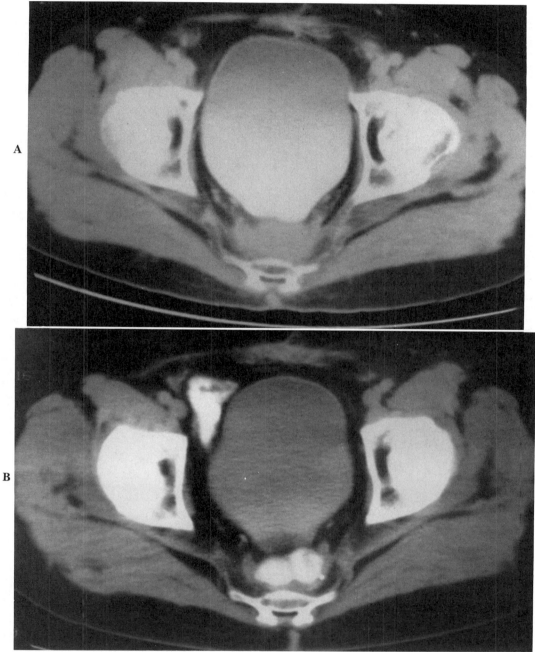

Fig. 1-7. Abdominal-perineal resection. **A,** Scan of patient following abdominal-perineal resection. A mass is seen in the presacral region that is indistinguishable from recurrent carcinoma. **B,** Repeat scan 15 minutes later than **A.** The "mass" represents two loops of small bowel.

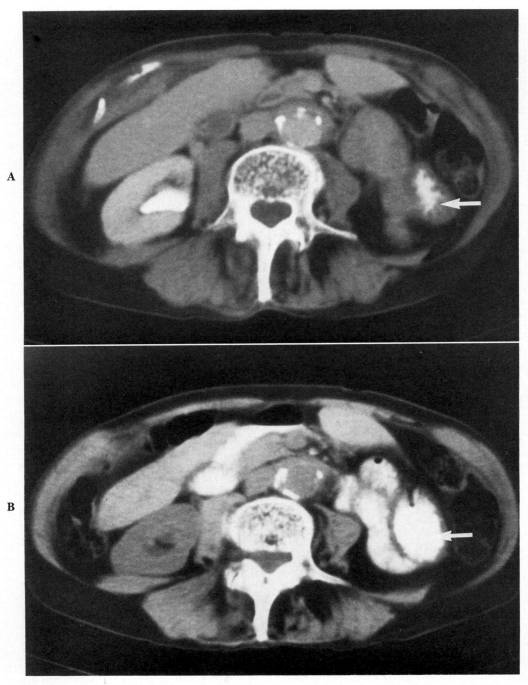

Fig. 1-8. False-positive retroperitoneal mass. **A,** Scan in 80-year-old patient with suspected abdominal neoplasm. The mass is noted adjacent to the aorta. Poor contrast filling of upper intestinal loops should increase the suspicion of unopacified loops. A small amount of contrast material is seen in the gastric fundus *(arrow)*. **B,** The patient was asked to return for additional scans with bowel flooding. Scan at the same level as **A** shows the "mass" accounted for by unfilled loops of jejunum. Note better filling of gastric fundus *(arrow)*.

Colon

The colon may be visualized by a variety of techniques. It is our belief that colonic opacification is best performed by retrograde installation of contrast material. Antegrade visualization of the colon may be obtained by pre-administration of oral contrast material 8 hours before the examination is undertaken.[24] Miller, et al. recommend that 3% water-soluble contrast material administered 12 hours before the scan will fill the rectosigmoid colon with streak artifacts in over 80% of patients. They recommend that this method be used routinely in all pelvic CT scanning.[25]

Most radiologists use rectal installation of dilute contrast solutions at similar concentrations as given the patient by mouth. These methods serve to identify the colon; but unless the bowel is cleansed, extension of pathological processes into the bowel wall cannot be appreciated and little is achieved over and above identification of the loops.

Colonic opacification is necessary in any patient with pelvic malignancy or pelvic mass.[26] The delayed opacification techniques using antegrade administration of contrast are used in patients in whom pelvic abscesses are suspected, particularly postoperative patients in whom retrograde colonic insufflation would not be advisable (Fig. 1-9).

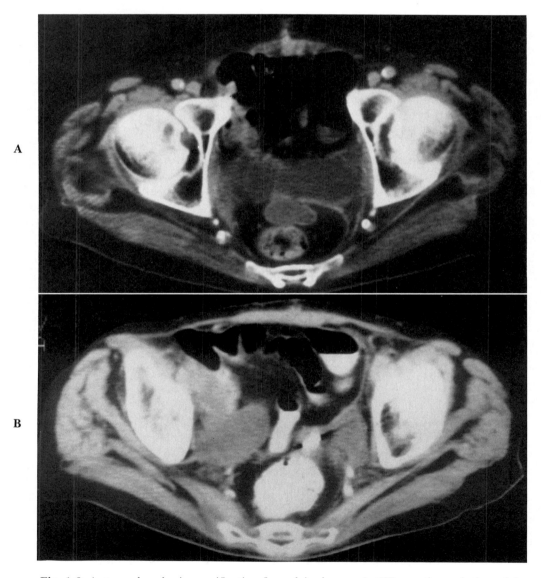

A

B

Fig. 1-9. Antegrade colonic opacification for pelvic abscess. **A,** CT scan through the pelvis of a patient who developed a fever 1 week following a radical cystectomy for bladder carcinoma. Fluid collections are seen, but the relation to the colon and bowel are not clearly demonstrated. **B,** Repeat scan 12 hours following administration of oral, water-soluble contrast material. The rectum and sigmoid are clearly shown, helping to delineate the true extent of the fluid collection.

Intravenous contrast agents

A full discussion of the techniques, pros, and cons of intravenous contrast agents is beyond the scope of this book. Our own belief is that intravenous contrast is an integral part of any CT examination of the abdomen, and we routinely administer it in the form of a rapid-bolus, rapid-infusion method coupled with dynamic incremental scanning. With the routine use of faster scanners and high-heat capacity tubes, dynamic sequential scanning is the procedure of choice for abdominal CT. By using rapid sequential scanning we are able to scan during the phase of maximal contrast difference between the intervascular and extracellular tissue compartments thus allowing maximal differences between enhanced organs and less enhanced pathologic processes.[32] Therefore we rarely perform noncontrast scans. In patients in whom liver metastases may be hyperdense or isodense to relative enhanced hepatic parenchyma, such as carcinoid tumors or islet cell tumors, noncontrast scans are performed initially. Intravenous contrast material is administered in all patients barring a history of myeloma, diabetes, renal failure, or allergy to contrast agents. Other uses of intravenous contrast agents in aiding differential diagnosis of bowel lesions is discussed in separate chapters. The reader is referred to the textbook by Bernardino and Sones for a more complete discussion of the use of intravenous contrast material in abdominal gastrointestinal CT.[33]

AIR CONTRAST TECHNIQUES

Alec J. Megibow
Elias A. Zerhouni

As stated in the previous section, bowel opacification should provide reliable visualization, distention, and definition of the given bowel loop. Visualization is based on the difference in attenuation between two adjacent structures. The great advantage of CT scanning is the ability to resolve attenuation differences between far greater scales of densities than in plain radiography. Nevertheless visualization depends on the density gradient between the pixels of one structure and the pixels of an adjacent structure. Oral contrast in the bowel has a CT number of approximately 150 Hounsfield units whereas perivisceral fat has a CT number of approximately −100 H units, providing a gradient of 250 H units. If the same viscus is filled with air (−900 H units), the gradient between adjacent pixels may be as high as 800 H units—considerably greater than positive contrast. Air reliably distends the viscus making analysis of subtler pathologic findings possible. Air insufflation provides a method by which the true thickness of the bowel wall may be ascertained.

Early attempts at air contrast techniques on the upper gastrointestinal tract were thwarted by the relatively long scan times (9.6 to 18 seconds) and by the large matrix that did not provide spatial resolution adequate to visualize the anatomic detail.[28] Hamlin reported exquisite detail in analysis of rectal tumors with rectally administered air and thin sections used to show the rectal wall as a guide for endocavitary irradiation.[28] Our experience with air contrast CT began in 1982 and these techniques have become the routine method of CT practice at our institutions.[30]

We first outline the techniques used in obtaining air contrast studies and then discuss particular detail relevant to specific segments of gastrointestinal tract. The principles related to positioning the patient that one utilizes when performing air contrast gastrointestinal CT scans are identical to those in positioning the patient for standard gastrointestinal fluoroscopy. With this basic fact in mind, extraordinary detail of the gastrointestinal wall is obtained.

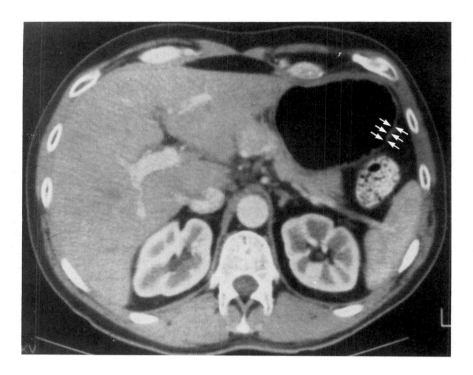

Fig. 1-10. Air distention of the stomach. This image indicates why we routinely use gas contrast of the stomach. The true thickness of the gastric wall can be measured *(arrows)*. There is superb differentiation of the greater curvature from the anterior border of the pancreatic body. The patient was studied with a dynamic scan using a rapid bolus of contrast medium. Because there may be a noticeable increase in the incidence of patient nausea as a result of the bolus, the advantage of an empty stomach is obvious.

Stomach

Air contrast has become the method of choice for visualizing the upper gastrointestinal tract in our practice. Aside from allowing visualization of the gastric wall, the air-filled stomach allows for more accurate delineation of the upper abdominal viscera, particularly the pancreas and adrenals. The technique has a further benefit in that the stomach is empty rather than filled with liquid. Thus aspiration secondary to vomiting as a result of a rapid infusion of contrast material is less of a problem with an air-filled stomach (Fig. 1-10). The "air" is produced by having the patient consume effervescent granules dissolved in 10 to 20 ml of water.* Because this actually produces carbon dioxide in the stomach, gas contrast is a more appropriate term. The effervescent is given to the patient *instead of the final cup* of oral contrast material as described in the previous section. Best results are achieved when the stomach is completely empty; thus patients are kept NPO approximately 3 to 5 hours before the scan. If residual oral, positive contrast material is present in the stomach, the air

*E-Z-GAS II manufactured by E-Z-EM Company, Westbury, New York.

contrast level produced may theoretically produce objectionable streak artifacts. Therefore approximately 10 minutes should pass from the time when the patient drinks the final cup of oral contrast material until the administration of the effervescent. With 2 second scanners, the streak artifact is not present. Water admixed with positive contrast material may degrade visualization of the most posterior portion of the fundus in the supine position. The smallest amount of water to dissolve the effervescent minimizes this effect. Positioning the patient is important to optimize the distention of the viscus. The body, antrum, and pyloric region are routinely distended in the supine position (Fig. 1-11). If a pathologic condition is suspected in the fundus or proximal stomach, scanning the patient in the right-side-down decubitus position allows air to rise into the relatively superior fundus and distends it. Thompson et al. have advocated left-side-down decubitus scanning of air insufflation to evaluate esophagogastric junction pathology.[30] While this positioning allows air to rise toward the relatively table far lesser curvature of the esophagogastric junction, less air than in a right-side-down position arises to the entire proximal portion of the stomach. Therefore we advocate a right-side-down decubitus position with air insufflation to evaluate esophagogastric junction pathology (Fig. 1-12). Conversely if distal (antral, pyloric, or duodenal) pathology is suspected, then left-side-down decubi-

tus positioning maximally distends the segment of the stomach (Fig. 1-13). One need only think of the cranial-caudad and anteroposterior relations of the stomach used in fluoroscopic examination to decide on the optimal patient position.

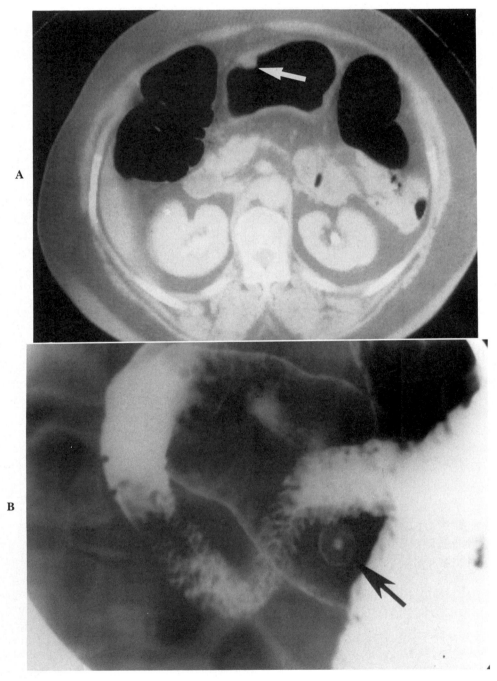

Fig. 1-11. Gastric polyp—air contrast. **A,** Gastrointestinal series reveals a mass along the non-dependent surface of the gastric wall (the anterior wall in the supine patient). A hanging droplet is present *(arrow)*. **B,** CT scan reveals the polyp along the anterior wall of the gastric body *(arrow)*. This portion is maximally distended in the supine patient.

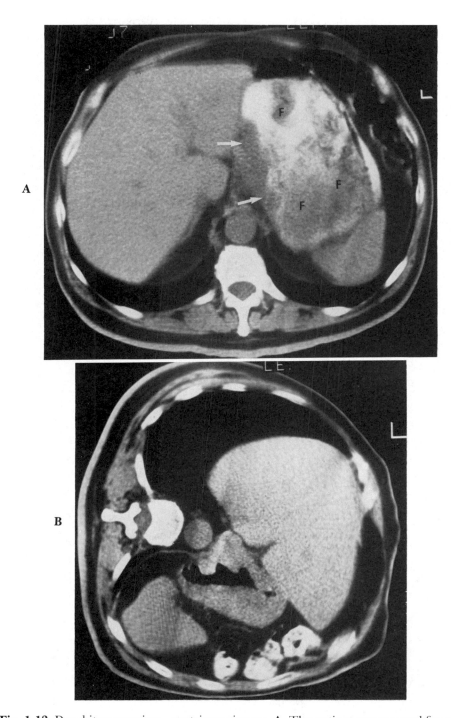

Fig. 1-12. Decubitus scanning—gastric carcinoma. **A,** The patient was scanned for weight loss. Notice the food *(F)* in the stomach. This makes it difficult to appreciate the significance of the soft-tissue density along the lesser curvature aspect of the esophagogastric junction *(arrows)*. **B,** Scan of the patient in the left-lateral decubitus position. The image is diagnostic of a lobulated carcinoma along the lesser curvature, with circumferential involvement of the stomach.   *Continued.*

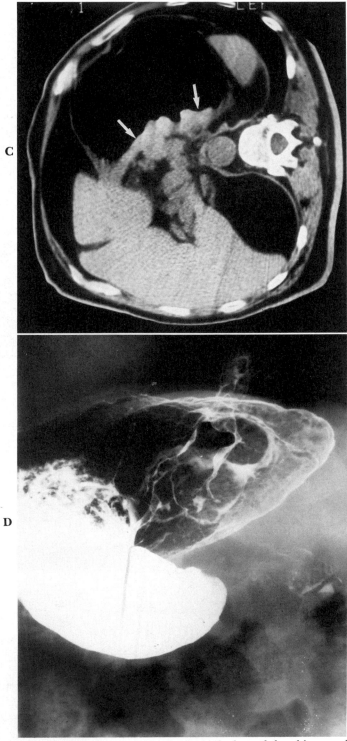

Fig. 1-12, cont'd. C, Scan of the patient in the right-lateral decubitus position. The tissue extent of the neoplasm is better shown. Note that the greater curvature is normal. The tumor mass is clearly visualized *(arrow)*. **D,** Gastrointestinal series. The tumor is shown at the esophagogastric junction with sparing of the greater curvature and posterior fundus. Note the film is obtained with the patient in a right-side-down decubitus position. The optimal patient positioning for air-contrast CT is based on the principles of double-contrast gastrointestinal fluoroscopy.

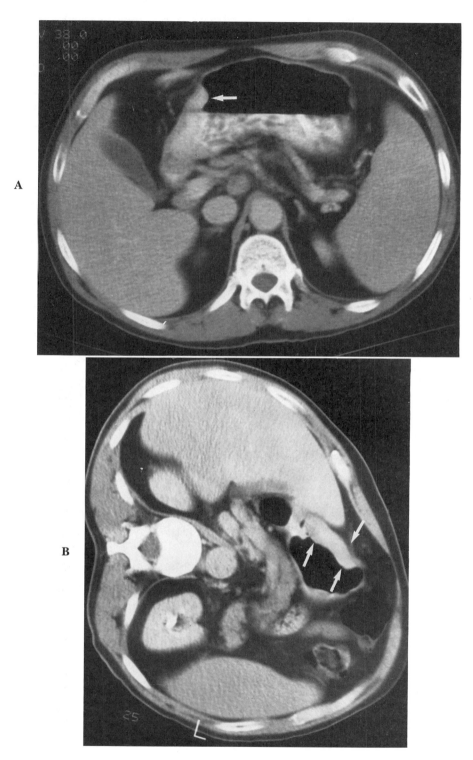

Fig. 1-13. Gastric carcinoma—antrum. **A,** Scan of patient in supine position. The patient was not NPO, therefore particulate material is seen in the stomach. There is a nodular fold seen along the greater curve of the antrum *(arrow).* **B,** Scan of patient in the left-side-down decubitus position clearly displays thickened, "rigid" wall of greater curvature. Extensive gastric carcinoma was present in this region *(arrows).*

Duodenum

As discussed in the previous section on positive contrast techniques, duodenal visualization is critical in CT diagnosis of upper abdominal pathology. Reasons making duodenal visualization difficult were outlined. Air techniques can aid in selected cases. When an effervescent is given in routine, supine, air contrast scanning, the proximal duodenum (bulb and first portion) is generally visualized, but the second and third portions generally are not air distended, although sufficient air is present to identify these segments adequately for routine work. By altering the patient's position, using a left-side-down decubitus position, air will rise into the now superiorly located duodenal sweep (Hampton's view). The use of glucagon (0.1 mg intravenous) is essential for optimal imaging. The air-distended sweep can be seen on the scout view, and therefore the axial sections can be easily localized (Fig. 1-14). We use this technique as an adjunct to routine scanning. It has been useful in identifying the duodenum in thin patients in whom the viscus may be mistaken for retroperitoneal mass and/or outlining the pancreatic head, especially when a mass is suspected within this region (Fig. 1-15). One major use has been in the jaundiced patient in whom an extrahepatic biliary obstruction is present without apparent etiology. Duodenal air accentuates the tissue contrast gradient between the common duct and the lumen, possibly improving detection of bile duct stones. We have seen the duodenal papilla and detected neoplastic distortion of this structure using this technique when other conventional scanning positions have failed. This technique works best with high resolution scanners with a 2-second scan time and a 512 × 512 reconstruction matrix. This technique has allowed for imaging of small lesions (Fig. 1-16).

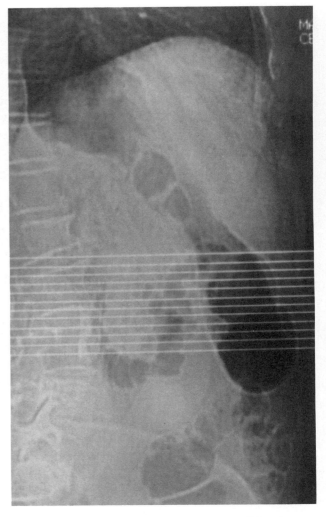

Fig. 1-14. Scout view for air contrast scan of duodenum. The gas-filled viscus allows visualization of the duodenal bulb and sweep, allowing for accurate indexing of images to evaluate the sweep. The patient is scanned in the left-side-down decubitus position.

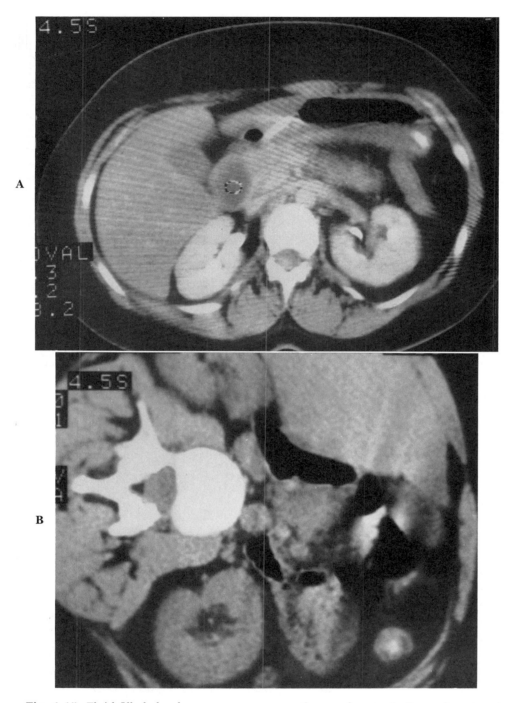

Fig. 1-15. Fluid-filled duodenum versus pancreatic pseudocyst. **A,** Scan of patient in supine position with acute pancreatitis. Note the nasogastric tube in the stomach. A rounded mass is seen near the pancreatic head. The possibility of a pseudocyst could not be excluded. These patients are generally NPO and may not be able to drink sufficient amounts of contrast for optimal bowel opacification. **B,** The same patient is scanned in the left-side-down decubitus position. The "pseudocyst" is actually a fluid-filled duodenum. Note the clear definition of the pancreatic head, uncinate process, and second duodenal portion.

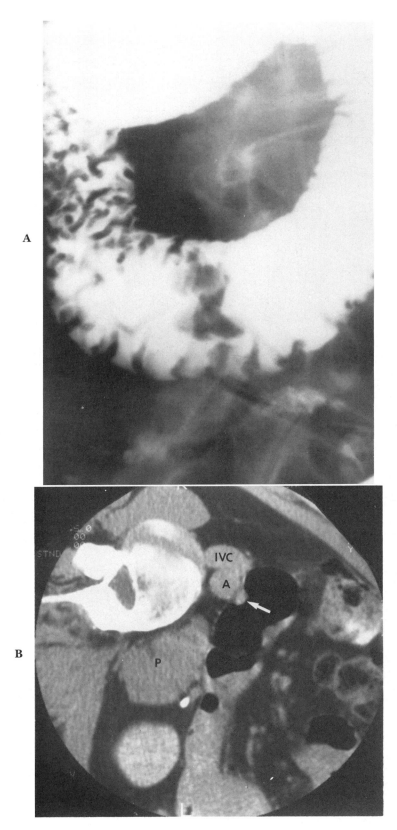

Fig. 1-16. Villous tumor of duodenum. **A,** Gastrointestinal series identifies a polypoid lesion in the third portion of the duodenum. **B,** CT scan with patient in left-lateral decubitus position. The tumor mass is seen on the lateral wall of the third portion of the duodenum *(arrow).* There is no evidence of infiltration into the duodenal wall or retroperitoneum. (*A,* Aorta; *IVC,* vena cava; *P,* left psoas.)

Small bowel

At the time of this writing we have not routinely used air contrast techniques to visualize the small bowel. One of us (E.A.Z.) is developing a system of enteric-coated tablets that would hopefully travel varying distances through the small bowel before effervescing, ultimately providing uniform distention of the whole small bowel with gas. These tablets are not yet commercially available.

Colon

Air contrast techniques are used routinely during CT scanning to visualize the colon for evaluation of pelvic masses and primary colonic pathology and in the follow-up of gynecologic surgery. This method has achieved clinical acceptance because it is safe, non-time consuming, and provides information achieved from positive contrast techniques as well as additional information that cannot be obtained from conventional methods.

All patients scheduled for CT examination of the pelvis for investigation of a pelvic mass, genitourinary neoplasm (except for testicular tumors), endometriosis, colon carcinoma, follow-up of colonic surgery, diverticulitis, and/or inflammatory bowel disease undergo air insufflation of the colon as part of the CT examination.[31] Maximal benefit is obtained when the colon has been previously prepared. All of our patients with the above indications are instructed to prepare their colons. We use an oral cathartic preparation.* This 12-hour preparation uses a low-residue diet and a high, oral fluid intake, (8 ounces of clear liquid per hour for 7 to 8 hours) followed by an oral cathartic (magnesium citrate or Phospho-soda) and an irritant agent (bisacodyl). If the patient does not prepare and if it is necessary for the performance of the CT examination, we have produced adequate colonic cleansing by administering a 2000 ml tap water enema containing 20 ml of liquid bisacodyl.* Scans may be performed immediately following the evacuation because mucosal drying is not critical as in barium studies.

Air is insufflated through a 14 French argyle red rubber catheter. Most patients can be relied on to give a verbal indication that their tolerance point has been reached. We are at present developing an administration set that will ensure the radiologist that the intercolonic pressure does not exceed 30 cm in water. This should provide an added safety feature and overcome trepidation of insufflating the colon without direct vision.

When insufflating air to visualize the rectosigmoid colon for evaluation of a pelvic mass (such as bladder carcinoma, endometrial carcinoma, etc.) the patient is placed in the prone position, allowing air to rise into the superiorly located rectosigmoid (Figs. 1-17 and 1-18). This produces maximal distention of the segment of bowel and helps outline the colonic relation to the pelvic mass. Intravenous glucagon, 0.5 to 1 mg, is used to relax the colon, minimize spasm, and facilitate retention. Scanning the patient from the symphysis to the iliac crest minimizes the time the patient must retain air. The use of 5 mm thick cuts (indexed at 10 mm intervals) increases the spatial resolution allowing a far more accurate assessment of the mass, bowel wall, and intervening pelvic fat.

---

*Fleet Kit One manufactured by CB Fleet Company, Lynchburg, Virginia; E-Z-Prep manufactured by E-Z-EM Company, Westbury, New York.

*CB Fleet Company, Lynchburg, Virginia.

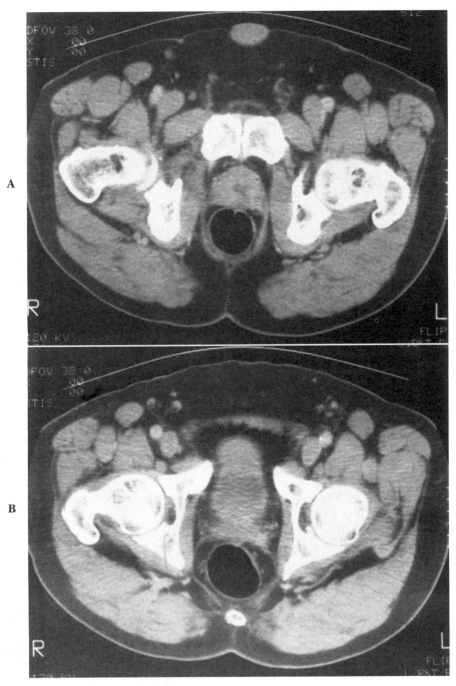

Fig. 1-17. Air-filled rectum—prostate carcinoma. **A,** The patient is scanned in the prone position to facilitate air rising to the relatively posterior rectum. The clear visualization of the wall allows assessment of the presence or absence of invasion. **B,** The same patient in the 10 mm cephalad position. The seminal vesicle angle is preserved. There is a clear fat plane between the air-filled rectum and seminal vesicles.

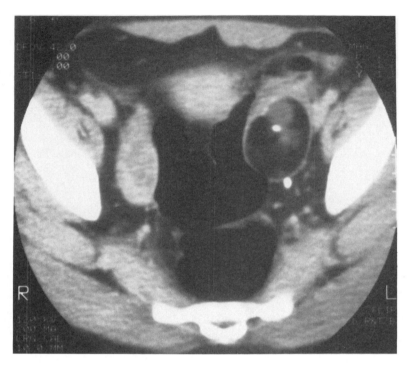

Fig. 1-18. Pelvic masses—air contrast of colon. This patient has an enlarged right ovary and a dermoid cyst of the left ovary. The borders of the air-filled rectosigmoid are seen clearly, as is the relationship of the colon to the masses.

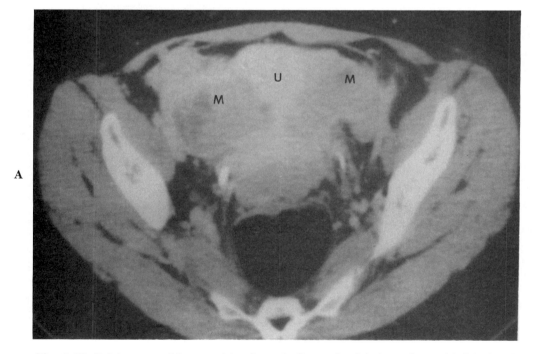

Fig. 1-19. Pelvic mass with serosal implant. **A,** Scan of pelvis in patient with lobulated, bilateral ovarian carcinoma *(M)*. The anterior wall of the gas-filled rectum abuts a tumor in the cul-de-sac. The uterus *(U)* appears as a homogeneous soft-tissue density surrounded by adnexal neoplasms. *Continued.*

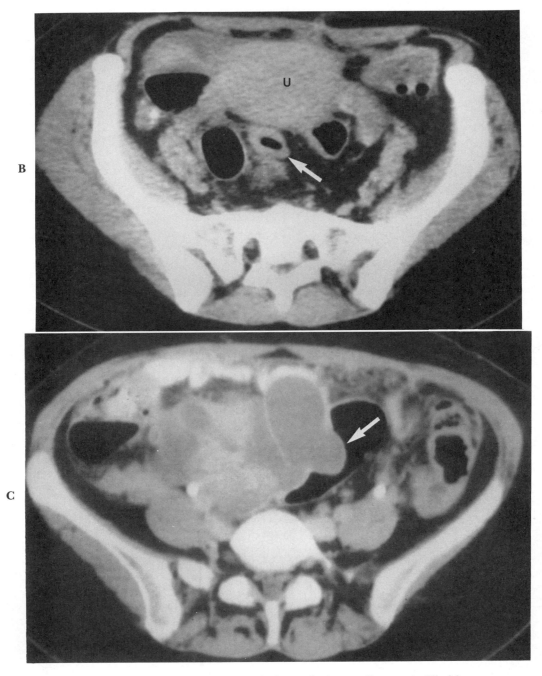

Fig. 1-19, cont'd. B, Scan slightly cephalad reveals three adjacent air-filled loops representing portions of the sigmoid colon indulating in the plane of section. The central loop is thickened and an ill-defined soft-tissue mass is seen adjacent to it *(arrow)*. Serosal implants were confirmed at surgery. Anteriorly, the homogeneous density of the uterus *(U)* is seen. **C,** Ovarian carcinoma with focal implant along mesenteric border of sigmoid colon *(arrow)*. (A different patient from that seen in **A** and **B**.)

Aside from marking the colon and showing its relationship to pelvic masses, the ability to see both sides of the bowel wall allows one to attempt to assess whether a contiguous mass is adjacent to or invading the wall of the bowel. Masses adjacent to the bowel wall will not produce visible bowel wall thickening in the air distended colon. However, if a mass does invade the serosa of the bowel, visible thickening of the wall can be seen (Fig. 1-19). This assessment is more difficult to make, if not impossible, with positive contrast and colonic opacification. This technique allows visualization of colonic neoplasms as well. Carcinoma appears as an area of focal wall thickening (Fig. 1-20). The increased contrast gradient allows for visualization of small polyps that may be obscured by the barium pool. As in all levels of the gastrointestinal tract, positioning the patient to achieve maximal distention is necessary to visualize various segments of the alimentary tube (Fig. 1-21). Submucosal neoplasms are rare but exert their effect by thickening the wall and sparing the mucosa. Barium examination is necessary for characterization (Fig. 1-22).

In patients with a history of inflammatory bowel disease and in whom the CT is requested to evaluate colonic pathology, a case-by-case decision must be made as to whether or not to administer air (Fig. 1-23). We do not insufflate the colon in patients with *acute* diverticulitis or ulcerative colitis or in patients with Crohn's disease when searching for abscess. In patients who have received pelvic irradiation, air should be administered judiciously, especially if there is a history of rectal bleeding (Fig. 1-24). In patients with clinical radiation proctitis, air should not be administered.

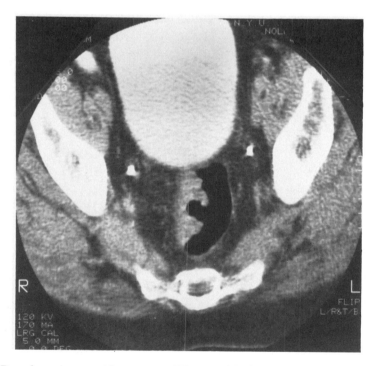

Fig. 1-20. Rectal carcinoma. Air-contrast CT scan with the patient in the prone position. There is an easily identifiable sessile lesion with a central ulcer noted along the right, lateral, rectal wall. There are changes in the pericolic fat indicative of tumor infiltration. Use of thin (5 mm) sections improves spatial resolution and assessment of the interface of the bowel wall and adjacent pericolic fat.

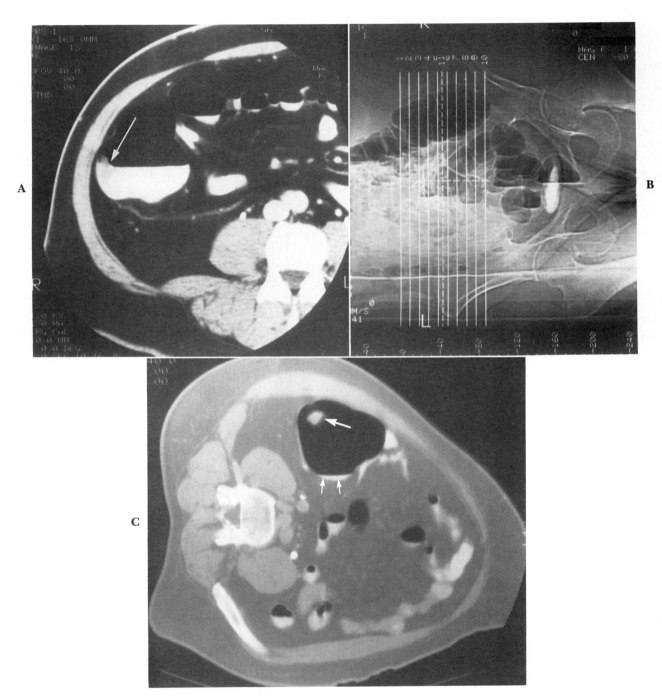

Fig. 1-21. Cecal polyp. **A,** A soft-tissue density is seen in the cecum but obscured by the barium pool *(arrow)*. There is no streak artifact from the air/barium level. **B,** Scout view with patient in the left-side-down decubitus position. The cuts are easily localized. **C,** CT of patient in the left-side-down decubitus position. The polyp and stalk are clearly visualized *(arrow)*. This positioning allows air to rise into the cecum and the barium pool to drop away from the lesion *(small arrows)*.

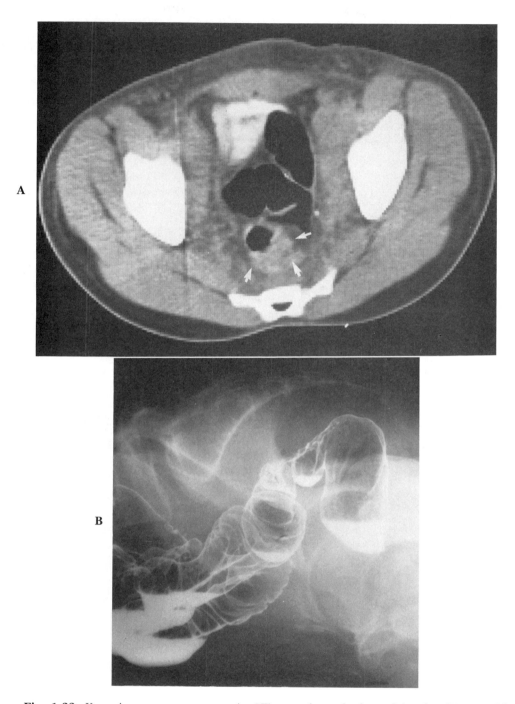

Fig. 1-22. Kaposi sarcoma—rectum. **A,** CT scan through the pelvis of a 35-year-old patient with AIDS and rectal bleeding. The dilated sigmoid loops have a normal wall. The rectum has a thick wall and a narrowed lumen *(arrow)*. The luminal surface is less distorted than in mucosa-based carcinoma (compare to Fig. 1-19). **B,** Barium enema. Submucosal mass affects posterior rectal wall and increases retrorectal space corresponding to level scanned in **A.**

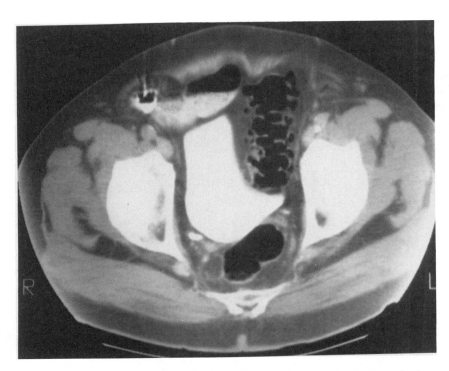

Fig. 1-23. Diverticular disease. The colonic wall is not significantly thickened—innumerable diverticulae are seen in the sigmoid. There is no evidence of inflammation in the pericolic fat. We do *not* recommend air insufflation in acute diverticulitis unless the patient can tolerate a contrast enema.

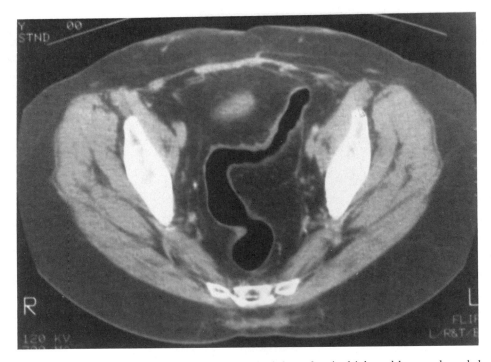

Fig. 1-24. Radiation colitis—chronic. The wall of the colon is thick and haustral, and the lumen is tubular. There is proliferation of the pelvic fat. The patient had been radiated 5 years previously for cervical carcinoma. She was asymptomatic at the time of the CT scan. Air should not be administered in a patient who has undergone pelvic irradiation with clinical symptoms (bleeding, diarrhea) that suggest radiation coloproctitis.

CONCLUSION

These techniques may initially appear cumbersome and unnecessary to adopt into a busy CT practice. We believe that because the patient pays a substantial sum of money for this examination, *all* information available should be obtained. The use of air contrast techniques opens new possibilities in bowel CT, improves the sensitivity or detection of small lesions, and because the bowel wall is accurately seen improves specificity of diagnosis as well.

REFERENCES

1. Kressel, H.Y., et al.: Computed tomography in the evaluation of disorders affecting the alimentary tract, Radiology 129:451-454, 1978.
2. Stanley, R.J., Sagel, S.S., and Levitt, R.G.: Computed tomography of the body: early trends in application and accuracy of the method, AJR 127:53-67, 1976.
3. Kirkpatrick, R.H., Wittenberg, J., Schaffer, D.L., et al.: Scanning techniques in computed body tomography, AJR 130:1069-1075, 1978.
4. Korobkin, M.: Use of contrast material in body CT, J. Comput. Assist. Tomogr. 3:556-559, 1979.
5. Megibow, A.J., and Bosniak, M.A.: Dilute barium solution as a contrast agent for abdominal CT scanning, AJR 134:1273-1274, 1980.
6. Hatfield, K.D., Segal, S.D., and Tait, K.: Barium sulfate for abdominal computer assisted tomography, J. Comput. Assist. Tomogr. 4:570-575, 1980.
6a. Ball, D.S., Radecki, P.D., Friedman, A.C., et al.: Contrast medium precipitation during abdominal CT, Radiology 158:258-260, 1986.
7. Federle, M.P., Goldberg, H.I., Kaiser, J.A., et al.: Evaluation of abdominal trauma by computed tomography, Radiology 138:637-644, 1981.
8. Jeffrey, R.B., Federle, M.P., and Wall, S.: Value of computed tomography in detecting occult gastrointestinal perforation, J. Comput. Assist. Tomogr. 7:825-827, 1983.
9. Cochran, D.O., Armond, C.H., and Shucart, W.A.: An experimental study of the effects of barium and intestinal content on the peritoneal cavity, AJR 89:883-885, 1963.
10. Davenport, H.W.: Physiology of the digestive tract, Chicago, 1966, Year Book Medical Publishers, Inc.
11. Hunt, J.N., and Knox, M.T.: Physiology—alimentary motility and transport and their relation to sensation. In Margulis, A.R., and Burhenne, H.J., editors: Alimentary tract roentgenology, ed. 2, St. Louis, 1983, The C.V. Mosby Co.
12. Eaton, S.B., and Ferrucci, J.T.: Radiology of the duodenum, Philadelphia, 1972, W.B. Saunders Co.
13. Moss, A.A., and Goldberg, H.I.: Pharmacoradiology in CT scanning. In Margulis, A.R., and Burhenne, H.J., editors: Alimentary tract radiology, St. Louis, 1979, The C.V. Mosby Co.
14. Moss, A.A., Kressel, H.Y., Korobkin, M., et al.: The effect of gastrograffin and glucagon on CT scanning of the pancreas: a blind clinical trial, Radiology 126:711-714, 1978.
15. Sones, P.J., and Steel, J.R.: Advances in CT examination of the pancreas, J. Comput. Assist. Tomogr. 2:514-518, 1978.
16. Feczko, P.J., Simms, S.M., and Iorio, J.: Gastroduodenal response to low dose glucagon, AJR 140:935-940, 1983.
17. Miller, R.E., Chernish, S.M., Greenman, G.F., et al.: Gastroduodenal response to minute doses of glucagon, Radiology 143:317-320, 1982.
18. Kaye, M.W., Young, S.W., and Hayward, R.: Gastric pseudotumor on CT scanning, AJR 135:190-193, 1980.
19. Marks, W.M.: Intestinal pseudotumors: a problem in abdominal CT solved by direct techniques, Gastrointest. Radiol. 5:155-157, 1980.
20. Baldwin, G.H.: Computed tomography of the pancreas: negative contrast medium, Radiology 128:827-828, 1978.
21. Kreel, L.: Contrast media for gastrointestinal examinations with computed tomography. In Felix, R., Kagner, E., and Wegener, O.H.: Contrast media in computed tomography, Berlin, 1981, Excerpta Medica.
22. Hamlin, D.J., and Burgener, F.A.: Positive and negative contrast agents in CT evaluation of the abdomen and pelvis, CT 5:81-90, 1981.
23. Haaga, J.R., Alfidi, R.J., Zelich, M.G., et al.: Computed tomography of the pancreas, Radiology 120:589-599, 1976.
24. Cranston, P.E.: Technical note: colon opacification by oral water soluble contrast medium administration the night prior to CT examinations, J. Comput. Assist. Tomogr. 6:413-415, 1982.
25. Miller, D.G., Bjorguinsson, E., Termeulen, D., et al.: Gastrografin vs. dilute barium for colonic CT examination: a blind, randomized study, J. Comput. Assist. Tomogr. 9:451-453, 1985.
26. Saunders, R.C., Mcneil, B.J., Freidberg, H.J., et al.: A preoperative study of computed tomography and ultrasound in the detection and staging of pelvic masses, Radiology 146:439-442, 1983.
27. Coin, J.T., and Coin, C.G.: "Nontoxic" contrast agents for computed tomography. In Felix, R., Kagner, E., and Wegener, O.H., editors: Contrast media in computed tomography, Berlin, 1981, Excerpta Medica.
28. Hamlin, D.J., Burgener, F.A., and Sicky, B.: A new technique to stage early rectal carcinoma by computed tomography, Radiology 141:539-540, 1981.
29. Megibow, A.J., Zerhouni, E.A., Schumacher, K.J., et al.: Air contrast techniques in gastrointestinal computed tomography, AJR 145:418, 1985.
30. Thompson, W.A., Halvorsen, R.A., and Williford, M.E.: Computed tomography of the gastroesophageal junction, Radiographics 2:179-194, 1982.
31. Megibow, A.J., Zerhouni, E.A., Hulnick, D.H., et al.: Air opacification of the colon as an adjunct in CT evaluation of the pelvis, J. Comput. Assist. Tomogr. 8:797-800, 1984.
32. Foley, W.D., Berland, L.L., Lawson, T.L., et al.: Contrast enhancement techniques for dynamic hepatic computed tomography, Radiology 147:797-803, 1983.
33. Bernardino, M.A., and Sones, P.J., editors: Hepatic radiology, New York, 1984, Macmillan Publishing Co.

Chapter Two

ESOPHAGUS

David P. Naidich

Considerable interest has focused on the use of computed tomography (CT) in evaluating esophageal disease. Although esophagography and endoscopy provide invaluable information concerning the esophageal mucosa, CT offers the potential advantage of identification of the entire thickness of the esophageal wall, as well as direct visualization of adjacent mediastinal structures. This basic principle was first described in 1978 by Kressel et al. who defined three categories of alimentary tract abnormalities most readily assessed by CT: (1) intramural masses; (2) diffuse bowel-wall thickening; and (3) extrinsic involvement.[1] Significantly, of the 43 patients originally described in this series, only two patients with esophageal lesions were included. Although subsequent reports have confirmed the role of CT in evaluating gastrointestinal pathology, convincing evidence of the value of CT in esophageal disease has been delayed. This in part is a consequence of the need for relatively fast scanning capability to adequately visualize thoracic anatomy. Additionally, reliable means for distending the esophagus for CT evaluation has proved elusive. However, experience with a wide range of esophageal lesions has been reported. It is the purpose of this chapter to review current knowledge about CT of the esophagus, as well as speculate on future applications.

INDICATIONS

CT should not be used as a screening examination for patients with suspected esophageal disease. Although a diagnosis of a primary esophageal abnormality will occasionally be made with CT, this is almost always serendipitous. Esophagography and endoscopy remain the initial choices for examining symptomatic patients.

In our experience CT is especially indicated in the following settings:

1. To evaluate and characterize lesions that appear intramural or extramural on esophagography
2. To evaluate esophageal perforations
3. To evaluate and stage patients with esophageal carcinoma, primarily to evaluate the mediastinum and upper abdomen

As discussed and illustrated throughout this chapter, CT frequently allows precise localization of pathology and may provide the additional benefit of detailed tissue characterization by use of attenuation coefficients. In select patients this may be of diagnostic value.

At the present time there is no convincing evidence that CT plays any substantial role in the evaluation of most benign esophageal disease. This includes: benign strictures, inflammatory disease of any etiology, and disorders of esophageal motility, such as achalasia or scleroderma. CT is useful in esophageal perforation to assess the extent of pleural and mediastinal fluid collections and to detect regions of loculation.

TECHNIQUE

There is no generally accepted technique for routine CT scanning of the esophagus. A variety of methods have been employed in an attempt to obtain uniform distention and opacification of the esophageal lumen, with only limited success reported.

This problem has been obviated to some degree by the recent development of a 3% barium paste that is now commercially available.* Cayea and Seltzer evaluated use of this paste in 31 patients and found that the esophageal lumen was well coated in a majority of patients (75%, 85%, and 60% of cases for the upper, mid, and, lower esophagus respectively).[2] In no case was esophageal anatomy obscured by streak artifacts. Our experience with this product has been equally positive, and its use or its equivalent is recommended in the evaluation of all cases with esophageal pathology.

The following guidelines are recommended for CT evaluation of the esophagus:

1. No attempt should be made to opacify or distend the esophageal lumen for routine thoracic CT. Uniformity of opacification is difficult in normal individuals, and in asymptomatic patients the use of specialized barium preparations is probably not cost-effective.

2. Correlation with esophagography or endoscopy should be considered mandatory in order to determine the specific area(s) of greatest interest before scanning.

3. Ten to fifteen minutes before the start of the CT examination each patient should be given a standard preparation of approximately 200 ml of oral contrast material in order to distend the stomach. In our practice dilute barium sulfate suspensions are preferred, since they are palatable and provide quality images without causing streak artifacts. Just before scanning, with the patient already in the CT gantry and the scout image obtained, the patient is given an additional ounce of high-density barium paste. Sequential 10 mm thick scans are then obtained from the thoracic inlet through the upper abdomen. Short scan times (usually in the range of 5 seconds) should be employed to minimize respiratory artifacts.

4. The initial scan sequence is reviewed while the patient is still on the table. Additional scans are then obtained as deemed necessary to improve anatomic definition. If the esophagus has been less than optimally opacified additional high-density oral contrast material should be given.

5. Intravenous contrast need not be administered routinely. Instead the initial noncontrast scans should be reviewed and, depending on the indication, a bolus of 50 ml of 60% diatrizoate meglumine (Renografin 60) or its equivalent can be given with images obtained through the region of maximum interest. Whenever possible, imaging should be performed with dynamic incrementation. This is especially valuable in identifying mediastinal vascular structures and in evaluating the liver and retroperitoneum. In select cases this technique may be of value in direct characterization of esophageal and periesophageal lesions themselves.

Modification of these guidelines are to be anticipated as determined by experience and as dictated by the exigencies of scanning. Ideally, each case should be individually monitored to maximize diagnostic accuracy.

*Esoph-O-Cat available from E-Z-EM Company, Inc., Westbury, New York.

ANATOMY

Accurate interpretation of CT scans requires detailed knowledge of normal cross-sectional anatomy. Thorough familiarity with normal CT anatomy is a prerequisite for confident recognition and interpretation of subtle pathologic change.

The esophagus is a muscular tube lined by squamous epithelium that extends inferiorly from the cricopharyngeus muscle at the level of the cricoid cartilage for a distance of approximately 25 cm to terminate at the gastric cardia. Brombart anatomically divided the thoracic esophagus into the following segments: (1) paratracheal; (2) aortic; (3) bronchial; (4) interaorticobronchial; (5) interbronchial (subcarinal); (6) retrocardiac; (7) epiphrenic; (8) intrahiatal; and (9) intraabdominal (submerged).[3] This classification has proved useful in the interpretation of esophagrams and with slight modification corresponds to most published CT-anatomic descriptions of the thoracic esophagus.[4,5] All of these classifications are based on recognition of representative or characteristic sections from the thoracic inlet to the upper abdomen and each is defined by the most prominant, adjacent, mediastinal landmarks.

Level 1: cervical esophagus— pharyngoesophageal junction (Fig. 2-1)

Anatomically the pharyngoesophageal junction is defined by the cricopharyngeous muscle at the level of the C6 vertebral body. This level is most easily localized in cross-section by identification of the cricoid cartilage, which is usually calcified and forms the lateral borders of the tracheal air column. The esophagus lies adjacent to the posterior wall of the trachea into which it may protrude slightly. Anterolaterally, the esophagus is close to both lobes of the thyroid gland. Posterolaterally, the esophagus may be distinguished from the adjacent prevertebral muscles (the longus colli and longus capitis muscles). It is infrequent to see air within the esophageal lumen at this level.

Level 2: thoracic inlet (Fig. 2-2)

This section marks the approximate level dividing the cervical from the thoracic esophagus and is easily identified by the characteristic cross-sectional appearance of the sternoclavicular joint spaces anteriorly. The esophagus continues to lie adjacent to the membranous portion of the trachea posteriorly, which it may normally indent to a slight degree. The esophagus may also lie immediately lateral and to the left of the trachea, a common normal variant. Mediastinal fat is usually sufficiently abundant in these sections to allow definition of the lateral borders of the esophagus.

Level 3: upper mediastinum (Fig. 2-3)

At this level the esophagus normally moves slightly to the left, lying posterolateral to the trachea and posteromedial to the subclavian artery. The esophagus may also lie directly lateral to the trachea, as noted earlier. No intervening fat plane separates the esophagus from the trachea although one can usually be defined between the esophagus and the subclavian artery.

It is often possible to identify a small amount of air within the esophagus as it passes through the thoracic inlet and upper mediastinum (Figs. 2-2 and 2-3). This has been documented to occur in 80% of scans in some series and may cause the esophagus to assume an irregular or odd-shaped configuration as a result of incomplete distention of the esophageal lumen.[5] A spurious impression of abnormal esophageal wall thickening may result (Fig. 2-3, A). As discussed in greater detail in the section on esophageal cancer, these variations should not be misconstrued as pathologic. Images obtained following additional contrast material administration are of value in dispelling doubt in equivical cases.

Occasionally, on sections through the upper mediastinum, the esophagus will lie close to the left lung. This relationship accounts for visualization of the posterior junction line identifiable on some posteroanterior radiographs (Fig. 2-3, B). The posterior junction line is usually most prominent when there is some degree of overinflation of the lungs as may occur with underlying chronic obstructive pulmonary disease, causing the esophagus to be in contact with both lungs simultaneously (Fig. 2-3, B).

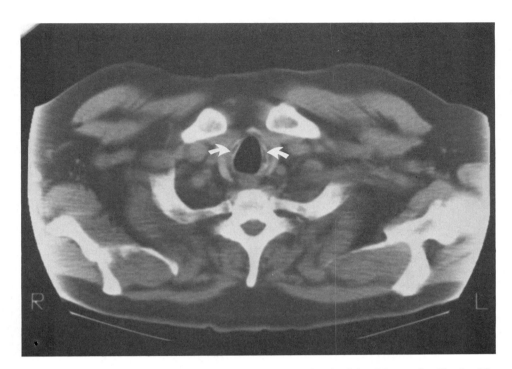

Fig. 2-1. Pharyngoesophageal junction. Section at the level of the C6 vertebral body. The cricoid cartilage is calcified and easily identified along the lateral borders of the tracheal air column *(curved arrows)*. The esophagus lies adjacent to the posterior wall of the trachea.

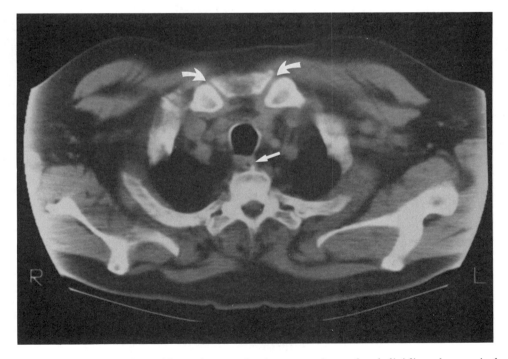

Fig. 2-2. Thoracic inlet. This section marks the approximate level dividing the cervical from the thoracic esophagus and is easily identified by the characteristic appearance of the sternoclavicular joints *(curved arrows)*. The esophagus lies posterior to the trachea and slightly to the left with no identifiable intervening fat plane *(arrow)*.

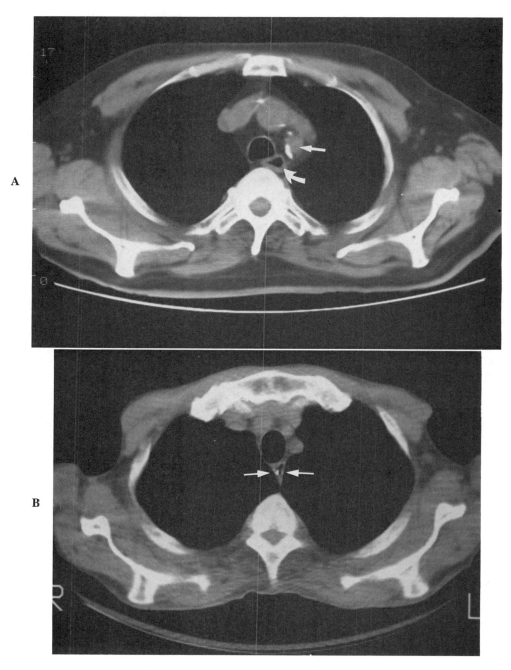

Fig. 2-3. Upper mediastinum. **A,** Section at the level of the great vessels. The esophageal lumen is partially distended by air *(curved arrow)*. This is a frequent and normal variant that may create the false impression of esophageal wall thickening (compare to Fig. 2-31). The lateral margins of the esophagus are well defined on the left side by fat, allowing for clear delineation of the left subclavian artery *(arrow)*. **B,** Section through the great vessels at approximately the same level shown in **A.** In this case there is hyperinflation of the lungs, which bilaterally approximate the esophagus *(arrows)*. These relationships account for the posterior junction line seen on posteroanterior chest radiographs.

Level 4: aortic arch (Fig. 2-4)

In this section, the esophagus continues to lie just to the left of and posterior to the trachea with no apparent intervening fat plane. Behind the trachea a portion of the right upper lobe may extend medially to lie adjacent to the right lateral wall of the esophagus. These relationships can be defined on plain radiographs and have been designated variously as the "posterior tracheal band" or the "tracheoesophageal stripe."

As described by Bachman and Teixidor, the posterior tracheal band is a thin, uniform line, 3 mm thick, which can be identified in up to 90% of normal individuals in properly positioned, lateral chest radiographs.[6] This line is defined anteriorly by air within the tracheal lumen and posteriorly by aerated lung in the retrotracheal recess (Fig. 2-4). A similar landmark, the tracheoesophageal stripe has been described by Palayew.[7] This is a sharply demarcated line that may be identified behind the cervical or thoracic portions of the trachea in lateral chest radiographs and that is formed by air within the tracheal lumen anteriorly and the esophageal lumen posteriorly. The potential significance of these lines as plain radiographic indicators of esophageal pathology is made obvious by correlation with cross-sectional images (Fig. 2-4).[8]

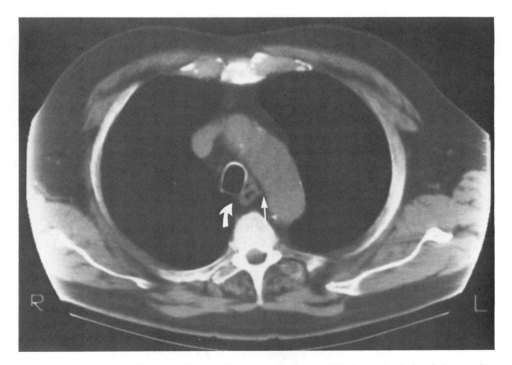

Fig. 2-4. Aortic arch. The esophagus lies posterior and slightly to the left of the trachea with no apparent intervening fat plane. Behind the trachea, a portion of the right upper lobe may extend medially to lie adjacent to the right lateral wall of the esophagus, posterior to the trachea *(curved arrow)*. The esophageal lumen is partially expanded by air (compare to Fig. 2-3, *A*). These features may be identified on lateral chest radiographs and have been termed the posterior tracheal band and the tracheoesophageal stripe, respectively. Note that in this patient a fat plane is present between the esophagus and the aorta *(arrow)*. This may not be present in less obese patients.

Level 5: carina—left main stem bronchus
(Fig. 2-5)

At and just below the carina the esophagus usually lies immediately posterior to the left main stem bronchus. As reported by Schneekloth, et al. in their evaluation of normal topographic relationships between the esophagus and airways in 20 normal patients, in no case could fat planes be established between the esophagus and either the trachea or left main stem bronchus.[5] This lack of an identifiable fascial plane has been documented by Samuelson et al. and accounts for the frequency with which esophagobronchial fistula occurs in esophageal carcinoma.[9,10]

Posteriorly, the esophagus lies adjacent to the azygos vein; laterally and to the right, the esophagus is in contact with aerated lung and pleura forming the azygoesophageal recess. Posteriorly and to the left, the esophagus approximates the descending thoracic aorta, which it will continue to parallel throughout the length of the thorax. These relationships, especially between the right lung, pleura, and azygos vein on the right, and the aorta posteriorly on the left usually can be identified with little significant variation from the level of the carina to the hemidiaphragms.

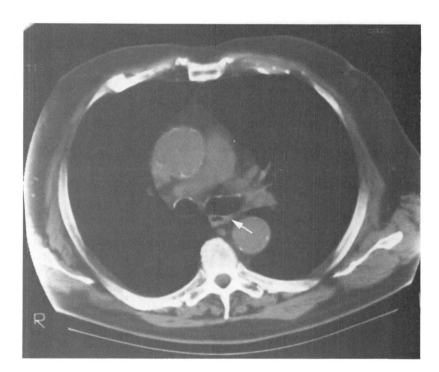

Fig. 2-5. Carina-left main stem bronchus. At and just below the carina the esophagus usually lies immediately posterior to the left main stem bronchus (*arrow*). The close relationship between structures at this level and higher, between the trachea and esophagus, accounts for the frequency with which esophagobronchial fistula occur in esophageal carcinoma (compare to Figs. 2-38 and 2-39).

Level 6: subcarinal space (Fig. 2-6)

In this section essential anatomic relationships between the esophagus, azygos vein, right lung and pleura, and aorta are similar to these already illustrated in Fig. 2-5. Anteriorly, the esophagus still lies adjacent to the left main stem bronchus. The esophagus will also lie adjacent to any enlarged subcarinal lymph nodes if present (Fig. 2-6). As shown by Levy-Ravetch et al., the uppermost portion of the oblique pericardial sinus lies close to the esophagus at this level, providing a potential pathway for spread of disease from the subcarinal space and esophagus to the pericardium.[11]

Level 7: retrocardiac—left atrial region
(Fig. 2-7)

Below the carina the esophagus lies adjacent to the posterior wall of the left atrium. As shown in Fig. 2-7, in obese or well-nourished individuals, a fat plane separating the posterior pericardial reflections and left atrium from the esophagus may be defineable. However, as reported by Samuelson, et al. it may not be possible to differentiate the esophagus from the left atrium, especially in aesthenic individuals.[9] In their series of 25 normal patients in no case could a fat layer be identified separating the esophagus from the left atrium at all levels.

On the right side, the esophagus may be adjacent to the medial aspect of the inferior pulmonary ligament (usually best defined on sections imaged with wide or lung windows). Posteriorly the esophagus maintains its close relationship to the descending thoracic aorta.

Level 8: lower mediastinal esophagus—the gastroesophageal region (Figs. 2-8 and 2-9)

From the vantage of cross-sectional imaging, the lower mediastinal esophagus and the gastroesophageal region are easiest to visualize if approached as a unit. The key to the anatomy of this region is identification of the esophageal hiatus and the gastrohepatic ligament.

The lower mediastinal esophagus maintains its position adjacent to the aorta posterolaterally and the azygos vein laterally (Fig. 2-9, *A*). At this level the esophagus lies between the medial portions of both lower lobes with their associated pleural reflections. Anteriorly the esophagus is still in contact with the posteroinferior pericardial reflections, as well as with the cephalic portion of the inferior vena cava and the coronary vein. Mediastinal fat is usually prominent at this level, aiding anatomic orientation.

Inferiorly, the esophagus courses through the esophageal hiatus (Fig. 2-9, *B* through *D*). The esophageal hiatus is an elliptical opening in the muscular portion of the diaphragm just to the left of the midline. The uppermost portion of the hiatus corresponds to the level of the tenth thoracic vertebral body. The margins of the hiatus are formed by the arms of the diaphragmatic crura, which are easily identified on cross-section. Variation in the normal appearance of the crura is common, especially nodular thickening that may be mistaken for either abnormally enlarged lymph nodes or rarely crural invasion by adjacent tumor. These variations have been well described.[12,13]

Throughout most of its course the esophagus lies just to the left of the midline and anterior to the descending aorta. As the esophagus passes through the upper margin of the hiatus, it assumes an oblique orientation, coursing in a posterior-to-anterior and right-to-left direction (Fig. 2-9, *B* through *D*). As the esophagus courses through the hiatus it is anchored anatomically by the phrenico-esophageal ligament. This ligament is formed from collagen and elastic fibers derived primarily from the endothoracic and endoabdominal fascia.[14] These attachments anchor the esophagus at, above, and below the hiatus and physiologically play an important role in preventing esophageal herniation (see the section that follows).

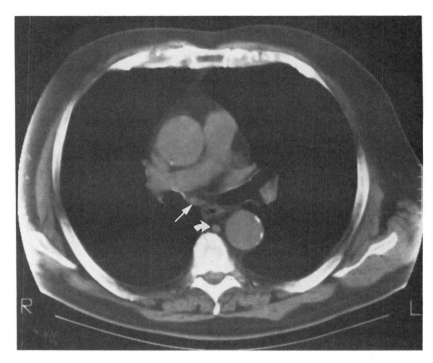

Fig. 2-6. Subcarinal space. Anatomic relationships at this level are similar to those illustrated in Fig. 2-5. Anteriorly, the esophagus lies adjacent to the posterior wall of the left main stem bronchus; to the right, a small subcarinal lymph node is present *(arrow)*. The proximity between subcarinal nodes and the anterior wall of the esophagus accounts for the frequent involvement of the esophagus in patients with tuberculous adenitis, the sequela of which may be a traction diverticulum (compare to Fig. 2-26). Posteriorly, the esophagus lies adjacent to the azygos vein *(curved arrow)* and the anteromedial surface of the aorta.

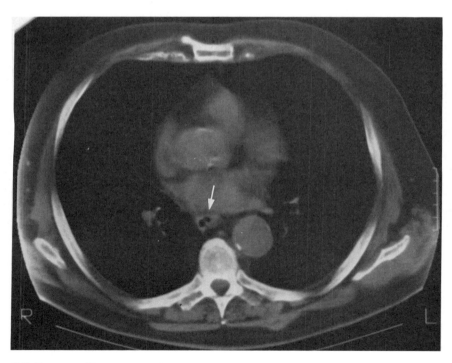

Fig. 2-7. Retrocardiac space. Below the carina the esophagus lies adjacent to the posterior wall of the left atrium *(arrow)*. A clearly defined fat plane is generally seen only in well-nourished or obese patients. On the right side the esophagus may lie in contact with the medial portion of the right lower lobe and its pleural reflections.

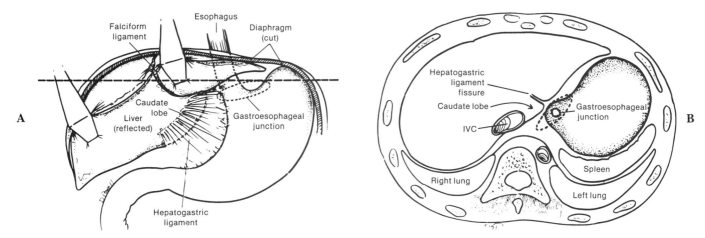

Fig. 2-8. Gastroesophageal junction. **A** and **B,** Schematic representation of the gastro-esophageal junction in the coronal and transverse planes, respectively. **A,** Note the relationship between the gastrohepatic ligament, the caudate lobe of the liver, and the medial wall of the gastroesophageal junction. **B,** A cross-section of the gastroesophageal region that corresponds to the level of the dotted line in **A.** Note that laterally the gastrohepatic ligament can be identified as a line separating the caudate lobe posteriorly from the lateral segment of the left lobe anteriorly. (Adapted from Thompson, W.M., et al.: Computed tomography of the gastroesophageal junction, Radiographics **2:**179-193, 1982.)

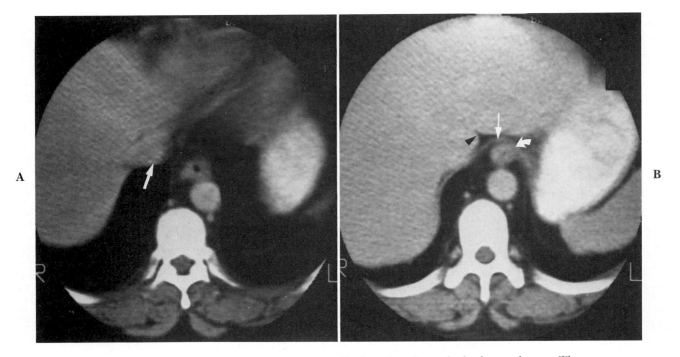

Fig. 2-9. Gastroesophageal region. **A,** Magnified section through the lower thorax. The esophagus lies between the medial portions of both lower lobes with their associated pleural reflections. Anteriorly the esophagus is in contact with the posteroinferior pericardial reflections as well as the cephalic portion of the inferior vena cava *(arrow).* Mediastinal fat is usually prominent at this level. **B,** Magnified section through the upper portion of the esophageal hiatus. The medial margin of the right crus is especially visible in this section, lying immediately anterior to the esophagus *(arrow).* The medial margin of the left crus also approximates the anterior wall of the distal esophagus; it is somewhat less well seen *(curved arrow).* Mediastinal fat still surrounds the esophagus. Oral contrast material is present within the stomach. The uppermost portion of the fissure for the gastrohepatic ligament is also identifiable at this level *(arrowhead).*

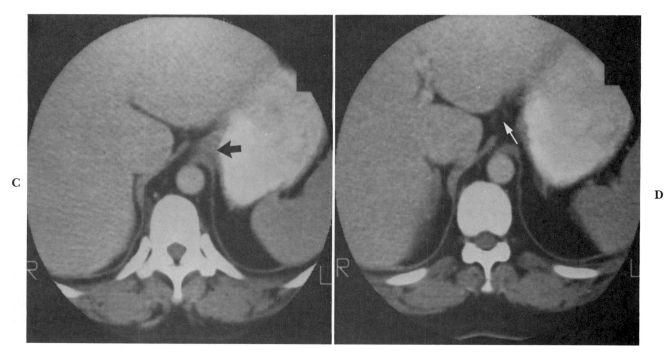

Fig. 2-9, cont'd. C, Section through the submerged or abdominal esophagus. At this level the esophagus is frequently cone-shaped with its base at the junction of the gastric fundus *(arrow)*. This appearance should not be misconstrued as pathologic. The medial margins of the crura are still readily identifiable. The fissure of the gastrohepatic ligament is easily identified, separating the caudate lobe posteriorly from the medial aspect of the left lobe anteriorly. **D,** Section through the lowest portion of the esophageal hiatus. The medial margins of the crura are still easily identified, as is the cleft of the gastrohepatic ligament. There is fat within the leaves of the ligament medially in which a few ill-defined densities can be identified, probably representing normal vascular and lymphatic structures *(arrow)*.

The gastroesophageal junction itself lies just below the diaphragm and in the context of this discussion represents the junction of the abdominal esophagus with the stomach. As it courses through the upper abdomen the distal esophagus is enveloped by the most cranial aspect of the gastrohepatic ligament. This originates from a deep cleft in the liver, separating the caudate lobe posteriorly from the lateral segment of the left lobe anteriorly and serves as a convenient reference point for identifying the esophagogastric junction.[15] As pointed out by Balfe et al., while the peritoneal surfaces lining the gastrohepatic ligament cannot be seen on CT, fat, vascular structures, and nodes within the leaves of the ligament routinely can be identified (Fig. 2-9, *D*).[16] Typically, the gastrohepatic lig-

ament appears as a triangular or crescentric area of fat density located between the liver on the right and the lesser curvature of the stomach on the left. This corresponds to the lowest portion of the esophageal hiatus (Fig. 2-9, *D*).

At the level of the gastrohepatic ligament the abdominal esophagus lies close to the posterior surface of the left lobe of the liver anteriorly, the caudate lobe of the liver laterally, and the fundus of the stomach to the left. On cross-section the abdominal or submerged portion of the esophagus is frequently cone-shaped with its base at the junction of the gastric fundus.[17] This segment is only rarely distended by air or oral contrast agents on routine supine scans, and as a consequence this appearance may be mistaken as pathologic. Marks

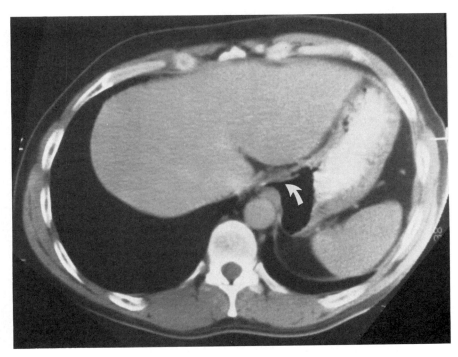

Fig. 2-10. Gastroesophageal junction—decubitus view. Section through the esophageal hiatus obtained with the patient in a decubitus position immediately following ingestion of 200 ml of standard oral contrast material, rotated 90 degrees for illustrative purposes. The submerged portion of the esophagus and the cardia are distended by air *(curved arrow),* allowing for accurate identification of the true thickness of the esophageal walls.

et al., in their retrospective series of 100 randomly selected cases, have drawn attention to the frequency of this pseudotumoral appearance by noting that a prominent soft-tissue density could be defined in the region of the gastroesophageal junction in 38% of cases.[18] In 12% the findings necessitated further CT evaluation. Particularly disturbing was the suggestion of a mass along the medial-cephalic aspect of the stomach in apparent continuity with the abdominal esophagus. As shown by Thompson et al., anatomic clarification is simply obtained by scanning patients in the left lateral decubitus position following ingestion of at least 200 ml of standard oral contrast material (Fig. 2-10).[19] Similar results may be obtained if the stomach is distended only by air.

HIATAL HERNIA

Thorough familiarity with the normal radiographic and cross-sectional appearance of the gastroesophageal region is a necessary prerequisite for accurate identification of hiatal hernias (see Figs. 2-8 and 2-9). As discussed previously the esophageal hiatus is formed by the decussation of muscle fibers originating from the diaphragm around the lower esophagus. The esophagus is fixed at the level of the hiatus by the phrenicoesophageal ligament, which is not routinely visible on CT scans. This is generally quite well defined in infants but with age shows a definite tendency toward loosening.[14] The most common anatomic abnormalities seen in individuals with sliding hiatal hernias are dehiscence of the diaphragmatic crura and stretching of the phrenicoesophageal ligament, which for all practical purposes ceases to exist in adults with long-standing hiatal hernias.

Widening of the esophageal hiatus can be diagnosed on cross-section whenever the medial margins of the diaphragmatic crura are not tightly apposed (Fig. 2-11). Ginalski et al., in a retrospective study of the anatomy of the esophageal hiatus in 320 patients, correlated the presence of dehiscense with patient's age and sex.[20] Widening of the hiatus was demonstrated in 122 patients (38%). This was never observed in 40 individuals under the age of 20, yet a steady increase in the incidence of widening could be documented with increasing age. These findings have been interpreted as supportive evidence that dehiscence of the diaphragmatic junction is an acquired malformation. Actual mea-

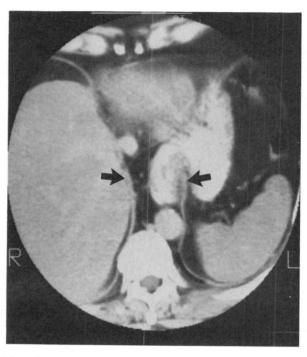

Fig. 2-11. Hiatal hernia. Magnified section through the esophageal hiatus in a patient with a sliding hiatal hernia. The medial margins of the crura are widely separated *(arrows)*. A portion of the contrast-filled stomach and peritoneal fat can be identified between the widened margins of the crura.

surements of the standard width of the esophageal hiatus have been reported by Schneekloth et al.[5] In a series of 20 normal patients between 46 and 76 years of age, the average width of the hiatus, defined as the distance between the medial club-like margins of the crura, was 10.66 mm (SD ± 2.43 mm) with a maximum width of 15 mm.

The relationship between a widened esophageal hiatus and findings at barium swallow has also been defined by Ginalski.[20] In his series, 34 of 43 patients (86.4%) with a widened hiatus on CT were found to have sliding hernias documented by corresponding upper gastrointestinal series. In 26 of 37 cases, the sliding hernia itself was detected by CT, defineable as an apparent pseudomass usually filled with oral contrast material lying within and above the esophageal hiatus (Figs. 2-11 and 2-12). Similar findings have been reported by Lindell and Bernardino.[21]

Sliding hiatal hernias are frequently associated with an apparent increase in mediastinal fat surrounding the distal esophagus (Figs. 2-11 and 2-12).[22] This appearance is secondary to herniation of omentum through the phrenicoesophageal ligament. The term "sliding" is applied to these her-

nias because a portion of the peritoneal sac always forms a part of the wall of the hernia.[14] This is easily identified with CT and may be present prior to actual herniation of the stomach itself (Fig. 2-12).[23] Occasionally, in the presence of massive ascites, it may also be possible to identify fluid within herniated peritoneum anterior to the contrast-filled stomach (Fig. 2-13).

Paraesophageal herniation, which occurs when a portion or all of the stomach is displaced superiorly into the thorax through a diaphragmatic defect, may also be defined with CT. The key to diagnosis is identification of the esophagogastric junction, which generally remains in a normal subdiaphragmatic position (Fig. 2-14).

Occasionally, tumors arise in hernias and may be suggested on CT examination by the finding of either eccentric thickening of the esophageal wall or of a discrete soft-tissue mass (Fig. 2-15). Correlation with esophagography or endoscopy is always necessary since incomplete filling of the lumen of an uncomplicated sliding hiatal hernia may mimic the appearance of carcinoma.[25] In select cases CT may play a role in evaluating complications of surgery performed in this region (Fig. 2-16).

Text continued p. 50.

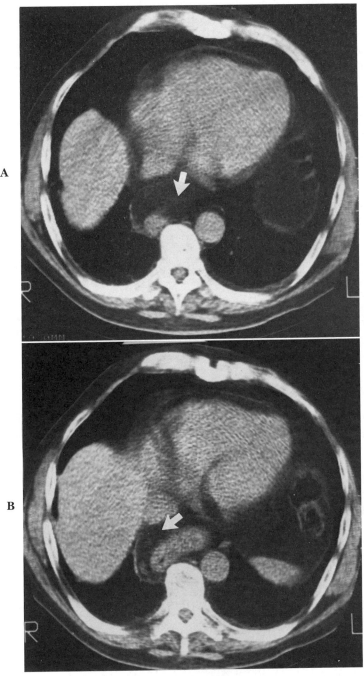

Fig. 2-12. Hiatal hernia. **A** and **B,** Sequential sections taken from above downward through the lower thorax. There is a marked increase in the amount of posterior mediastinal fat *(arrow)* anterior to the esophagus (compare to Fig. 2-9, *A*), representing herniated peritoneal fat, which may occasionally be identified before visualizing actual herniation of the stomach itself.

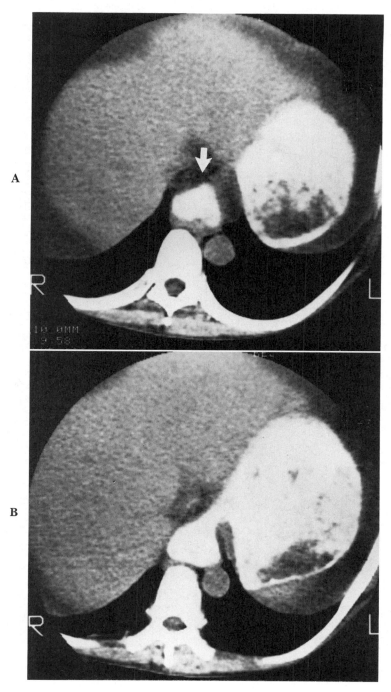

Fig. 2-13. Hiatal hernia. **A** and **B,** Scans through the lower thorax and esophageal hiatus, respectively, show a large contrast-filled, sliding hiatal hernia. Note that in both scans there is a large quantity of ascites surrounding both the liver and spleen. **A,** Fluid present anterior to the contrast-filled esophagus represents fluid in a portion of the peritoneal sac that anteriorly forms a part of the wall of the hernia *(arrow).*

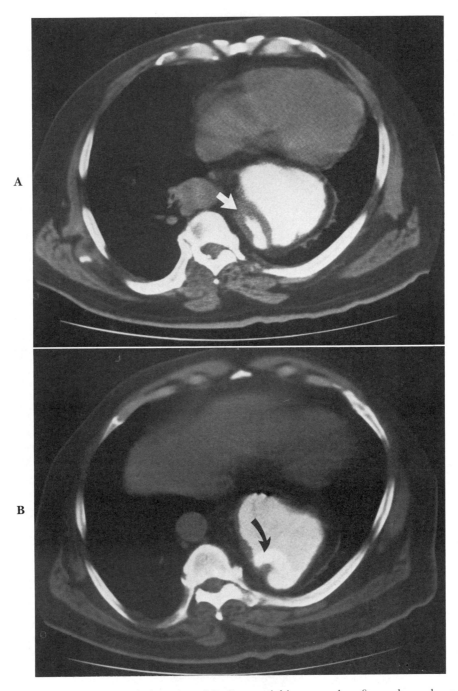

Fig. 2-14. Complex herniation. **A** and **B,** Sequential images taken from above downward through the lower thorax in a patient with a hiatal hernia. Note that a portion of the hernia sac has come to lie anterolateral to the distal esophagus (*arrow* in **A**). Inferiorly, the esophagogastric junction is well defined due to a streaming effect of contrast material as it leaves the esophagus and enters the stomach (*curved arrow* in **B**). Identification of the gastroesophageal junction above the esophageal hiatus confirms that this is essentially a sliding hiatal hernia with a paraesophageal component. Note the large quantity of associated fat that surrounds the hernia both anteriorly and laterally within the peritoneal reflections, which can actually be identified medially (*curved arrow* in **B**).

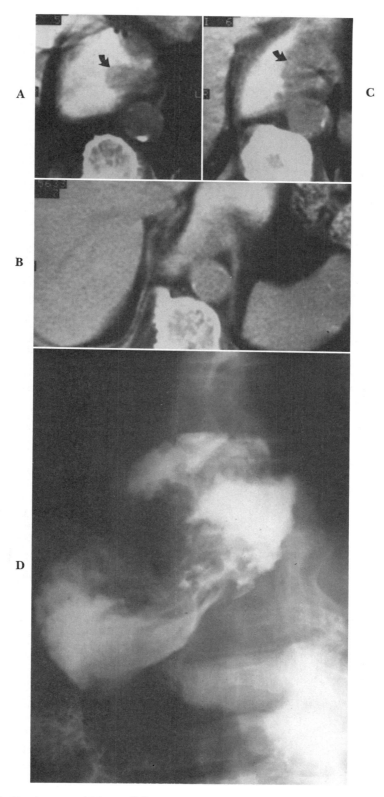

Fig. 2-15. Carcinoma within a sliding hiatal hernia. **A, B,** and **C,** Magnified sections through a sliding hiatal hernia. The stomach is distended with oral contrast material. There is a nodular soft-tissue density along the left lateral wall of the stomach that proved to be a result of adenocarcinoma of the stomach *(arrows)*. **D,** Corresponding esophagram documents large filling defect within the hernia.

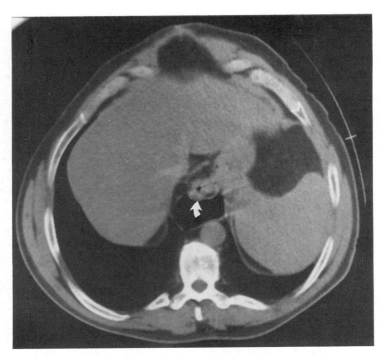

Fig. 2-16. Gastroesophageal region—postoperative evaluation. Section through the esophageal hiatus in a patient following Nissen fundoplication. The esophagus *(curved arrow)* lies anterior to the stomach, which is distended by air.

Intramural lesions

Tumors arising in the wall of the esophagus are rare, accounting for less than 0.5% of all esophageal lesions.[26] They are usually detected on upper gastrointestinal series where they characteristically appear as smooth, rounded, filling defects with clearly defined edges. Differential diagnosis most commonly includes leiomyomas, duplication cysts, neurofibromas, lipomas, myoblastomas, and, rarely, metastases or sarcomas.

The most common benign lesion of the esophagus is a leiomyoma. These may be asymptomatic, although if sufficiently large they can cause dysphagia, or rarely, hematemesis.[27] The CT appearance of both leiomyomas and leiomyosarcomas has been described by Megibow et al.[28] (Fig. 2-17). Leiomyomas typically are smooth, well-defined lesions, causing eccentric thickening of the bowel

wall and deformity of the adjacent bowel lumen. On rare occasions calcification may be defineable. Most leiomyomas are of uniform, soft-tissue density and show diffuse enhancement following intravenous contrast material administration (Fig. 2-18). In the series reported by Megibow, the average CT number of enhanced lesions was 49 Hounsfield units when studied using a continuous infusion with a reported range of 30 to 63 H units.[28] In general, maximal enhancement within lesions averaged 1 to 1.5 times the base-line precontrast-enhanced values. Although suggestive, these patterns of enhancement are of only limited diagnostic value. As shown in Fig. 2-19, the findings of a smooth, well-defined lesion with uniform density may not always signify a benign etiology. From a practical standpoint, isolated mural lesions of the esophagus usually require surgical resection.

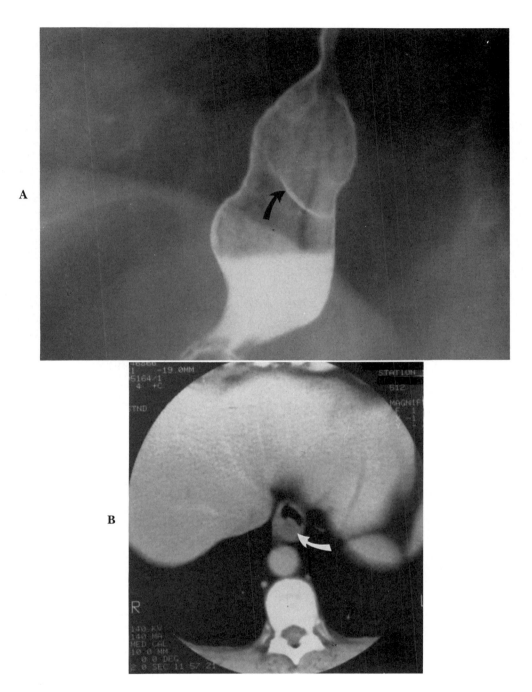

Fig. 2-17. Leiomyoma. **A,** Coned-down view of distal esophagus shows smooth filling defect in distal esophagus *(curved arrow)*. **B,** Magnified section through the distal esophagus at the level indicated by the *arrow* in **A.** There is a smooth, soft-tissue mass arising within the posterior wall of the esophagus, causing deformity of the adjacent air-filled lumen *(curved arrow)*. Leiomyoma was proved surgically.

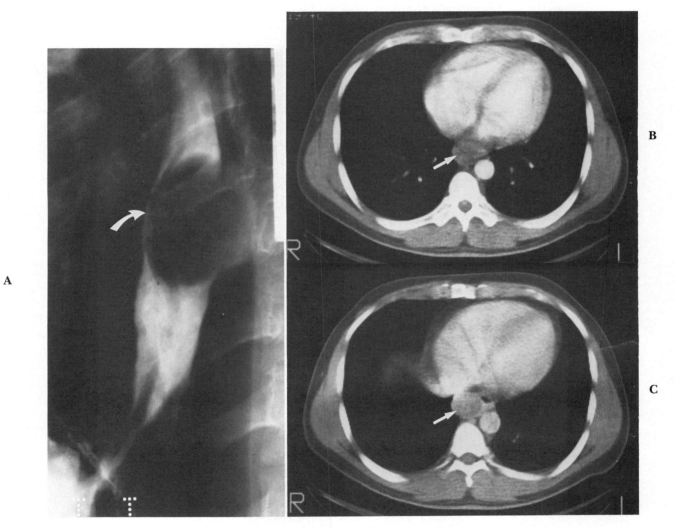

Fig. 2-18. Effect of contrast enhancement on leiomyoma. **A,** Coned-down view of distal esophagus shows a mass with characteristic features of a typical intramural lesion *(curved arrow)*. **B** and **C,** Sections at approximately the same level obtained through the distal esophagus following a bolus of intravenous contrast material. **B,** During the phase of maximal arterial enhancement, the lesion appears relatively lucent *(arrow)*. **C,** A time delayed scan obtained approximately 45 seconds later demonstrates uniform enhancement within this lesion *(arrow)*, which is readily apparent on visual inspection alone (compare to **B**). Leiomyomas are vascular lesions that can be enhanced, especially when in the capillary phase and following a bolus of intravenous contrast medium.

An important exception to the usual lack of histologic specificity encountered with most mural lesions is the role of CT in the evaluation of esophageal and bronchogenic duplication cysts.[29,30,31] These are included together because their radiologic and CT appearances overlap to a considerable degree. Sixty percent of esophageal duplication cysts are located in the lower esophagus, with the rest being distributed between the upper and middle thirds. These cysts are either intramural or, more commonly, may be attached to the esophagus in a paraesophageal location. As shown in Fig. 2-20, duplication cysts are well-defined lesions that are easily diagnosed on CT examination when they can be shown to be of water density (−5 to 20 H units). Even those lesions that have higher density resulting from the presence of debris or previous infection still characteristically show no evidence of enhancement following a bolus of intravenous contrast material. Recently, interest has focused on the potential role of CT for localization and documentation of the cystic nature of these lesions prior to esophagoscopy and diagnostic transesophageal needle aspiration.[32]

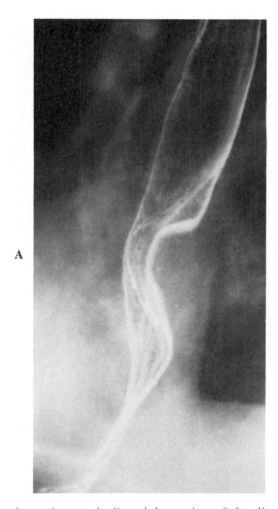

Fig. 2-19. Metastatic carcinoma. **A,** Coned-down view of the distal esophagus shows a smooth-bordered lesion deforming the esophageal lumen and compatible with either a mural or extramural lesion.

Continued.

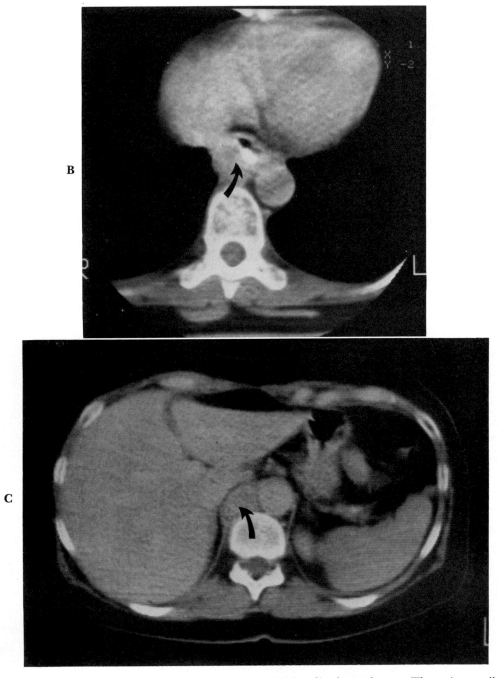

Fig. 2-19, cont'd. B, Magnified section through the distal esophagus. There is a well-defined soft-tissue mass of uniform density distorting and displacing the contrast-filled esophageal lumen *(curved arrow).* The appearance is similar to that of a leiomyoma (compare to Figs. 2-17 and 2-18). **C,** Section through the upper abdomen. *Curved arrow* points to a mass of retrocrural nodes secondary to metastatic breast carcinoma that had metastasized to the wall of the esophagus (biopsy proven).

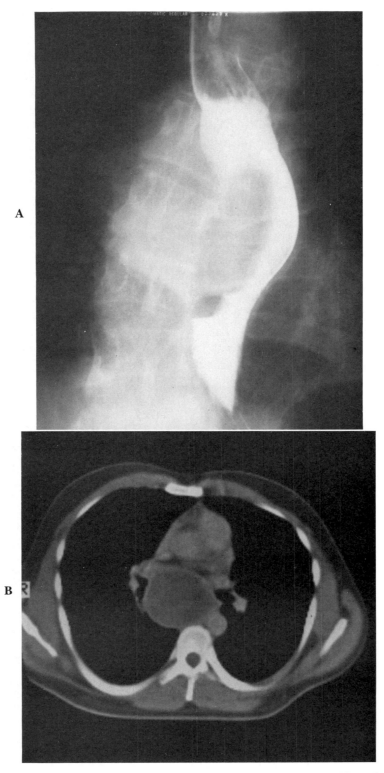

Fig. 2-20. Esophageal duplication cyst. **A,** Coned-down view of the midesophagus shows features typical of extrinsic displacement resulting from a large, well-defined mediastinal mass. **B,** Section at the level of the subcarinal space. There is a large, well-defined, fluid-filled mediastinal mass displacing the origins of the middle and lower lobe bronchi on the right. These features are typical of either an esophageal or bronchial duplication cyst (surgically proven).

ESOPHAGEAL VARICES

The role of CT in the evaluation of both gastric and esophageal varices has been well defined by numerous authors, including the demonstration of "downhill" varices associated with superior vena caval obstruction.[33,34,35] CT is especially valuable in the detection of paraesophageal varices. Ishikawa, et al. have shown in a study of 352 patients with documented portal hypertension that paraesophageal varices could be identified on routine films in 17 cases (4.8%).[36] Typically these paraesophageal varices appear as either right-sided or left-sided soft-tissue masses, necessitating their differentiation from enlarged periesophageal lymph nodes or other posterior mediastinal or paraspinal masses (Figs. 2-21 and 2-22). Although esophagography and endoscopy are accurate in confirming the presence of esophageal varices, paraesophageal varices have previously required angiography for definitive diagnosis. As documented by Clark et al. CT can obviate the need for invasive procedures by showing characteristic serpiginous, paraesopha-geal, and perigastric densities that show marked enhancement following dynamic CT (Fig. 2-23).[33] Varices within the wall of the esophagus itself may also be defined by CT when there is adequate distention of the esophageal lumen. These too can appear enhanced following a bolus of intravenous contrast material (Fig. 2-23, B).

In addition to detection, CT may be of use in the follow-up evaluation of patients with esophageal varices treated with endoscopic sclerotherapy. Haldin et al. have reported an apparently characteristic postsclerotherapy appearance of a thickened esophagus that on bolus scans showed enhancement of only the outer rim of the esophageal wall as a result of nonenhancement of thrombosed submucosal varices.[37]

Perhaps of greater interest is the potential role of CT in evaluating complications resulting from endoscopic sclerotherapy. Acutely, these include necrosis of the esophageal wall, pleural effusions, and mediastinitis—abnormalities easily diagnosed by CT.[38]

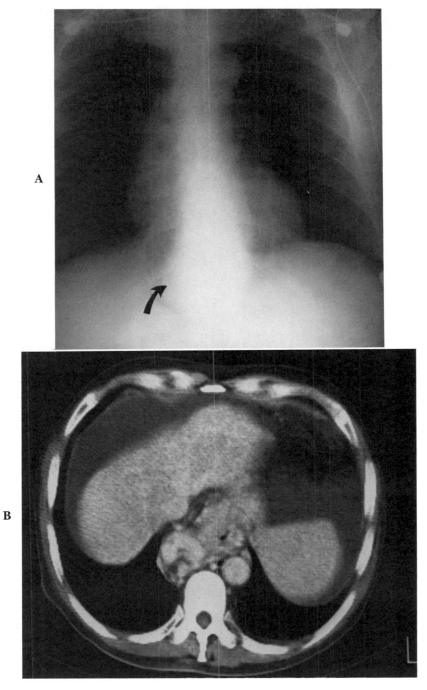

Fig. 2-21. Esophageal varices. **A,** Posteroanterior radiograph shows paraspinal widening *(curved arrow)* most prominent on the right side. **B,** Section through the lower thorax followng contrast enhancement. The paraspinal mass seen in **A** is caused by serpiginous mediastinal vascular structures that lie predominantly along the right side of the esophagus. Note that the esophagus itself appears to have thickened walls. This appearance is nonspecific, however, as the esophagus has been incompletely distended. There is a significant amount of ascites surrounding the spleen and a small contracted liver (biopsy proven cirrhosis with associated varices).

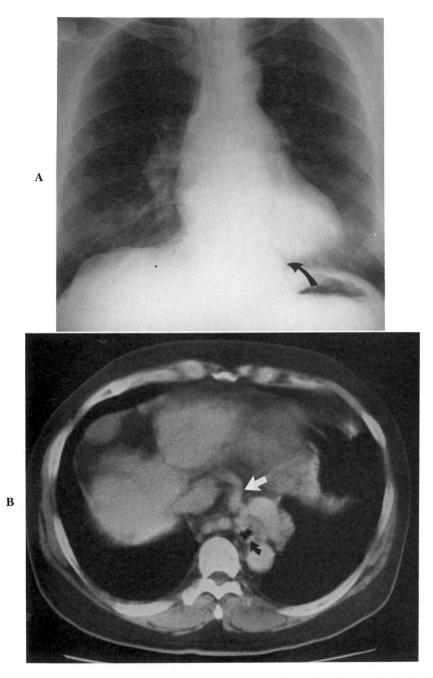

Fig. 2-22. Esophageal varices. **A,** Posteroanterior radiograph shows a left-sided paraspinal mass with no other apparent abnormalities *(curved arrow)* (compare to Fig. 2-21). **B,** Contrast-enhanced scan through the lower thorax demonstrates enlarged, tortuous mediastinal varices extending predominantly to the left and communicating anteriorly with the coronary vein *(arrow)*. The esophagus is partially distended by air and has a nodular appearance along its inner surface *(curved arrow)*. The enhancement of the esophageal wall is apparent even on visual inspection due to enlarged, submucosal, contrast-filled varices.

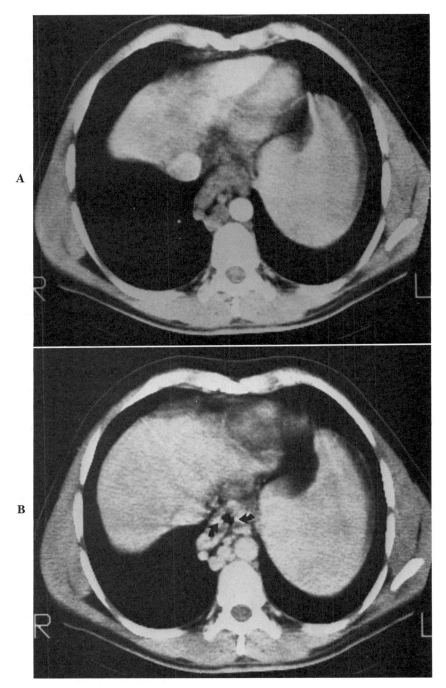

Fig. 2-23. Effect of contrast enhancement on esophageal varices. **A** and **B,** Sections at approximately the same level during and immediately after the injection of a bolus of intravenous contrast (note dense opacification of the aorta in **A**). There is marked enhancement of the periesophageal densities noted in **A,** confirming their vascular origin. Submucosal varices in the wall of the esophagus are also enhanced (*curved arrows* in **B**).

EXTRAMURAL LESIONS

There are innumerable causes for extrinsic compression of the esophagus. Although these are usually easily detected by barium swallow, differentiation between the various etiologies is frequently problematic. In select cases CT may prove diagnostic, especially when the underlying abnormality proves benign.[39,40]

In the upper mediastinum CT is especially helpful in the diagnosis of vascular abnormalities involving the aorta and great vessels. The CT diagnosis of aneurysmal dilation of the aorta usually obviates the need for aortography.[41] A variety of vascular anomalies causing compression or displacement of the esophagus have also been reported, including aberrant right and left subclavian arteries, double aortic arch anomalies, and even the CT diagnosis of a pulmonary vascular sling (Fig. 2-24).[42-45] Day has recently suggested routine preoperative CT evaluation of neonates with esophageal atresia and tracheoesophageal fistulas.[46] In 5% of these cases, infants will have an associated right-sided aortic arch, making a left-sided thoracotomy mandatory. Preoperative localization of the aortic arch on routine radiographs may be difficult if there is associated volume loss or consolidation secondary to the bronchial fistula.

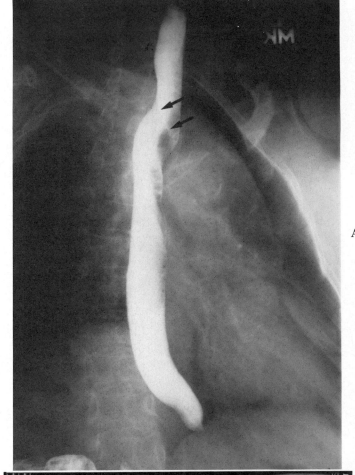

A

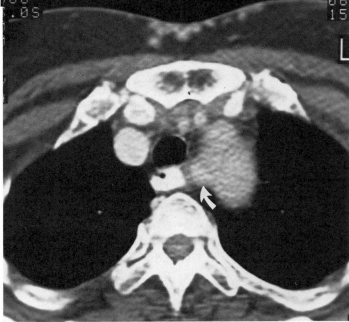

B

Fig. 2-24. Aberrant right subclavian artery. **A,** Typical oblique indentation of the esophagus running from below-upwards, from left to right caused by an aberrant right subclavian artery *(arrows).* **B, C,** and **D,** Sequential magnified views from below-upward through the upper portion of the aortic arch and great vessels documenting the course of an aberrant right subclavian artery *(curved arrows).*

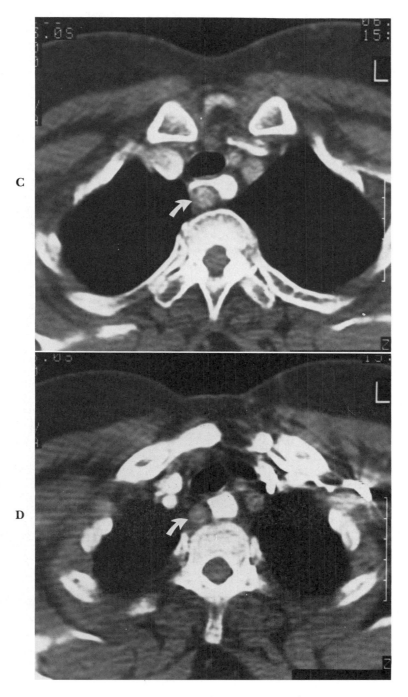

Fig. 2-24, cont'd. For legend see opposite page.

Another common cause of benign extrinsic displacement of the upper thoracic esophagus is a substernal thyroid. The CT characteristics of intrathoracic goiters, including the relatively unusual appearance of posterior mediastinal extension, have been thoroughly reviewed by numerous authors (Fig. 2-25).[47-49] In general these lesions are easy to identify because they are well defined, often contain punctate foci of calcification, and characteristically have a precontrast-enhanced density slightly greater than adjacent muscle tissue. Sequential images through the thoracic inlet and neck are diagnostic when they establish continuity between the "mass" and the cervical thyroid gland.[50]

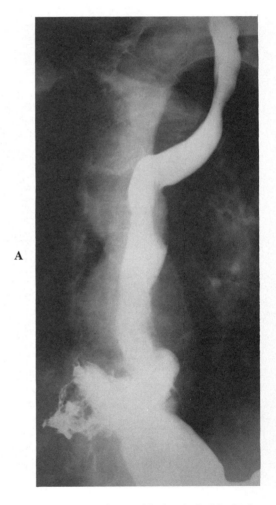

Fig. 2-25. Substernal thyroid gland. **A,** Marked anterior displacement of the upper portion of the esophagus documented on esophagography.

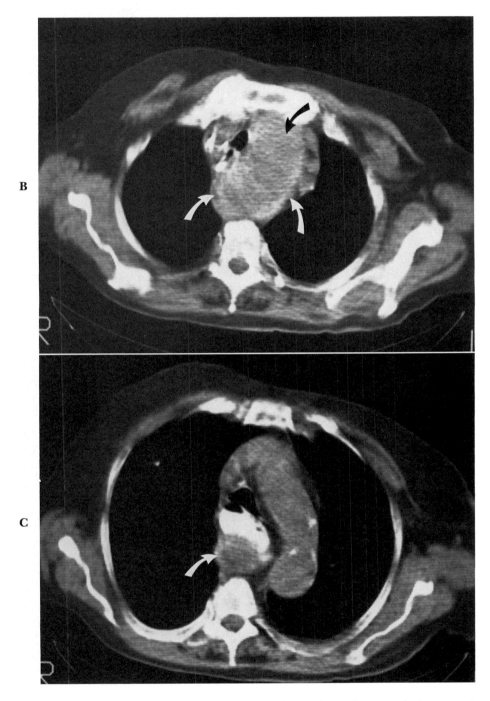

Fig. 2-25, cont'd. B and **C,** Sequential sections from above-downward, documenting a large substernal thyroid insinuated between the trachea and esophagus and the great vessels and aortic arch *(curved arrows).* **C,** Inferiorly, the most caudal portion of the thyroid lies posterior to the contrast-filled esophagus *(curved arrow).* Superiorly, sections confirmed continuity with the cervical thyroid gland.

Throughout the entire length of the mediastinum the esophagus may be displaced by enlarged
lymph nodes. These result from a wide variety of
both benign and malignant causes and their appearance is usually nonspecific. In select cases, CT
may allow a presumptive diagnosis especially when
images are carefully correlated with the clinical
presentation. Williford et al. have reported the CT
appearance of esophageal involvement secondary
to mediastinal tuberculous lymphadenitis.[51] Extensive tuberculous adenopathy often appears as a
heterogeneous, low-density, mediastinal mass following a bolus of intravenous contrast material
(Fig. 2-26). The extent of disease is usually well
defined in cross-section, including extension of
adenopathy into both hilar regions, as well as associated distortion of the adjacent esophagus. Significantly, CT may disclose the presence of miliary
lung disease prior to detection on corresponding
chest radiographs, leading to prompt diagnosis
and treatment (Fig. 2-22, B).

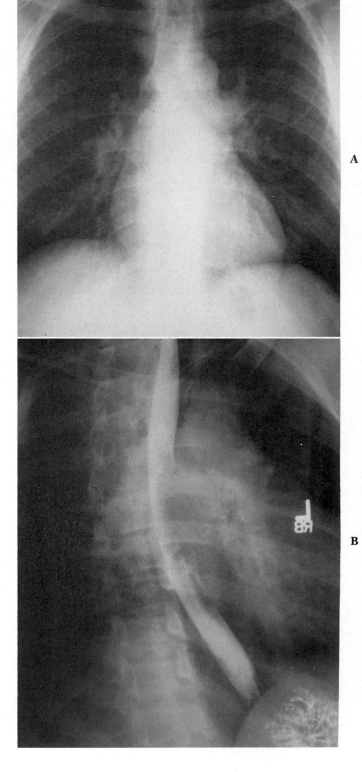

A

B

Fig. 2-26. Tuberculous esophagitis. **A,** Posteroanterior
chest radiograph shows a large, subcarinal, soft-tissue density. The hila appear slightly enlarged bilaterally. The pulmonary parenchyma is normal. **B,** Barium swallows show
abnormal configuration and some irregularity of the anterior aspect of the midesophagus.

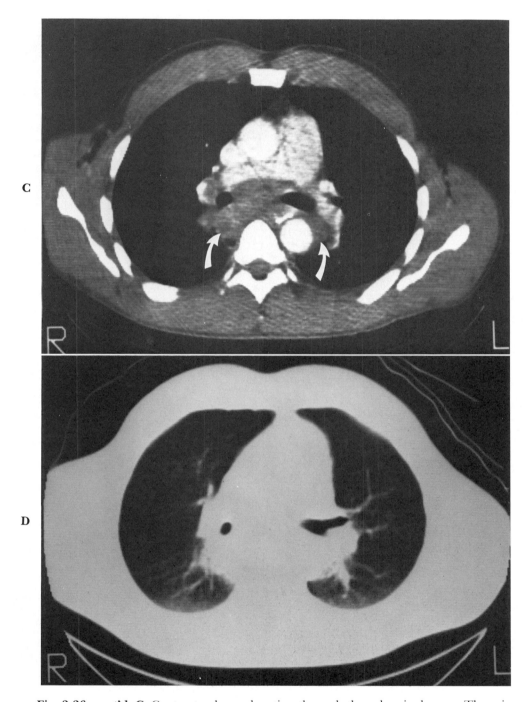

Fig. 2-26, cont'd. C, Contrast enhanced section through the subcarinal space. There is a heterogeneous soft-tissue density within the mediastinum that extends into the posterior aspects of both hila *(curved arrows)*. The esophagus is displaced posteriorly, and the right main pulmonary artery is draped against this soft-tissue mass anteriorly. **D,** Same section as in **C** imaged with wide windows. There is a subtle miliary pattern in both lung fields that is slightly more apparent in the lower lobes. Together these findings are characteristic of tuberculous mediastinitis with secondary involvement of the esophagus. In this case miliary disease was first noted with CT.

In the lower thorax, lymphadenopathy is most often malignant in etiology. Because of the close association between lower mediastinal nodes and abdominal and pelvic neoplasia, the finding of enlarged lower thoracic periesophageal nodes should lead to thorough CT evaluation of the abdomen (Fig. 2-27).

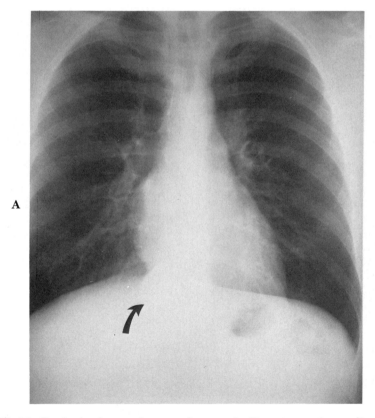

Fig. 2-27. Mediastinal adenopathy—seminoma. **A,** Posteroanterior radiograph shows right paraspinal mass *(curved arrow)* (compare to Figs. 2-21 and 2-22).

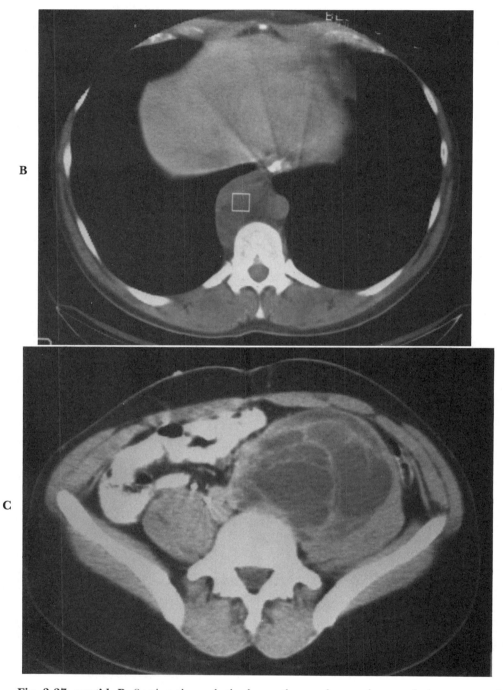

Fig. 2-27, cont'd. B, Section through the lower thorax shows a large soft-tissue mass of uniform density in the posterior mediastinum causing some anterior displacement of the contrast-filled esophagus. **C,** Section at the level of the aortic bifurcation. There is a large, multiseptated tumor mass on the left that on sequential sections extended into the pelvis. This case emphasizes the need to scan through the entire abdomen when evaluating patients with enlarged lower thoracic periesophageal nodes. Surgery confirmed benign teratomatous tissue in a patient with previously-documented malignant disease.

ESOPHAGEAL PERFORATION

Esophageal perforation is a potentially lethal condition that is frequently complicated by the rapid onset of severe mediastinitis, empyema, and overwhelming sepsis.[52] In addition to its association with esophageal carcinoma, perforation may be spontaneous (associated with excessive strain—Boerhaave syndrome), post-traumatic, or, increasingly, iatrogenic in etiology, complicating endoscopy, esophageal dilation, or attempted intubation. Plain radiographic findings of esophageal perforation have been well documented and include a widened mediastinum, subcutaneous emphysema, pneumomediastinum, and hydrothorax. As documented in a recent review by Han et al., plain films may be normal in as many as 12% of patients with esophageal perforation.[53] Although definitive diagnosis is usually established by an esophagram, CT may provide invaluable information concerning the extent of mediastinal, pleural, and parenchymal disease (Fig. 2-28).[54] In select cases this information may be helpful in determining which patients require immediate surgical intervention as opposed to those that could be managed conservatively by confirming the presence of mediastinal fluid collections (Fig. 2-29).

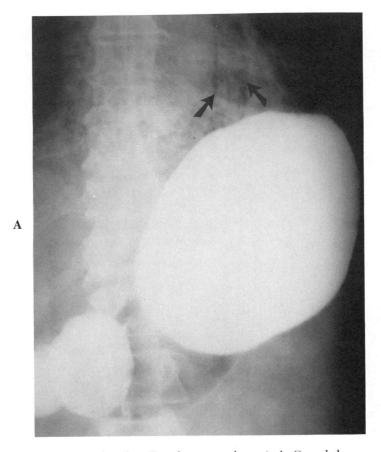

Fig. 2-28. Esophageal perforation (Boerhaave syndrome). **A,** Coned-down radiograph of the left upper quadrant and left lower lobe in a patient suspected of esophageal perforation. Note mottled appearance of the mediastinum due to air *(arrows)*. There is no evidence of extravasation of oral contrast material.

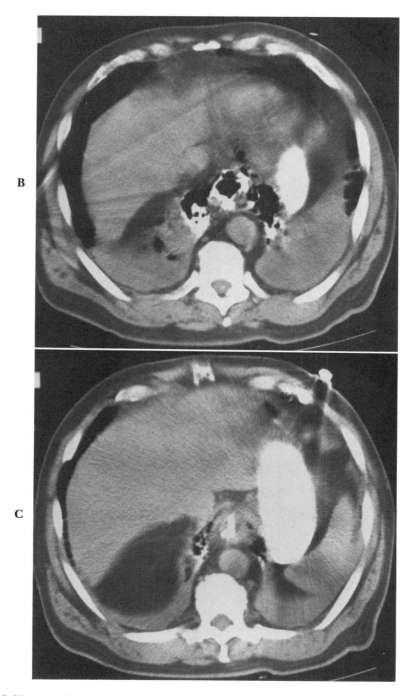

Fig. 2-28, cont'd. B and **C,** Sequential sections from above down through the lower thorax, documenting extravasation of oral contrast material into the mediastinum and bilateral pleural effusions. (Case courtesy of Dr. R. Meisell, Booth Memorial Hospital, New York, New York.)

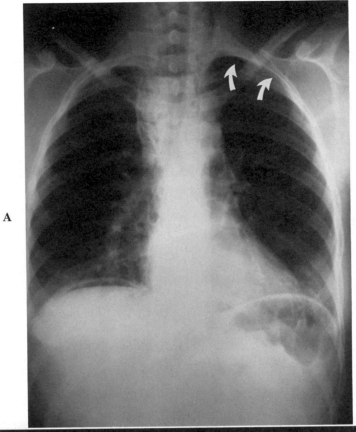

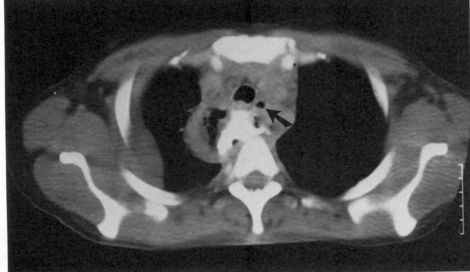

Fig. 2-29. Esophageal perforation. **A,** Posteroanterior radiograph shows widening of the mediastinum, mediastinal and cervical emphysema, and a left apical pneumothorax *(curved arrows)*. This film was obtained immediately following abdominal surgery to evaluate postoperative fever. The presence of air underneath the right diaphragm is secondary to the recent surgery. **B,** Section at the level of the great vessels shows a large mediastinal abscess partially filled with air and oral contrast material and separated from the esophageal lumen that lies to the left of the trachea *(arrow)*. There is a loculated pleural fluid collection on the right side as well.

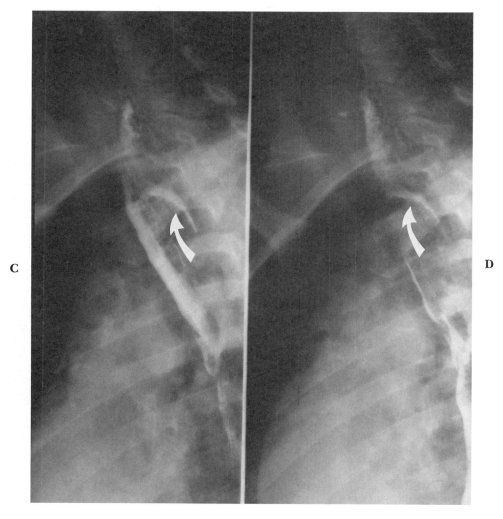

Fig. 2-29, cont'd. C and **D,** Sequential spot films taken during a barium swallow confirm posterior esophageal perforation with fistulization into the mediastinum *(curved arrows).*

ESOPHAGEAL CARCINOMA

Carcinoma of the esophagus represents approximately 10% of all cancers of the gastrointestinal tract. Excluding adenocarcinomas of gastric origin with secondary extension to the esophagus, between 90% and 95% of all esophageal lesions are squamous cell carcinomas. Most of the remaining 5% represent primary adenocarcinomas that arise either from the esophageal mucosal or submucosal glands, heterotopic gastric mucosa, or columnar-lined epithelium (Barrett esophagus).[26,55]

The incidence of esophageal cancer varies widely in different parts of the world. High-risk regions include Iran, parts of Africa (including South Africa), Italy, and especially China where the risk of esophageal carcinoma has been estimated to be as high as 100/100,000 in Henan Province alone.[56] Epidemiologically the United States is considered a low-risk region, with about 9000 cases reported annually. This is considered too low to justify attempts at mass screening, despite the proven efficacy of cytologic evaluation in early detection.[57]

Predisposing factors include heavy use of tobacco and alcohol, chronic strictures following lye ingestion or other corrosives, celiac disease, a previous history of head and neck cancer, and Barrett esophagus. An increased risk of developing esophageal carcinoma has also been documented in patients with the Plummer-Vinson syndrome and in those patients with tylosis, a rare congenital disorder characterized by thickening of the skin of the palms and soles.[55]

Esophageal carcinoma generally presents in an advanced stage. Despite significant improvements in surgical techniques, there has been little recent change in overall prognosis. As reported by the American Joint Committee on Cancer (AJCC), 5-year survival rates vary between 3% and 20%.[26] This poor prognosis is a result of rapid submucosal extension of tumor and early transmural invasion facilitated by the lack of an esophageal serosa. The result is early spread to regional and distal lymphatics, associated most frequently with hepatic, adrenal, and pulmonary metastases (Fig. 2-30). Unfortunately, dysphagia and anorexia, the most common presenting symptoms, are usually manifestations of extensive disease resulting from tumor that has already grown circumferentially. Some investigators have questioned whether esophageal carcinoma should not be considered a systemic disorder from the outset.[58]

Accurate presurgical assessment of the extent of disease has proved elusive. Despite evaluation with esophagography, endoscopy, bronchoscopy, mediastinoscopy, azygography, lymphography and radioisotopic scanning, accurate determination of the true extent of disease, both regional and metastatic, has been poor when compared to findings at surgical exploration.[59-62] It is for this reason that considerable recent interest has focused on the potential role of CT in preoperative staging.

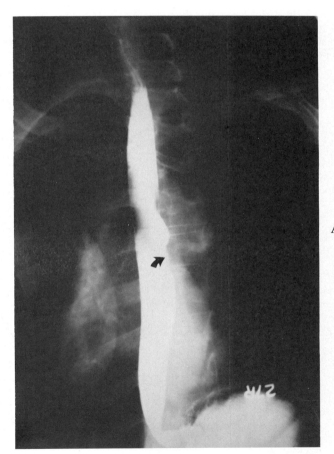

Fig. 2-30. Esophageal carcinoma—retroperitoneal metastases. **A,** Barium swallow shows subtle irregularity along lateral wall of esophagus, which was later confirmed at endoscopy to be squamous cell carcinoma (*curved arrow*).

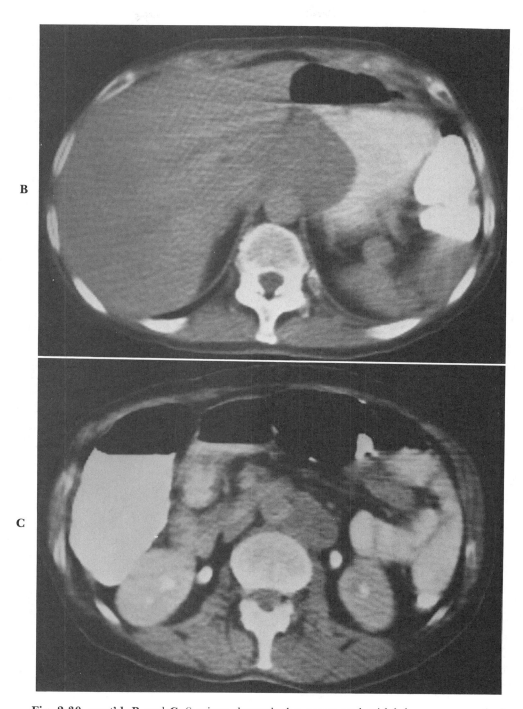

Fig. 2-30, cont'd. B and **C,** Sections through the upper and midabdomen, respectively, document extensive extranodal gastrohepatic and retroperitoneal metastases. Note the marked disproportion in the size and appearance of the primary tumor versus the extent of lymphatic disease.

Table 2-1. TNM staging of esophageal carcinoma

Primary tumor	T_1	Tumor 5 cm or less in length with no evidence of circumferential involvement, extraesophageal spread, or obstruction.
	T_2	Tumor greater than 5 cm in length without extraesophageal spread, or tumor of any size that is circumferential or causes obstruction in the absence of extra-esophageal spread.
	T_3	Any tumor with evidence of extraesophageal spread.
Nodal involvement	N_1	Nodal involvement
Distant metastases	M_1	Metastases: especially those involving abdominal and retroperitoneal lymph nodes; liver; adrenals; lungs; pleura; and diaphragm.

Post surgical resection—pathologic classification

Stage 1	$T_1N_0M_0$
Stage 2	$T_2N_0M_0$
Stage 3	$T_3N_0M_0$
	Any T, N_1, M_0
Stage 4	Any T_1, Any N, M_1

Adapted from Beahrs, O.H., and Myers, M.H.: Manual for staging of cancer, ed. 2, Philadelphia, 1983, J.B. Lippincott Co.

CLINICAL-PATHOLOGIC STAGING

Traditionally, esophageal carcinoma has been staged according to the TNM classification of the AJCC (Table 2-1).[63] Moss et al. have proposed an alternative staging classification based on CT scanning.[64] As modified by Reinig et al., esophageal carcinoma can be divided into four stages: Stage 1—lesions that are either intraluminal or that cause localized wall thickening of between 3 and 5 mm; Stage 2—esophageal wall thickening, localized or circumferential, greater than 5 mm; Stage 3—esophageal wall thickening associated with evidence of contiguous spread or tumor into adjacent mediastinal structures including the trachea, main stem bronchi, aorta, or pericardium; and Stage 4—any locally defineable disease associated with distal metastases (Table 2-2).[65]

Table 2-2. CT staging of esophageal carcinoma

Stage 1	Intraluminal tumor or localized esophageal wall thickening between 3 and 5 mm.
Stage 2	Localized or circumferential esophageal wall thickening greater than 5 mm.
Stage 3	Esophageal wall thickening with evidence of contiguous spread into adjacent mediastinal structures, including the trachea, main stem bronchi, aorta, or pericardium.
Stage 4	Any locally defineable disease associated with distal metastases.

Adapted from Moss, A.A., Schnyder, P., Thoeni, R.F., et al.: Esophageal carcinoma: pretherapy staging by computed tomography, AJR **136:**1051-1056, 1981.

Initial reports concerning the accuracy of CT have been extremely enthusiastic.[64,66] Moss et al. evaluated 52 patients, 17 of whom had surgical confirmation of the extent of disease. In all verified cases, CT staging correlated precisely with surgical findings, including local extension, regional adenopathy, and size of tumor mass.[64]

Thompson et al., in the largest series reported to date, evaluated a total of 76 patients—12 with carcinomas of the gastroesophageal junction and 64 with esophageal carcinoma.[67] CT scans were analyzed using both the staging system advocated by Moss et al. and the TNM classification. CT correctly identified 61 of 64 patients with esophageal carcinoma, 49 of whom had surgical confirmation. Of the 49 patients, 42 (86%) were correctly staged using the Moss et al. classification; 46 (94%) were accurately staged using the TNM system. CT was 88% accurate in evaluating regional extent of disease, correctly identifying 40 of 44 patients with mediastinal invasion and 11 of 15 patients without invasion (sensitivity of 90%; specificity of 79%). Additionally, CT correctly identified 15 of 19 patients with distant abdominal metastases and 28 of 39 patients without metastatic disease (overall accuracy of 88%). Similar results have been reported by others, although differences in patient population, interpretive criteria, numbers of surgically verified cases, and staging classifications limit the extent of comparability.[5,10,68]

Unfortunately, the value of CT in staging esophageal malignancy has not been universally documented. Quint et al. evaluated preoperative CT scans of 33 patients with esophageal cancer all of whom subsequently underwent transhiatal esophagectomies.[69] Using a modification of the TNM clinical-diagnostic staging system, only 13 tumors (33%) were staged accurately. Thirteen of 33 cases were understaged, primarily as a result of inaccurate assessment of tumor invasion through the muscular layer of the esophagus with contiguous mediastinal soft-tissue extension; 7 cases were overstaged largely as a result of false-positive CT diagnoses of metastatic celiac adenopathy. Similar poor results have been reported by Samuelson et al.[9]

PRESURGICAL EVALUATION

It cannot be overemphasized that the clinical efficacy of CT in evaluating esophageal cancer depends solely on its impact on patient management. Recent improvements in surgical techniques and a corresponding decline in operative mortality have caused a significant change in approach to patients with esophageal carcinoma.[70] Because of extremely low rates of survival despite various forms of therapy, a philosophy strongly favoring palliative surgical intervention has evolved. This trend has been further stimulated by the frequent failure of radiotherapy to improve survival or provide adequate palliation by eliminating dysphagia.[71]

In most institutions patients are considered unresectable a priori only if there is documentation of one of the following: evidence of tumor extension into the trachea or left main stem bronchus; invasion of the thoracic aorta, pericardium, or left atrium; evidence of metastatic disease to the liver, adrenals, lung, or perigastric lymph nodes (especially if the latter interferes with operative mobilization of the stomach); or finally, if a patient is considered inoperable for medical reasons. Mediastinal adenopathy and clinical, radiographic, or surgical evidence of transmural periesophageal invasion are no longer considered contraindications to resection.[72] Even when a patient is considered unresectable, a bypass procedure with esophageal exclusion may be indicated to provide palliation.[73]

Using the criteria defined above, Piccone et al. were able to perform esophagectomies on 81 of 89 patients for a resectability rate of 93%, despite evidence of invasion of contiguous mediastinal structures and nodal involvement in 60% and 75% of cases, respectively.[74] In a series reported by Ellis et al. of 167 patients, esophagectomies were successfully performed in 149 patients (89.2%), regardless of the extent of tumor, providing the procedure could be performed safely.[75] In 25 of these cases (16.8%) tumor was knowingly left behind. The overall adjusted survival rate at 5 years was 21.7%, the operative mortality rate was 1.3%, and satisfactory palliation of dysphagia was achieved in 82.7% of patients—convincing evidence for the role of palliative surgery for an otherwise incurable disease. More recently, Orringer has obtained similar results, including comparable survival rates, with transhiatal esophagectomies.[76]

These changes in the approach to management of patients with esophageal carcinoma have obvious implications for the potential diagnostic value of CT. Rather than provide a means for identifying patients who are potentially curable, the role of CT is to avoid denying patients potentially successful palliation. This necessitates a critical in-depth review of all CT criteria for staging esophageal carcinoma and especially for determining unresectability.

ESOPHAGEAL WALL THICKNESS

The efficacy of CT in staging esophageal cancer is predicted on its ability to evaluate the full thickness of the esophageal wall and directly visualize periesophageal fascial planes. In the most complete assessment of the accuracy of CT in detecting abnormalities of the esophageal wall to date, Reinig et al., using 3 mm as the upper limit of normal, evaluated 200 consecutive thoracic CT scans (Fig. 2-31).[65] Seventy patients (35%) had CT evidence of thickened esophageal walls. In all cases the esophagus was subsequently proven to be abnormal, although thickening per/se was etiologically nonspecific (Figs. 2-32 and 2-33). In addition to esophageal carcinoma, other mediastinal malignancies, in particular metastatic lung carcinoma, as well as benign inflammatory, vascular, and fibrotic conditions can result in esophageal wall thickening making conclusive differentiation between benign and malignant disease difficult (Fig. 2-34). The high incidence of esophageal pathology cited in this study is presumed to be a consequence of inadvertent preselection bias.

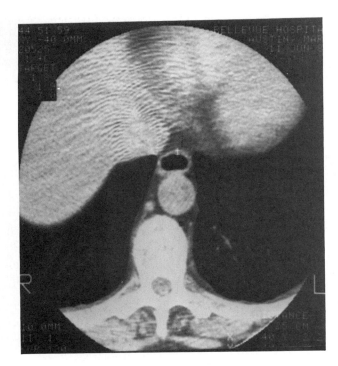

Fig. 2-31. CT appearance of normal esophageal wall. Enlargement of a section through the distal esophagus distended by air. Cursors bracket the anterior esophageal wall, which measures precisely 2.25 mm in thickness.

Fig. 2-32. Esophageal carcinoma. **A,** Barium swallow documents presence of esophageal cancer with dilation of the upper portion of the esophagus.

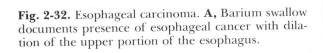
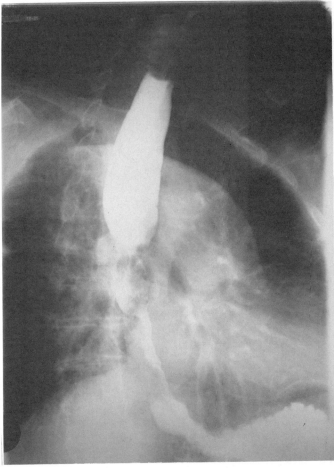

A

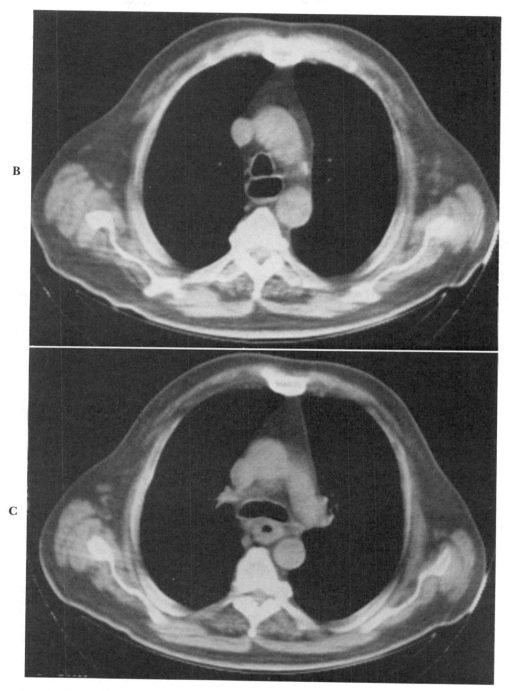

Fig. 2-32, cont'd. B, Section at the level of the aorticopulmonary windows shows a dilated, thin-walled esophagus with a dependent fluid level within. **C,** Section at the level of the carina, just below that section shown in **B.** The esophageal walls are circumferentially thickened and the esophageal lumen is narrowed. Note that the periesophageal fascial planes are well visualized (compare to Figs. 2-35 and 2-36).

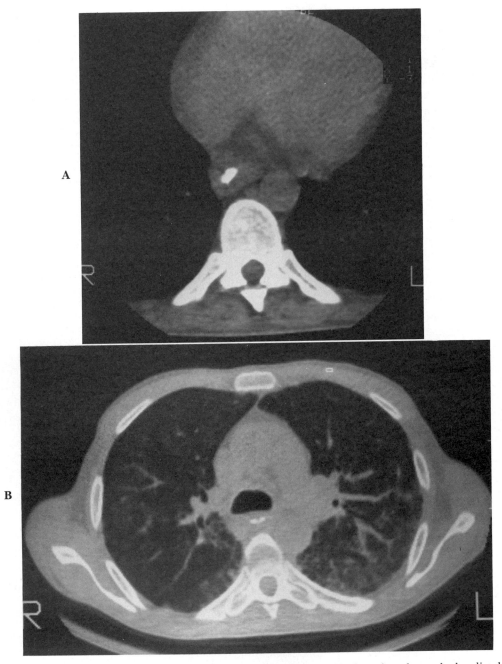

Fig. 2-33. Esophageal wall thickening—candida. **A,** Magnified section through the distal esophagus shows circumferential wall thickening with narrowing of the esophageal lumen that is well visualized as a result of the presence of oral contrast material (compare to Fig. 2-32, **B**). **B,** Section through the carina imaged with lung windows in the same patient as above. There is extensive bilateral parenchymal disease as a result of biopsy-proven *Pneumocystis carinii* pneumonia in this patient with documented AIDS.

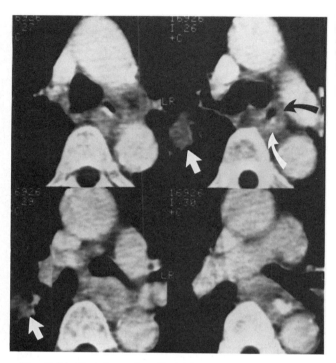

Fig. 2-34. Esophageal wall thickening—metastatic lung cancer. Sequential magnified sections from the carina through the subcarinal space. There is increased soft-tissue density surrounding the esophagus, the walls of which appear abnormally widened *(curved arrows)*. In addition, there is a tumor mass present in the posterior segment of the right upper lobe *(arrows)*. Biopsy-proven, large cell, undifferentiated carcinoma.

PERIESOPHAGEAL INVASION

Although periesophageal invasion is no longer considered a priori evidence of unresectability, deep invasion of periesophageal fascial planes by tumor may be a significant factor in determining resectability for patients who are otherwise considered marginally operable (Fig. 2-35).[72,73] Unfortunately, there is little consensus concerning the reliability of CT in predicting mediastinal invasion. Halber et al., in their review of 197 thoracic scans, concluded that the thoracic esophagus is easily demonstrated throughout its entire length and that fascial planes separating the esophagus from adjacent mediastinal structures are normally distinct.[4] Similar findings have been reported, leading investigators to equate loss of visualization of the periesophageal fat planes with periesophageal invasion.[64,65]

However, Reinig et al. have reported inadequate visualization of the esophagus in 27 of 200 consecutively scanned patients (13.5%), despite the use of 4 grams of citrocarbonate in 20 ml of water given orally via a nasogastric tube.[65] In 14 of 27 cases, the esophagus could not be evaluated due either to a lack of mediastinal fat or to the inability to distend the esophagus with air during the scan.

Samuelson et al. have documented that loss of visualization of periesophageal fat planes may prove insignificant at surgery.[9] In their series of 26 patients with esophageal carcinoma, a broad area of contact without an intervening fat plane between the tumor and adjacent mediastinal structures was present in 19 cases; despite this, 10 cases proved easily resectable (Fig. 2-36).

Similar difficulties have been encountered by Freeny and Marks.[77] In their study of tumors involving the gastroesophageal junction both the presence and absence of clearly defined periesophageal soft-tissue planes proved to be unreliable signs for predicting the extent of tumor, with CT incorrectly assessing the significance of the loss of soft-tissue planes in 6 of 12 cases (50%) documented surgically. These findings suggest that poor visualization of mediastinal fat planes is a nonspecific finding and should be interpreted cautiously.

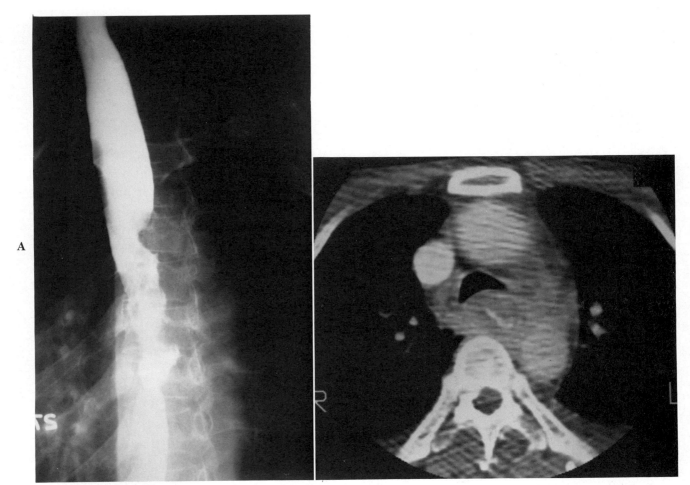

Fig. 2-35. Esophageal carcinoma—periesophageal invasion. **A,** Barium swallow shows typical features of midesophageal carcinoma. **B,** Enlargement of a section through the carina. There is extensive, poorly-defined, mediastinal tumor irregularly infiltrating the aorticopulmonary window and narrowing and displacing the trachea. Unresectable infiltrating esophageal carcinoma.

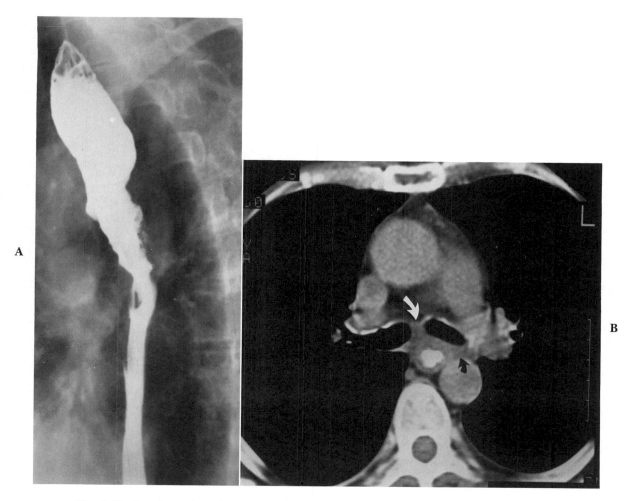

Fig. 2-36. Esophageal carcinoma—periesophageal infiltration. **A,** Barium swallow shows typical features of midesophageal cancer. **B,** Magnified section through the carina. The esophageal walls are thickened circumferentially; there is also abnormal increased soft-tissue density in the subcarinal space anteriorly and lateral to the esophagus between the aorta and left main stem bronchus posteriorly *(curved arrows)*. Periesophageal fascial planes are well visualized posteriorly between the azygos and posterolateral aspect of the aorta (compare to Figs. 2-32 and 2-35). At surgery this lesion proved resectable although there was histologic evidence of periesophageal invasion.

AORTIC INVASION

In an attempt to define prognostic signs of aortic invasion, Picus et al. correlated CT scans with surgical and autopsy findings in 30 patients with esophageal cancer.[78] All 11 patients in whom a fat plane could be defined between the aorta and adjacent tumor proved to have surgically resectable disease. The remaining 19 patients were divided into three groups depending on whether or not the area of contact between the aorta and adjacent tumor was less than 45 degrees, between 60 and 75 degrees, or greater than 90 degrees. None of the nine patients with an area of contact less than 45 degrees proved to have evidence of invasion, while four of five patients with an area of contact greater than 90 degrees proved surgically or at autopsy to have aortic invasion (Fig. 2-37). Areas of contact between 60 to 75 degrees were deemed indeterminate as only two of five patients were documented to have aortic invasion.

Similar results have been reported by Thompson et al. using a modification of the criteria proposed by Picus; although in their series of 51 cases, only eight had surgical or autopsy confirmation.[67] Unfortunately, others have found these same criteria inaccurate. Of six patients with greater than 90 degree contact between the tumor and adjacent aorta reported by Quint et al. only two proved to have tumor invasion at surgery.[69] Similar difficulties have been reported by Samuelson et al. who concluded that it is difficult to anticipate surgical findings of aortic invasion at CT.[9]

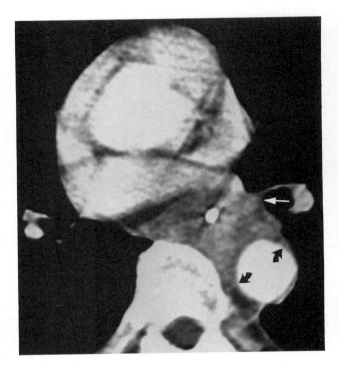

Fig. 2-37. Esophageal carcinoma—aortic invasion. Magnified view of the mediastinum following administration of a bolus of intravenous contrast material in a patient with distal esophageal carcinoma. There is an area of contact greater than 90 degrees apparent between the tumor and the adjacent aorta *(curved arrows)*. Additionally, tumor can be defined entering into the inferior pulmonary ligament on the left side *(arrow)*. The left atrium is eccentrically compressed on the left side, and there is a corresponding loss of the otherwise normal intervening fat plane seen on the right side.

TRACHEOBRONCHIAL INVASION

In most reported series, diagnosis of tracheobronchial invasion is based on the CT findings of displacement or compression of the airways by an adjacent esophageal mass (Fig. 2-38). Less frequently, the diagnosis of esophagotracheal or bronchial communication may be confirmed by direct visualization of a fistula.[79] Using these signs, the overall accuracy of CT has been reported to vary between 93% and 100%, in those series with bronchoscopic, surgical, or autopsy confirmation.[10,64,67,69,78]

However, Schneekloth et al. have documented that tumors of the upper and mid-esophagus may cause an impression or actually displace the trachea or left main stem bronchus and still be surgically resectable.[5] Only 7 of 14 patients with CT evidence of displacement of the tracheobronchial tree were documented to have invasive tumors, leading these investigators to conclude that dislocation of the airways is nonspecific, unless the degree of displacement or narrowing is marked (Fig. 2-39).

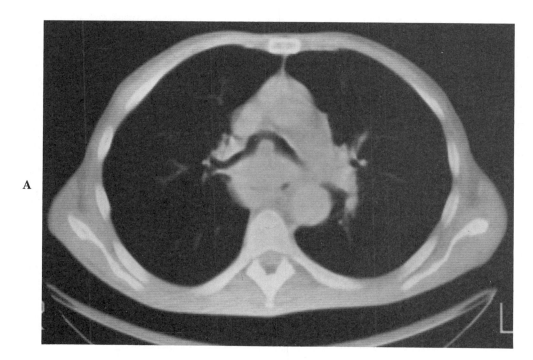

Fig. 2-38. Esophageal carcinoma—tracheobronchial invasion. **A,** Section through the carina imaged with wide windows to emphasize bronchial anatomy. There is marked displacement and irregular narrowing of both the right and left main stem bronchi by a large posterior mediastinal soft-tissue mass. *Continued.*

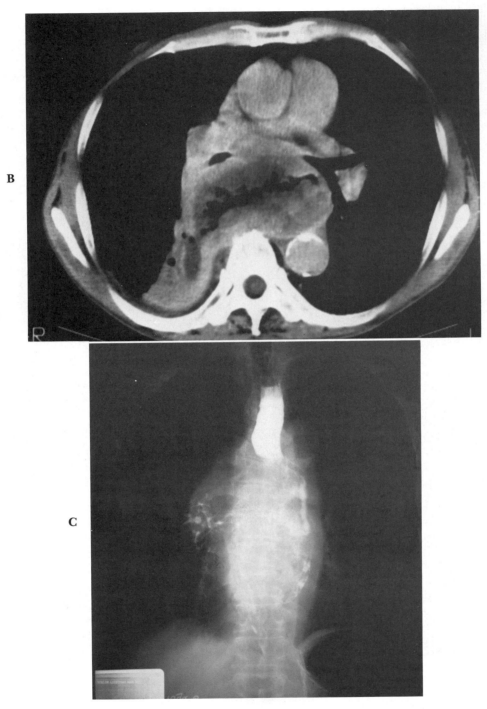

Fig. 2-38, cont'd. B, Section approximately 5 cm below that shown in **A** imaged with narrow windows. There is a large, necrotic posterior mediastinal tumor mass, containing both fluid and air, in direct communication with the right lower lobe, which is collapsed. Both the bronchus intermedius and the left main stem bronchus are narrowed and splayed apart. **C,** Esophagram confirms presence of an esophagobronchial fistula.

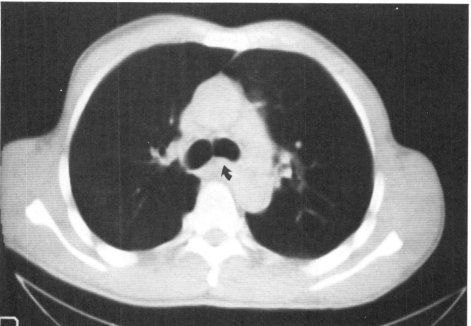

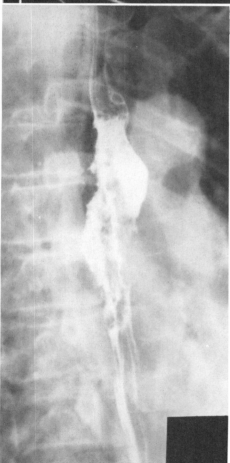

Fig. 2-39. Esophageal carcinoma—false-positive bronchial invasion. **A,** Section through the carina imaged with wide windows. There is a soft-tissue mass posterior to the carina that is compressing and distorting the posterior wall of the left main stem bronchus *(curved arrow)*. **B,** Barium swallow in same patient documents presence of midesophageal carcinoma. Radiographically, the lower esophagus appears normal. At surgery, this tumor was easily resected, with no evidence of fixation to the airways. However, histologic evaluation revealed submucosal extension along the entire length of the esophagus with invasion of the gastric cardia. This case emphasizes the difficult problem of accurate radiographic staging of esophageal cancer.

DISTANT METASTASES

Using 1 cm as the upper limit of normal, Thompson et al. reported a sensitivity of 69%, a specificity of 94%, and an overall accuracy of 82% in evaluating abdominal lymph node metastases in 61 patients with cancers of the esophagus and gastroesophageal junction.[67] Using the same criteria, Quint et al. have reported similar results with an overall accuracy of 85%.[69] This lack of correlation between lymph node enlargement and histology is typical for CT staging of most abdominal and pelvic malignancies. Limitations in the accuracy of CT for evaluating thoracic and abdominal lymphadenopathy in patients with esophageal carcinoma has been particularly well documented by Picus et al.[78] In their series of 29 patients presurgically staged with CT, 28 had no evidence of mediastinal lymph node enlargement either on CT nor on gross inspection of lymph nodes removed either at surgery or autopsy. Nonetheless, 12 of these patients (41%) proved to have metastatic carcinoma disclosed histologically, involving for the most part nodes measuring less than 7 mm in size. In this same report, nine patients had histologically verified abdominal lymph node metastases, only five of which were detected presurgically even though 5 mm was used as a criterion for lymph node enlargement. In practice, in the absence of massive confluent extranodal disease, the diagnosis of metastatic lymphadenopathy necessitates percutaneous or surgical biopsy.

Unlike metastatic adenopathy, CT is of proven efficacy in the evaluation of hepatic metastases. It must be emphasized, however, that accurate evaluation of the liver requires meticulous attention to technique.[80] The liver is best evaluated by use of dynamic incremental scanning following a bolus of intravenous contrast material. Significantly, this technique has not been used routinely in most reported series, rendering interpretation and comparison of results difficult.

Less commonly, tumor may directly invade the pulmonary parenchyma or erode an adjacent vertebral body.[81] CT is extremely sensitive in detecting these modes of spread, as well as detecting pulmonary metastases. Tumor may also involve the pleura or peritoneum; unfortunately, in the absence of associated pleural effusions or ascites, this mode of spread may be impossible to detect.[82] In a series reported by Terrier et al. of 15 patients with esophageal tumors found to be in contact with the adjacent pleura, in only one case was local pleural

invasion documented at surgical exploration.[10] In this same series, peritoneal carcinomatosis was detected at surgery in four patients but was diagnosed preoperatively only once.

CT OF ESOPAGHEAL CANCER: OVERVIEW

It has been suggested that routine CT evaluation of patients with esophageal carcinoma be discouraged because of low prevalence and the low accuracy of CT in detecting complications that could preclude surgery.[69] It is apparent on reviewing published series that there are significant limitations in the ability of CT to accurately predict the extent of tumor. On the basis of available data the following conclusions appear justified:

1. Esophageal wall thickening is a nonspecific finding indicative equally of benign and malignant disease.
2. Patients in whom clearly delineated periesophageal fascial planes can be demonstrated should be considered potential candidates for transthoracic resection, even though a significant percentage of these patients will prove to have invasive carcinoma histologically. Inadequate visualization of periesophageal soft-tissue planes, however, is nonspecific and should not be misconstrued necessarily as evidence of unresectability. Unfortunately CT has not been proved efficacious in predicting which patients are potential candidates for transhiatal esophagectomies.
3. The diagnosis of aortic, pericardial, and pleural invasion is difficult. Determining the extent of contact with adjacent tumor is suggestive only and therefore not a reliable sign of unresectability.
4. The diagnosis of tracheobronchial invasion can be made with CT provided there is marked displacement or narrowing of the adjacent airways or direct evidence of fistualization. Moderate displacement is not a reliable sign of unresectability; these cases will require bronchoscopic evaluation.
5. CT is inaccurate in detecting lymphatic metastases unless there is considerable enlargement or evidence of extranodal disease. CT is of value in detecting hepatic and adrenal metastases.

Ultimately, precise definition of the role of CT in the evaluation of patients with esophageal carcinoma will have to await further refinements of both technique and interpretation. Thompson et al. for example, have recently suggested that local mediastinal invasion should be diagnosed only if there is a loss of fat planes documented in two contiguous slices with normal fascial planes present in scans immediately above and below.[67] Documentation of the accuracy of these and other criteria will require considerably greater clinical experience than has now been reported. Despite the limitations outlined above and pending developments with newer imaging modalities, thoracoabdominal CT is of value in the overall assessment of patients with esophageal carcinoma for whom palliative surgery is contemplated.[83]

POSTSURGICAL EVALUATION

In addition to presurgical staging, CT may play an indispensible role in the evaluation of abnormalities arising in the postoperative period (Fig. 2-40). As shown by Heiken et al., CT may be of use in detecting early postoperative complications of esophagogastrectomies, including anastomosic leaks with associated mediastinitis, parenchymal consolidation, pleural empyema, and subphrenic abscesses (Fig. 2-41).[84] CT may also be of value in guiding percutaneous drainage of mediastinal, pleural, or intraabdominal fluid collections, especially in patients who are considered poor surgical candidates postoperatively (Fig. 2-42).[85]

Of equal interest is the potential role of CT in detecting the presence of recurrent tumor. Although esophagography is a sensitive method for detecting mucosal recurrence, before the advent of CT extramucosal disease had proved difficult to document. Gross et al. have reported detecting locally recurrent mediastinal neoplasia in 7 of 21 patients following transhiatal esophagectomies; in only four of these cases could recurrence be documented by corresponding barium studies (Fig. 2-43).[85]

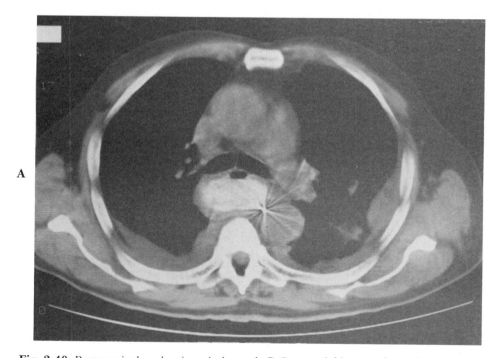

A

Fig. 2-40. Postsurgical evaluation. **A** through **C,** Sequential images from the carina to the esophageal hiatus in a patient following esophagectomy and subsequent esophagogastrostomy performed in the native esophageal bed. The esophagogastrostomy, which is filled with oral contrast material, is well seen despite the presence of innumerable surgical clips. There is no evidence of residual or recurrent extramucosal tumor. Note the presence of bilateral, partially loculated pleural effusions. *Continued.*

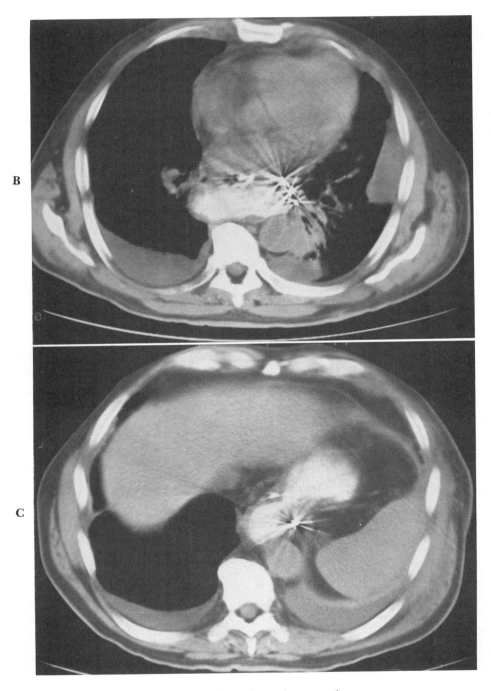

Fig. 2-40, cont'd. For legend see previous page.

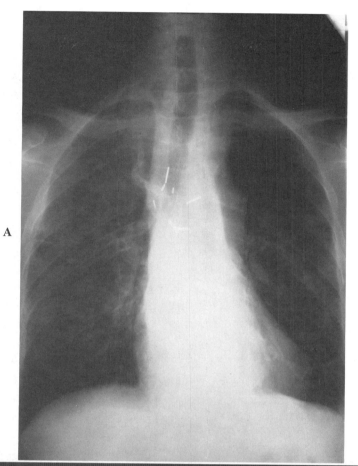

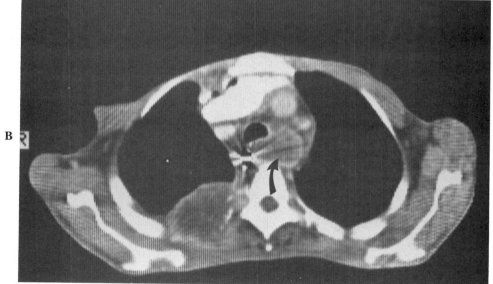

Fig. 2-41. Postsurgical evaluation—mediastinitis. **A,** PA radiograph of a patient following esophagectomy and substernal esophagogastrostomy. The mediastinum is widened; there is no obvious mediastinal abscess, or pleural disease. **B,** Section through the lower trachea. Oral contrast material is present substernally within the esophagogastrostomy. There is a well-defined mediastinal fluid collection posterolateral to the trachea *(curved arrow)*. There is also a large, loculated fluid collection in the pleural space posteriorly on the right that is extending into the chest wall. These fluid collections proved to be in communication on subsequent images; this was further confirmed at surgery.

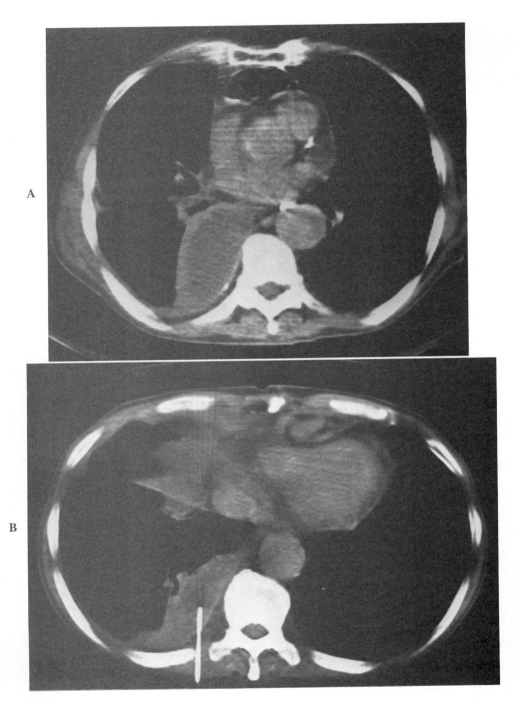

Fig. 2-42. Postsurgical evaluation—CT guided aspiration. **A,** Sections through lower thorax in a patient following esophagectomy with a retrosternal esophagogastrostomy. There is a large, loculated pleural fluid collection on the right side. **B,** Section somewhat lower than that shown in **A,** showing CT guided aspiration of what proved to be a sterile postoperative fluid collection.

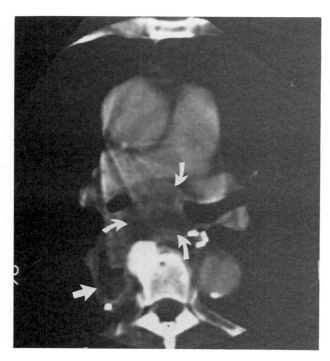

Fig. 2-43. Postsurgical evaluation of recurrent tumor. Enlargement of a section through the subcarinal space in a patient following esophagectomy and posterior mediastinal esophagogastrostomy. The stomach lies to the right of the spine and is partially filled with air and fluid *(arrow)*. Medially, there is a large, low-density, soft-tissue mass occupying the entire subcarinal space *(curved arrows)*. While mucosal recurrence is best detected with a barium swallow, extramucosal tumor is most easily assessed with CT.

ATYPICAL ESOPHAGEAL NEOPLASIA

In addition to squamous cell carcinoma and adenocarcinoma, a large variety of unusual tumors, both benign and malignant, may arise from the esophagus. Especially intriguing are so-called spindle cell squamous carcinomas.[86] These are rare epithelial tumors that have variously been designated carcinosarcomas or pseudosarcomas because they are compromised of both carcinomatous and sarcomatous elements.[87] Radiologically these lesions appear as large polypoid masses that usually arise in the middle third of the esophagus and are generally smooth, lobulated, or scalloped in appearance. These tumors rarely cause constriction or narrowing as a result of infiltration of the esophageal wall (Fig. 2-44). Differential diagnosis includes benign lesions such as fibrovascular polyps, lipomas, and leiomyomas; and mesenchymal malignancies, such as leiomyosarcomas, fibrosarcomas, and melanoma.[88] Rarely, oat cell carcinoma may arise from the argyrophil cells of the esophageal mucosa and closely mimic the appearance of other esophageal epithelial malignancies (Fig. 2-45).[89]

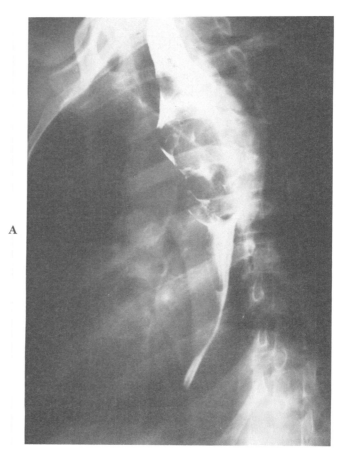

A

Fig. 2-44. Spindle-cell squamous carcinoma. **A,** Esophagram shows a large, polypoid lesion in the midesophagus causing expansion of the lumen and minimal obstruction.   *Continued.*

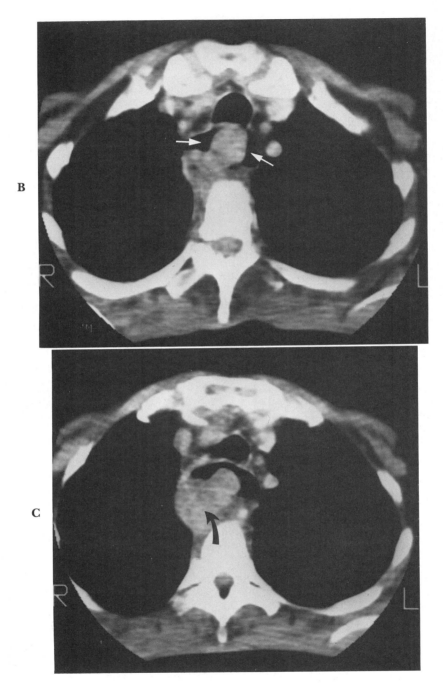

Fig. 2-44, cont'd. B and **C,** Sections at the level of the great vessels show a lobulated polypoid soft-tissue mass eccentrically located within the esophagus and outlined by air anterolaterally (*arrows* in **B** and **C**). There is considerable enhancement within this mass following administration of intravenous contrast material (*curved arrow* in **C**), confirming the presence of tumor (compare to Fig. 2-46).

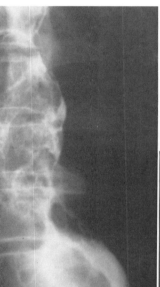

A

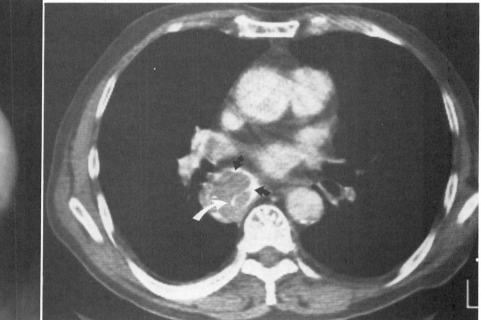

B

Fig. 2-45. Oat cell carcinoma of the esophagus. **A,** Coned-down view from an esophagram shows lobular mass with central ulceration *(curved arrow)* deforming the esophageal lumen. **B,** Section through the midthorax shows a lobular soft-tissue mass filling most of the esophageal lumen outlined by oral contrast material *(small arrows)*. Note the presence of contrast material within the mass due to central ulceration *(curved arrow)*. Biopsy proved oat cell carcinoma.

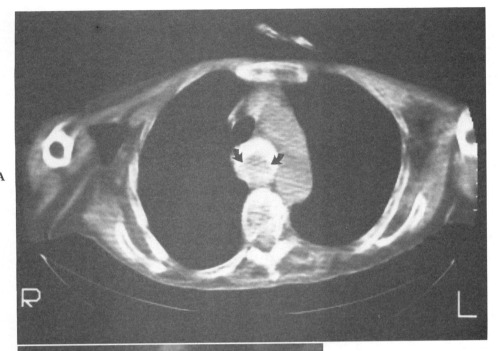

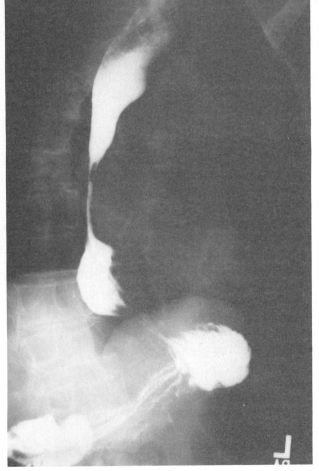

Fig. 2-46. Benign esophageal stricture. **A,** Section at the level of the aortic arch shows a dilated esophagus. Oral contrast material outlines a smooth filling defect anteriorly whose margins are sharply defined bilaterally *(curved arrows).* **B,** Corresponding esophagram shows a sliding hiatal hernia and a midesophageal stricture resulting from reflux. There is no evidence of a polypoid filling defect. The defect shown in **A** proved to be the result of debris, not present at the time of the esophagram. Endoscopy proved benign stricture resulting from peptic esophagitis.

Occasionally, the presence of impacted food, debris, or even a foreign body may mimic the appearance of a polypoid esophageal maligancy (Fig. 2-46).[90] Care should be exercised in excluding this potential pitfall in diagnosis by careful correlation with ancillary studies, especially a barium swallow, if available. Although the radiologic appearance of most epithelial esophageal lesions is frequently suggestive, definitive diagnosis almost invariably requires biopsy (Fig. 2-47).

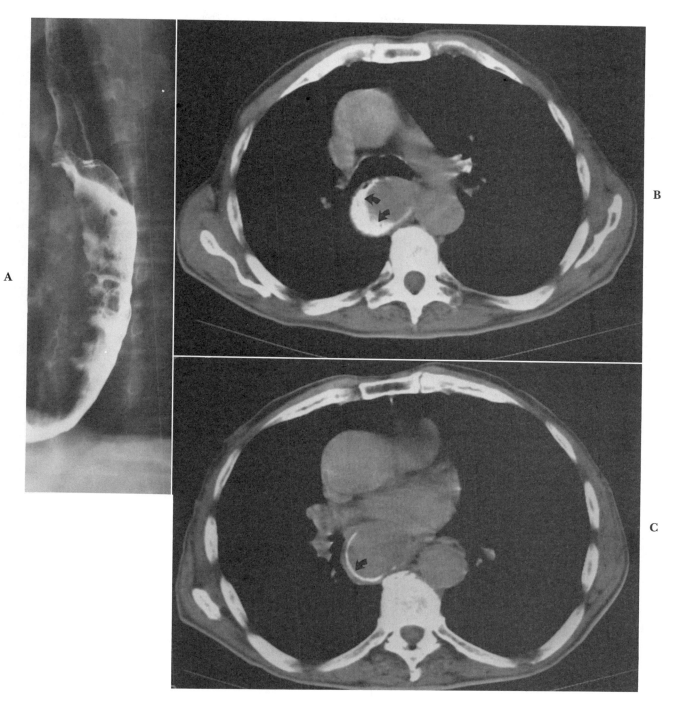

Fig. 2-47. Waldenström's macroglobulinemia. **A,** Esophagram shows lobulated filling defects deforming the lower esophagus. **B** and **C,** Sections through the carina and lower thorax respectively show smooth filling defects deforming the contrast-filled esophageal lumen *(curved arrows)*. Endoscopy verified Waldenström's macroglobulinemia infiltrating the esophageal wall.

REFERENCES

1. Kressel, H.Y., Callen, P.W., Montagne, J.P., et al.: Computed tomographic evaluation of disorders affecting the alimentary tract, Radiology 129:451-455, 1978.

2. Cayea, P.D., and Seltzer, S.E.: A new barium paste for computed tomography of the esophagus, J. Comput. Assist. Tomogr. 9:214-216, 1985.

3. Brombart, M.R.: Roentgenology of the esophagus. In Margulis, A.R., and Burhenne, H.J., editors: Alimentary tract radiology, ed. 2, vol. 1, St. Louis, 1973, The C.V. Mosby Co.

4. Halber, M.D., Daffner, R.H., and Thompson, W.M.: CT of the esophagus: normal appearance, AJR 133:1047-1050, 1979.

5. Schneekloth, G., Terrier, F., and Fuchs, W.A.: Computed tomography in carcinoma of esophagus and cardia, Gastrointest. Radiol. 8:193-206, 1983.

6. Bachman, A.L., and Teixidor, H.S.: The posterior tracheal band: a reflector of local superior mediastinal abnormality, Br. J. Radiol. 48:352-359, 1975.

7. Palayew, M.J.: The tracheo-esophageal stripe and the posterior tracheal band, Radiology 132:11-13, 1979.

8. Cimmino, C.V.: The esophageal-pleural stripe: an update, Radiology 140:609-613, 1981.

9. Samuelson, L., Hambraeus, G.M., Mercke, C.E., et al.: CT staging of esophageal carcinoma, Acta Radiol. Diagn. 25:7-11, 1984.

10. Terrier, F., Schapira, C.L., and Fuchs, W.A.: CT assessment of operability in carcinoma of the esophagogastric junction, Eur. J. Radiol. 4:114-117, 1984.

11. Levy-Ravetch, M., Auh, Y.H., Rubenstein, W.A., et al.: CT of the pericardial recesses, AJR 144:707-714, 1985.

12. Callen, P.W., Filly, R.A., and Korobkin, M.: Computed tomographic evaluation of the diaphragmatic crura, Radiology 126:413-416, 1978.

13. Naidich, D.P., Megibow, A.J., Ross, C.R., et al.: CT of the diaphragm: normal anatomy and variants, J. Comput. Assist. Tomogr. 7:633-640, 1983.

14. Gray, S.W., Rowe, J.S., and Skandalakis, J.E.: Surgical anatomy of the gastroesophageal junction, Am. Surg. 45:575-587, 1979.

15. Thompson, W.M., Halvorsen, R.A., Williford, M.E., et al.: Computed tomography of the gastroesophageal junction, Radiographics 2:179-193, 1982.

16. Balfe, D.M., Mauro, M.A., Koehler, R.E., et al.: Gastrohepatic ligament: normal and pathologic CT anatomy, Radiology 150:485-490, 1984.

17. Govoni, A.F., Whalen, J.P., and Kazam, E.: Hiatal hernia: a relook, Radiographics 3:612-644, 1983.

18. Marks, W.M., Callen, P.W., and Moss, A.A.: Gastroesophageal region: source of confusion on CT, AJR 136:359-362, 1981.

19. Thompson, W.M., Halvorsen, R.A., Foster, W., et al.: Computed tomography of the gastroesophageal junction: value of the left lateral decubitus view, J. Comput. Assist. Tomogr. 8:346-349, 1984.

20. Ginalski, J.M., Schnyder, P., Moss, A.A., et al.: Incidence and significance of a widened esophageal hiatus at CT scan, J. Clin. Gastroenterol. 6:467-470, 1984.

21. Lindell, M.M., and Bernardino, M.E.: Diagnosis of hiatus hernia by computed tomography, Comput. Radiol. 5:16-19, 1981.

22. Rohlfing, B.M., Korobkin, M., and Hall, A.D.: Computed tomography of intrathoracic omental herniation and other mediastinal fatty masses, J. Comput. Assist. Tomogr. 1:181-183, 1977.

23. Naidich, D.P., Zerhouni, E.A., and Siegelman, S.S.: Computed tomography of the chest, New York, 1984, Raven Press.

24. Payne, W.S., and Ellis, F.H.: Esophagus and diaphragmatic hernias. In Schwartz, S.I., editor: Principles of surgery, New York, 1969, McGraw-Hill Book Co.

25. Pupols, A., and Ruzicka, F.F.: Hiatal hernia causing a cardia pseudomass on computed tomography, J. Comput. Assist. Tomogr. 8:699-700, 1984.

26. Robbins, S.L., Coltran, R.S., and Kumar, V., editors: Pathologic basis of disease, ed. 3, Philadelphia, 1984, W.B. Saunders Co.

27. Solomon, M.P., Rosenblum, H., and Rosato, F.E.: Leiomyoma of the esophagus, Ann. Surg. 199:246-248, 1984.

28. Megibow, A.J., Balthazar, E.J., Hulnick, D.H., et al.: CT evaluation of gastrointestinal leiomyomas and leiomyosarcomas, AJR 144:727-731, 1985.

29. Nakata, H., Nakayama, C., Kimoto, T., et al.: Computed tomography of mediastinal bronchogenic cysts, J. Comput. Assist. Tomogr. 6:733-738, 1982.

30. Weiss, L.M., Fagelman, D., and Warhit, J.M.: CT demonstration of an esophageal duplication cyst, J. Comput. Assist. Tomogr. 7:716-718, 1983.

31. Maroko, H., Hirsch, M., Sharon, N., et al.: Calcified mediastinal enterogenous cyst, Gastrointest. Radiol. 9:105-106, 1984.

32. Kuhlman, J., Fishman, E.K., Wang, K.P., et al.: Esophageal duplication cyst: CT and transesophageal needle aspiration, AJR 145:531-532, 1985.

33. Clark, K.E., Foley, W.D., Lawson, T.L., et al.: CT evaluation of esophageal and upper abdominal varices, J. Comput. Assist. Tomogr. 4:510-515, 1980.

34. Balthazar, E.J., Megibow, A., Naidich, D.P., et al.: Computed tomographic recognition of gastric varices, AJR 142:1121-1125, 1984.

35. Hirose, J., Takashima, T., Suzuki, M., et al.: Case report: "downhill" esophageal varices demonstrated by dynamic computed tomography, J. Comput. Assist. Tomogr. 8:1007-1009, 1984.

36. Ishikawa, T., Saeki, M., Tsukune, Y., et al.: Detection of paraesophageal varices by plain films, AJR 144:701-704, 1985.

37. Halden, W.J., Harnsberger, H.R., and Mancuso, A.A.: Computed tomography of esophageal varices after sclerotherapy, AJR 140:1195-1196, 1983.

38. Saks, B.J., Kilby, A.E., Dietrich, P.A., et al.: Pleural and mediastinal changes following endoscopic injection sclerotherapy of esophageal varices, Radiology 149:639-642, 1983.

39. Pugatch, R.D., Faling, L.J., Robbins, A.H., et al.: CT diagnosis of benign mediastinal abnormalities, AJR 134:685-694, 1980.

40. Sones, P.J., Torres, W.E., and Colvin, R.S.: Effectiveness of CT in evaluating intrathoracic masses, AJR 139:469-475, 1982.

41. Baron, R.L., Koehler, R.E., and Gutierrez, F.R.: Clinical and radiographic manifestations of aortoesophageal fistulas, Radiology 141:599-605, 1981.

42. Srinivasan, M.K., and Scholz, F.J.: Hemiazygos vein as a cause of posterior indentation of the esophagus: a case report, Gastrointest. Radiol. **5:**13-15, 1980.

43. Schlesinger, A.E., Leiter, B.E., and Connors, S.K.: Computed tomography diagnosis of right aortic arch with an aberrant left inominate artery, Comput. Radiol. **8:**81-87, 1984.

44. Webb, W.R., Gamsu, G., Speckman, J.M., et al.: CT demonstration of mediastinal arch anomalies, J. Comput. Assist. Tomogr. **6:**445-451, 1982.

45. Moncada, R., Demos, T.C., Churchill, R., et al.: Case report: chronic stridor in a child: CT diagnosis of pulmonary vascular sling, J. Comput. Assist. Tomogr. **7:**713-715, 1983.

46. Day, D.L.: Aortic arch in neonates with esophageal atresia: preoperative assessment using CT, Radiology **155:**99-100, 1985.

47. Bashist, B., Ellis, K., and Gold, R.P.: Computed tomography of intrathoracic goiters, AJR **140:**455-460, 1983.

48. Morris, U.L., Colletti, P.M., Ralls, P.W., et al.: Case report: CT demonstration of intrathoracic thyroid tissue, J. Comput. Assist. Tomogr. **6:**821-824, 1982.

49. Binder, R.E., Pugatach, R.D., Faling, J., et al.: Case report: diagnosis of posterior mediastinal goiter by computed tomography, J. Comput. Assist. Tomogr. **4:**550-552, 1980.

50. Silverman, P.M., Newman, G.E., Korobkin, M., et al.: Computed tomography in the evaluation of thyroid disease, AJR **141:**897-902, 1984.

51. Williford, M.E., Thompson, W.M., Hamilton, J.D., et al.: Esophageal tuberculosis: findings on barium swallow and computed tomography, Gastrointest. Radiol. **8:**119-122, 1983.

52. Michel, L., Grillo, H.C., and Malt, R.A.: Collective review: esophageal perforation, Ann. Thorac. Surg. **33:**203-210, 1982.

53. Han, S.Y., McElvein, R.B., Aldrete, J.S., et al.: Perforation of the esophagus: correlation of site and cause with plain film findings, AJR **145:**537-540, 1985.

54. Brown, B.M.: Case report: computed tomography of mediastinal abscess secondary to posttraumatic esophageal laceration, J. Comput. Assist. Tomogr. **8:**765-767, 1984.

55. Faintuch, J., Shepard, K.V., and Levin, B.: Adenocarcinoma and other unusual variants of esophageal cancer, Semin. Oncol. **11:**196-202, 1984.

56. Lightdale, C.J., and Winawer, S.J.: Screening diagnosis and staging of esophageal cancer, Semin. Oncol. **11:**101-112, 1984.

57. Shu, Y.U.: Cytopathology of the esophagus: an overview of esophageal cytopathology in China, Acta Cytol. **27:**7-16, 1983.

58. Skinner, D.B.: Surgical treatment for esophageal carcinoma, Semin. Oncol. **11:**136-143, 1984.

59. Moss, A.A., Koehler, R.E., and Margulis, A.R.: Initial accuracy of esophagograms in detection of small esophageal carcinoma, AJR **127:**909-913, 1976.

60. Koehler, R.E., Moss, A.A., and Margulis, A.R.: Early radiographic manifestations of carcinoma of the esophagus, Radiology **119:**1-5, 1976.

61. Kondo, M., Hashimoto, S., Kubo, A., et al.: [67]Ga scanning in the evaluation of esophageal carcinoma, Radiology **131:**723-726, 1979.

62. Mori, S., Kasai, M., Watanable, T., et al.: Preoperative assessment of resectability for carcinoma of the thoracic esophagus, Ann. Surg. **190:**100-105, 1979.

63. Beahrs, O.H., and Myers, M.H., editors: Manual for staging of cancer, ed. 2, Philadelphia, 1983, J.B. Lippincott Co.

64. Moss, A.A., Schnyder, P., Thoeni, R.F., et al.: Esophageal carcinoma: pretherapy staging by computed tomography, AJR **136:**1051-1056, 1981.

65. Reinig, J.W., Stanley, J.H., and Schabel, S.I.: CT evaluation of thickened esophageal walls, AJR **140:**931-934, 1983.

66. Daffner, R.H., Halber, M.D., Postlethwait, R.W., et al.: CT of the esophagus. II. Carcinoma. AJR **133:**1051-1055, 1979.

67. Thompson, W.M., Halvorsen, R.A., Foster, W.L., et al.: Computed tomography for staging esophageal and gastroesophageal cancer: reevaluation, AJR **141:**951-958, 1983.

68. Kron, I.L., Cantrell, R.W., Johns, M.E., et al.: Computerized axial tomography of the esophagus to determine the suitability for blunt esophagectomy, Ann. Surg. **49:**173-174, 1984.

69. Quint, L.E., Glazer, G.M., Orringer, M.B., et al.: Esophageal carcinoma: CT findings, Radiology **155:**171-175, 1985.

70. Drucker, M.H., Mansour, K.A., Hatcher, C.R., et al.: Esophageal carcinoma: an aggressive approach, Ann. Thorac. Surg. **28:**133-138, 1979.

71. Beatty, J.D., Deboer, G., and Rider, W.D.: Carcinoma of the esophagus: pretreatment assessment, correlation of radiation treatment parameters with survival, and identification and management of radiation treatment failure, Cancer **43:**2254-2267, 1979.

72. Gatzinsky, P., Berglin, E., Dernevik, L., et al.: Resectional operations and long-term results in carcinoma of the esophagus, J. Thorac. Cardiovasc. Surg. **89:**71-76, 1985.

73. Orringer, M.: Esophageal tumors. In Cameron, J., editor: Current surgical therapy 1984-1985, B.C. Decker, Inc, Publisher.

74. Piccone, V.A., LeVeen, H.H., Ahmed, N., et al.: Reappraisal of esophagogastrectomy for esophageal malignancy, Am. J. Surg. **137:**32-38, 1979.

75. Ellis, F.H., Gibb, S.P., and Watkins, E.: Esophagogastrectomy, Ann. Surg. **198:**531-540, 1983.

76. Orringer, M.B.: Transhiatal esophagoectomy without thoracotomy for carcinoma of the thoracic esophagus, Ann. Surg. **200:**282-288, 1984.

77. Freeny, P.C., and Marks, W.M.: Adenocarcinoma of the gastroesophageal junction: barium and CT examination, AJR **138:**1077-1084, 1982.

78. Picus, D., Balfe, D.M., Koehler, R.E., et al.: Computed tomography in the staging of esophageal carcinoma, Radiology **146:**433-438, 1983.

79. Berkmen, Y.M., and Auh, Y.H.: CT diagnosis of acquired tracheoesophageal fistula in adults, J. Comput. Assist. Tomogr. **9:**302-304, 1985.

80. Smith, D.F., Lawson, T.L., Foley, W.D., et al.: Abstract: dedicated dynamic hepatic versus combined thoracohepatic CT in patients with carcinoma of the lung, Radiology **153:**196, 1984.

81. Wippold, F.J., Schnapf, D., Bennet, L.L., et al.: Case report: esophagosubarachnoidal fistula: an unusual complication of esophageal carcinoma, J. Comput. Assist. Tomogr. **6:**147-149, 1982.

82. Reddy, S.C.: Clinical images: esophagopleural fistula, J. Comput. Assist. Tomogr. **7:**376-378, 1983.

83. Quint, L.E., Glazer, G.M., and Orringer, M.B.: Esophageal imaging by MR and CT: study of normal anatomy and neoplasms, Radiology **156:**727-731, 1985.

84. Heiken, J.P., Balfe, D.M., and Roper, C.L.: CT evaluation after esophagogastrectomy, AJR **143:**555-560, 1984.

85. Gross, B.H., Agha, F.P., Glazer, G.M., et al.: Gastric interposition following transhiatal esophagectomy: CT evaluation, Radiology **155:**177-179, 1985.

86. Agha, F.P., and Keren, D.F.: Spindle-cell squamous carcinoma of the esophagus: a tumor with biphasic morphology, AJR **145:**541-544, 1985.

87. Olmsted, W.W., Lichtenstein, J.E., and Hyams, V.J.: Polypoid epithelial malignancies of the esophagus, AJR **140:** 921-925, 1983.

88. Balthazar, E.J.: Gastrointestinal leiomyosarcoma—unusual sites: esophagus, colon and portal hepatis, Gastrointest. Radiol. **6:**295-303, 1981.

89. Reid, H.A.S., Richardson, W.W., Corrin, B., et al.: Oat cell carcinoma of the esophagus, Cancer **45:**2342-2347, 1980.

90. Gamba, J.L., Heaston, D.K., Ling, D., et al.: CT diagnosis of an esophageal foreign body, AJR **140:**289-290, 1983.

Chapter Three

STOMACH

Alec J. Megibow

For computed tomography (CT) to compete with the other established radiographic modalities of investigation of the stomach, specifically barium studies and endoscopy, it should provide clinically useful data unobtainable from these examinations. Furthermore the procedure should be safe and cost effective. CT has the potential to offer both complementary and unique diagnostic information in patients with diseases of the stomach. This is a result of the ability of CT to directly visualize the thickness of the gastric wall, the perigastric tissues, and the supporting structures of the stomach. This imaging capability allows assessment of the presence of disease within the wall of the stomach, its local extension, and sites of distant spread. These features make CT particularly useful in the radiographic assessment of patients with malignant disease.

Barium examinations are restricted to evaluation of the alteration of the mucosal pattern and contour in the stomach. Extension of a pathological process outside the serosa of the stomach can only be indirectly inferred by visualizing gross changes in the caliber of the adjacent bowel loops or displacement of the stomach and adjacent bowel loops from their predicted normal position. Because of the variability of patient body habitus, muscular tone, and mesenteric attachments, extrinsic lesions may reach large proportions before these displacements can be recognized. Endoscopy definitively establishes the histological diagnosis, but as a single procedure it cannot determine the full extent of the given disease. The spatial resolution of present day CT scanners is not sufficient to provide the fine detail of the gastric mucosal pattern that can be seen with high-quality barium studies. CT and barium studies provide information that is complementary. In patients who have clinical symptoms that may result from primary mucosal disease, specifically gastrointestinal bleeding or dyspeptic symptoms, barium examinations are the initial procedure of choice. If these studies reveal a malignancy, then CT can add a further dimension by not documenting only the presence of the malignant lesion but also local and distant spread.

As CT equipment becomes more readily available and as its use becomes more routine as a result of a decrease in price and increased patient throughput, unsuspected gastric pathology may be detected on CT examination performed for less specific indications. Keeping this possibility in mind, the radiologist must examine the stomach during CT procedures as he would examine the solid abdominal organs. Accurate identification of disease requires meticulous attention to reliable, adequate, and complete distention of the stomach. This is not only important in gastric evaluation but also in the evaluation of other structures in the upper abdomen, specifically the pancreas, adrenal glands, and liver.

Pathological states are recognized by increased thickness of the gastric wall as well as the presence of alterations in its density or the presence of abnormal masses in the perigastric tissues. Specificity in diagnosis is furthered by appreciation of the contours of the thickened wall and distribution of the extra gastric abnormalities. Specific radiographic features of the thickened wall, such as its CT number and presence or absence of contrast enhancement, may contribute to differential diagnosis but to a lesser extent than the entire constellation of findings.

TECHNIQUES

All CT examinations of the stomach should be performed with the thought of maximizing identification of the areas of the gastric wall thickened by disease. This requires adequate distention of the stomach during the period of scanning. Positive contrast agents have traditionally been used. We prefer 1% to 4% suspensions of barium sulfate* or 3% to 4% solutions of water-soluble iodinated oral contrast media. Regardless of the agent used, 8 ounces of contrast agent should be ingested immediately before the commencement of the scan of the upper abdomen. This provides distention necessary to fill the stomach, particularly the fundus, and allows accurate assessment of the gastric wall. This also facilitates separation of the stomach from the adjacent organs and allows for identification of the duodenum. When combined scans of the thorax and abdomen are performed, it is particularly important to remember to stop the scan sequence at the diaphragm and have the patient consume 8 ounces of contrast material regardless of the amount consumed before the examination.

If gas contrast techniques are used, 400 ml of carbon dioxide generated from one packet of effervescent granules in approximately 20 ml of water is substituted. This is administered in place of the final cup of contrast material. Specifics of techniques to both positive and negative contrasts are discussed in Chapter One.

ANATOMY

The important anatomical features for the radiologist attempting to evaluate the stomach on CT are: the appearance and thickness of the normal gastric wall, cross-sectional representation of the gastric curvatures, the relation of the gastric surfaces to the greater and lesser peritoneal cavities, the sites of attachment of supporting ligaments that contain the gastric blood supply and lymph nodes, the location of the major lymph node groups, and the perigastric vessels.

*E-Z Cat manufactured by E-Z Company, Westbury, Long Island; Tomo CAT, manufactured by Lafayette Company, Indiana; BARO-CAT, manufactured by Mallinckrodt Corporation, St. Louis, Missouri.

The gastric wall

Lee[1] and Balfe[2] found the gastric wall to be less than 1 cm thick in 90% of individuals. The average thickness is 5 mm. In Komaki's series the thickness ranges from 1.2 to 13 mm (5 mm average).[3] These series were performed after distending the stomach with positive contrast material.

We have examined by air contrast technique the appearance of the gastric wall in 50 consecutive patients in whom there is no clinical evidence of gastric disease. Our findings indicate the average thickness of the gastric wall to be 1.5 to 2.5 mm. These measurements were all obtained at a window of 500 Hounsfield (H) units to standardize contrast levels between the air in the lumen of the stomach, the soft-tissue density of the gastric wall, and the perigastric fat (Fig. 3-1). The routine visualization of the gastric wall probably reflects the fact that its thickness is produced by the three bands of smooth muscle within the muscular coats of the stomach. The same perceptible thickness is routinely noted in the rectum, which also has three muscular coats. The remainder of the alimentary tube from duodenal bulb to the rectum, which has only two smooth muscle coats, has significantly less perceptible thickness in a normal patient and appears as a thin (almost invisible) border.

Increased contrast resolution provided by the gas contrast techniques allows routine visualization of the rugal folds in the normal stomach. These are more prominent in the proximal stomach and decrease in number toward the antrum. These appear as well-defined sharp intraluminal protrusions usually measuring approximately 6 mm from their apex to the serosal aspect of the gastric wall. They are *evenly* distributed around the circumference of the distended stomach. At least 1 to 2 rugal folds were seen in 46 of the 50 cases. In 35 cases, multiple rugal folds could be visualized symmetrically distributed around the circumference of the stomach (Fig. 3-1). Routine visualization of rugal folds adds another parameter in the diagnostic evaluation of the stomach.

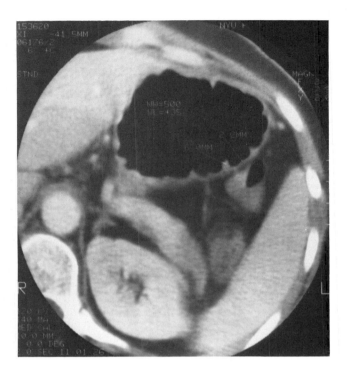

Fig. 3-1. Normal gastric wall—air contrast CT. The scan is imaged at a window of 500 and a level of 35. The mucosal and serosal aspects of the wall are clearly identifiable. This allows an accurate measurement of a 2.2 mm thickness. The rugae are clearly seen and are symmetrically distributed around the circumference. The wall measures 6 mm when the rugal fold is included. The constancy of this appearance of the air-filled stomach should increase sensitivity, allowing detection of subtler indications of gastric pathology.

In two areas of the stomach the wall is normally thickened. The pylorus and pyloric canal displays focal thickening. Occasionally the thin gastric lumen can be seen traversing the pyloric canal. The location and the symmetrical positioning of the gastric lumen traversing the pyloric canal helps eliminate confusion in identifying this wall thickening from a pathologic condition (Fig. 3-2). The thickening of the pylorus is a result of the presence of thick oblique muscle fibers in the region of the pyloric sphincter. The other region of thickening that may be normal is at the level of the esophago-gastric junction. This will be considered in more detail subsequently.

Cross-sectional representation of gastric curvatures and supporting ligaments

The position of the adult stomach is derived from a complex series of rotations of the primitive foregut during embryogenesis. The foregut begins as cephalocaudad-oriented tube anchored by a ventral and dorsal mesentery. Following rotation, the ventral mesentery becomes oriented cephalad, toward the right, and slightly posteriorly. The portion of the foregut in contact with the ventral mesentery becomes the lesser curvature. The ventral mesentery gives rise to a hepatic diverticulum that ultimately will form the liver itself. In doing so, the ventral mesentery becomes divided into an anterior and posterior portion. The anterior portion of the mesentery, which is now anterior to the liver, fuses with the ventral abdominal wall and becomes the falciform ligament. The posterior portion of the ventral mesentery remains in contact with the stomach at the lesser curvature and becomes the gastrohepatic ligament and the lesser omentum. The gastrohepatic ligament enters the liver anterior to the caudate lobe in the fissure of the ligament venosum, representing the point of origin of the hepatic diverticulum. This mesenteric attachment fans along the lesser curvature of the stomach to the duodenal bulb. The free edge of the ligament forms the roof of the entrance to Winslow's foramen (the hepatoduodenal ligament).

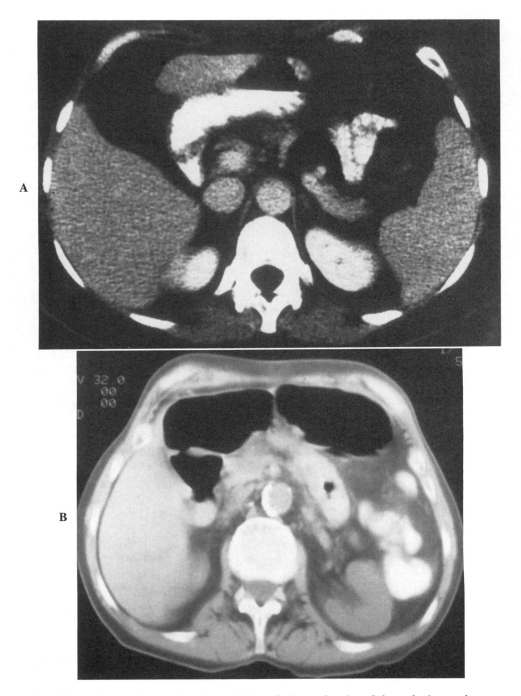

Fig. 3-2. A, Normal stomach pylorus. The soft-tissue density of the pyloric canal appears as a symmetric region with the lumen seen between the muscle bundles. The duodenal bulb is clearly seen immediately beyond the canal. **B,** Pyloric canal—air contrast CT. The narrow pyloric canal is seen between the thick pyloric musculature.

The dorsal mesentery rotates in an opposite direction, ultimately becoming the greater curvature of the stomach, facing the left, caudally, and somewhat anteriorly. That portion of the dorsal mesentery remaining in contact with the stomach, the dorsal mesogastrium, balloons to the left forming the omental bursa. The posterior wall of the omental bursa fuses to the pancreas and transverse colon, resulting in formation of the gastrocolic ligaments. The anterior portion of the omental bursa ultimately forms the greater omentum. The spleen forms within the greater omentum as well.[4,5] The most posterior portion of the greater omentum is the gastrosplenic ligament. As this peritoneal fold courses anteriorly along the greater curvature of the stomach, it continues as the gastrocolic ligament (see Fig. 3-5). The gastrocolic ligament fuses with the transverse mesocolon along the anterior border of the transverse colon to form the greater omentum.

On CT images, it becomes evident that the lesser curvature aspect of the stomach lies more posteriorly and to the right than the greater curvature aspect of the stomach. The esophagogastric junction can be seen in a relatively posterior location along the lesser curvature. The stomach arches anteriorly and to the right from the relatively posterior fundus and cardia on the left side of the abdomen to the anterior aspect of the body and antrum of the stomach on the right side of the abdomen. Anteriorly, the stomach is related to the undersurface of the lateral segment of the left lobe of the liver and the anterior abdominal wall and left anterior subphrenic space. Posteriorly the stomach is separated from the anterior surface of the pancreas by the lesser sac (Fig. 3-3). The fundus of the stomach is adjacent to the tail of the pancreas and is close to the left adrenal gland. Failure to distend the stomach may result in the false impression of a left adrenal mass or a mass in the tail of the pancreas.[6,7]

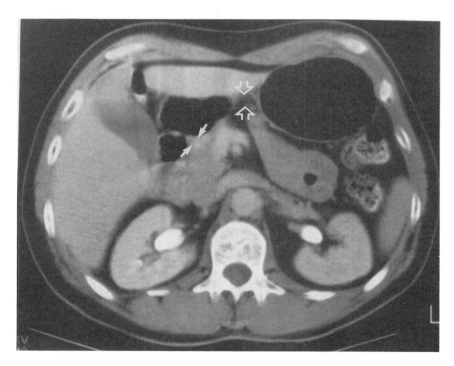

Fig. 3-3. Relations to the stomach. Scan through distral antrum and celiac region. The lesser curvature is located posterior to and abuts the anterior aspect of the pancreas, separated from it by the lesser sac (a potential space). The *closed arrows* show the region of the hepatoduodenal ligament coursing posterior to the duodenal bulb. The *open arrows* indicate structures in the midportion of the lesser omentum.

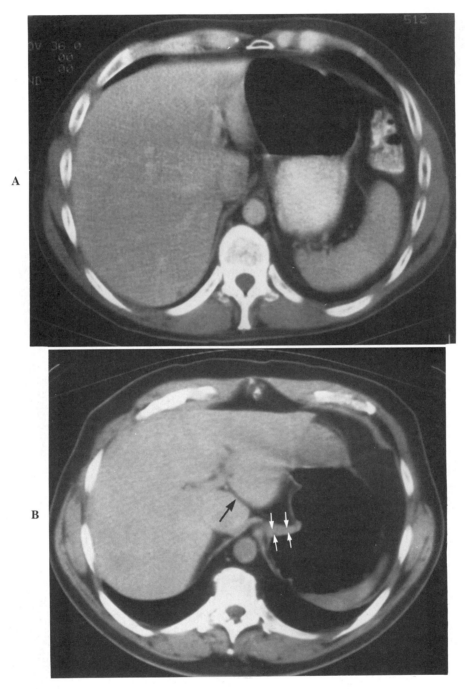

Fig. 3-4. A, Wall thickening at the esophagogastric junction. A focal thickening is noted along the lesser curvature portion of the stomach adjacent to the diaphragmatic crura. Note the smooth contour, lack of lobulation, and gentle zone of transition with the adjacent gastric wall. Note also the fissure for the ligamentum venosum "pointing" toward the level of the esophagogastric junction. **B,** Esophagogastric junction—air contrast. The submerged segment (the abdominal esophagus) can be seen exiting between the diaphragmatic crura (esophageal hiatus) and continuous with the lesser curvature aspect of the stomach (arrows). Note the relation to the fissure of the ligamentum venosum (single arrow).

Esophagogastric junction

The abdominal portion of the esophagus, the so-called submerged segment, is tethered to the diaphragm by a circumferential reflection of the inferior diaphragmatic fascia on to the fascia propria of the esophagus forming the phrenoesophageal ligament. This ligament fuses with the most cranial extension of the lesser omentum at the gastroesophageal junction. The fusion of the fascial layers of the distal esophageal fibers of the lesser omentum and the diaphragmatic fascia can result in apparent thickening of the gastric wall at the level of the esophagogastric junction (Fig. 3-4). Marks et al. found thickening to be present in 38% of normal patients studied by CT.[8] Confident recognition that this thickening is related to normal anatomy can be achieved by over-distention of the stomach with resultant flattening of the region. Furthermore the relation of the gastrohepatic ligament to the fissure of the ligament venosum can be confirmed on the images. Decubitus positioning of the patient along with air insufflation may be necessary to evaluate the contour of the gastroesophageal junction, particularly when the esophagus appears distended or when a hiatal hernia is present (Fig. 3-4, B). Methods of optimal distention are discussed in Chapter One, and a more detailed anatomic description of this region may be found in Chapter Two.

Ligamentous attachment

The important peritoneal ligaments related to the stomach include the hepatoduodenal ligament, gastric colic ligament, gastrosplenic ligament, and gastrohepatic ligament. The hepatoduodenal ligament is identified as that region containing the portal vein, common bile duct, and common hepatic artery. This can be visualized on high-quality dynamic scans and when sufficient fat is present to separate these vessels within the porta hepatis. This ligament extends from the porta hepatis to the postbulbar duodenum, representing the free edge of the lesser omentum (gastrohepatic ligament) (Fig. 3-5). The gastrohepatic ligament originates from the fissure of the ligament venosum of the liver at the gastroesophageal junction and fans along the lesser curvature aspect of the stomach, ending in the hepatoduodenal ligament. The branches of the right and left gastric arteries, the coronary vein, and the right and lesser curvature lymph nodes are located in this ligament. Structures smaller than 6 cm can be recognized within the gastrohepatic ligament in 85% of patients[9] (Fig. 3-5).

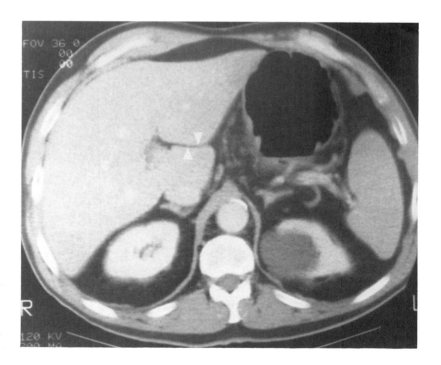

Fig. 3-5. Gastrohepatic ligament. Branches of the left gastric artery, coronary vein, lymph nodes, and short gastric veins are seen as streaklike densities in the fat between the liver and lesser curvature of the stomach. Note the relation to the fissure of the ligamentum venosum (*arrowheads*).

The gastrocolic ligament connects the stomach and transverse colon. The left border of the gastrocolic ligament merges with the gastrosplenic ligament. The right border ends at the gastroduodenal junction as a free edge. The gastrocolic ligament contains the gastroepiploic vessels. The gastrosplenic ligament is at the left extent of the greater omentum and relates the greater curvature of the stomach to the spleen. This ligament is particularly well visualized in patients with gastric varices because short gastric vessels within the ligament are engorged from increased portal venous pressure.[10] The gastrosplenic ligament continues to its posterior insertion on the diaphragm. This ligament serves as the lateral border of the left inferior subphrenic space. Medially, this space is delineated by the left triangular ligament of the liver (Fig. 3-6).

Lymph nodes

Lymph nodes are clustered along the vessels in each of these ligaments. Normal lymph nodes are not discernible from small vessels on enhanced CT scans. The ligamentous attachments define areas that should be carefully scrunitized for the presence of enlarged lymph nodes in patients with neoplasms of the stomach. The lymphatic channels draining the stomach follow the arterial blood supply. The flow of lymph is in reverse direction to the flow of arterial blood. Coller divided perigastric nodes into four groups based on dissection of the patients with metastatic disease from gastric carcinoma.[11] The zones correspond to four zones of arterial supply.

A more clinically practical classification of gastric lymph nodes is described by Sunderland.[12] Five nodal zones are identified. Zone 1 (paracardial) nodes are adjacent to the esophagogastric junction. This zone is further subdivided into Ia (lesser curvature) and Ib (greater curvature). Zone II nodes are the superior gastric nodes adjacent to the right and left gastric arteries within the lesser omentum. The nodes in zone III, the subpyloric nodes, are seen in the distal lesser curvature. Zone IV nodes, inferior gastric nodes, are found along the greater curve within the greater omentum. Pancreaticolienal nodes, zone V, are located at the hilum of the spleen, the tail of the pancreas, and along splenic arteries. All node groups drain into the celiac axis nodes (middle suprapancreatic node) and from there into the cisterna chyli. Retroperitoneal anastomoses are present at this level as well.[12]

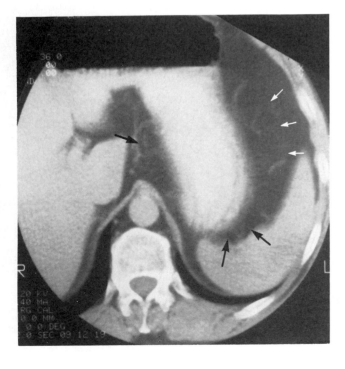

Fig. 3-6. Gastrocolic and gastrosplenic ligament. Loops of the gastroepiploic vessels can be seen coursing in the fibrofatty tissue that makes up the greater omentum. The most posterior portion, the gastrosplenic ligament (*black arrows*) courses anteriorly and to the left, becoming the gastrocolic ligament (*white arrows*). The branches of the left gastric artery are seen in the lesser omentum (*single arrow*).

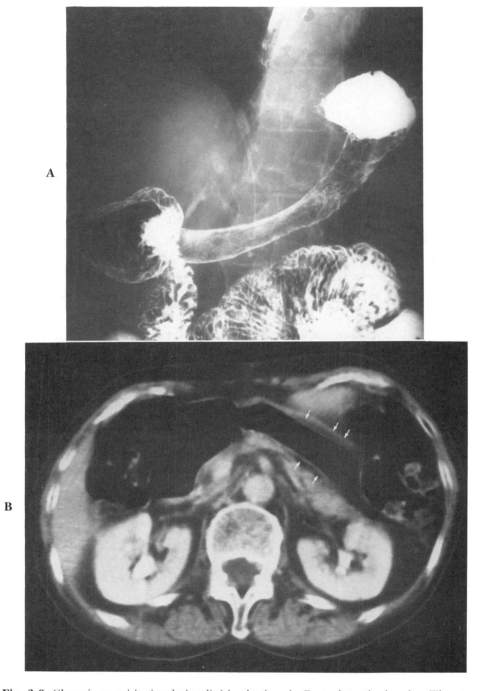

Fig. 3-9. Chronic gastritis simulating linitis plastica. **A,** Gastrointestinal series. The stomach is diminished in size. There is a loss of mucosal pattern. The findings mimic linitis plastica. **B,** CT scan shows the lumen to be narrowed. *No* wall thickening is seen; in fact there appears to be an excess of fat *(arrows)*. The patient was operated on because of diminished gastric reserve. No tumor was present. The patient had similar radiologic findings for 6 years.

Hypertrophic gastritis is the result of a variety of etiologies and can be seen as a manifestation of several systemic diseases, including Ménétrièr's disease, eosinophilic gastritis, and Zollinger-Ellison syndrome.[13] These diseases all display thickening of the rugal folds that results in thickening of the gastric wall. In Zollinger-Ellison syndrome peripancreatic lymph nodes, as well as liver metastases, may be visualized, suggesting the diagnosis. Changes of hypersecretion and fold thickening of the small bowel can be recognized as well. Fishman et al., in describing the CT finding in a single case of Ménétrièr's disease, called attention to the smooth, lobulated, clearly defined folds.[14] Williams et al. has reported a case of adenocarcinoma of the stomach associated with Ménétrièr's disease and called attention to 20 other reported cases.[15] We have no CT experience with the association. In two cases of hypertrophic gastritis studied in our institution we have also seen lobulated, thickened folds arranged symmetrically along the circumference of the proximal stomach as seen in cross section

(Fig. 3-8). We have seen one case of severe, chronic, atrophic gastritis appearing as diffuse narrowing and scarring of the stomach similar to linitis plastica (Fig. 3-9). Although the barium radiographic picture of this stomach is identical to that of linitis plastica, CT examination in this patient failed to reveal thickening of the gastric wall. In fact, the wall was infiltrated with fat. This finding may help differentiate this form of disease from neoplasm. We have seen antral gastritis detected by CT as an area of slight thickening of the distal stomach with preservation of the mucosal folds. We have made this observation in two patients and confirmed the CT findings with barium radiography (Fig. 3-10). Although we do not believe that CT is a necessary examination in these patients, both patients were studied for other indications and the observation of the CT could be included in part of the patients' overall diagnostic evaluation. Localized hypertrophy of the folds may present a CT picture identical to a primary neoplasm (Fig. 3-11).

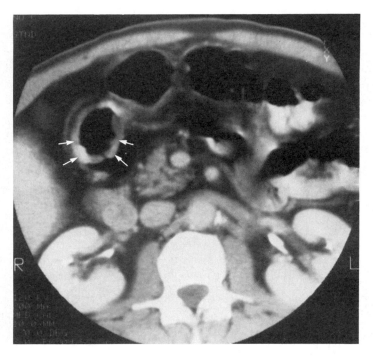

Fig. 3-10. Antral gastritis. There is focal, symmetric thickening at the gastric antrum *(arrows)*. The pyloric canal is central in location. Endoscopically thickened antral folds with small erosions were seen indicative of antral gastritis.

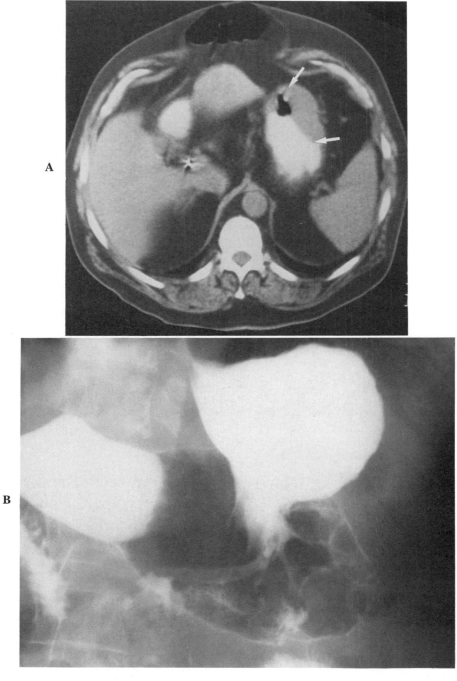

Fig. 3-11. Localized hyperugosity—greater curvature. **A,** CT suggests focal neoplasm *(arrows)* along the greater curvature. **B,** Gastrointestinal series. Thickened folds are seen. No tumor was seen at endoscopy nor at surgical full thickness biopsy obtained during cholecystectomy.

Crohn's disease of the stomach generally involves the gastric antrum and may produce antral duodenal fistulas.[16] In one patient with gastric Crohn's disease the findings on the CT examination were similar to gastric carcinoma in that the wall was asymmetrically thickened and mass-like in configuration (Fig. 3-12). Large ulcerations within this mass with fistulization to the duodenum were detected. A sinus tract leading to a peripancreatic abscess could also be shown. In light of the known clinical history, the findings were characteristic enough to be considered Crohn's disease. On barium radiography, this patient displayed the "rams horn" configuration described by Farman.[17] We have seen a patient with gastric amyloidosis who also demonstrated thickening of the wall of the stomach and increased edema in the perigastric fat. At the time of the CT examination this was thought to represent gastric carcinoma. Diagnosis was made at the time of gastrojejunostomy.

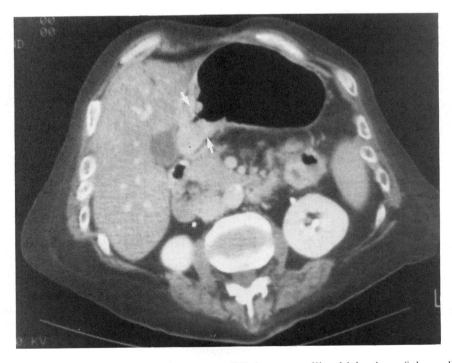

Fig. 3-12. Crohn's disease—gastric antrum. CT shows masslike thickening of the wall of the antrum (*arrows*). The appearance is compatible with carcinoma; however, this patient has a long history of severe Crohn's disease (see also Fig. 4-10).

Gastric varices

The diagnosis of gastric varices may be difficult with conventional barium studies, especially when esophageal varices are not present. Detection is difficult since varices may be confused with the rugal fold thickening or even tumor.[18] Gastric varices result from elevated portal venous pressure due to hepatic disease (cirrhosis) or extrahepatic occlusive disease (pancreatic carcinoma or pancreatitis)[19] (Fig. 3-13).

We studied 13 consecutive patients with proven gastric varices by CT and correlated the results with angiography and/or gastroscopy. In 11 of 13 patients studied, characteristic features could be defined. These included (1) well-defined clusters of rounded and tubular soft-tissue densities within the posterior and posteromedial wall of the stomach; (2) tubular structures running along the circumference of the gastric fundus, particularly in the posteromedial wall; (3) significant enhancement of the above mentioned abnormalities equal to that of an enlargement of a normal vessel; and (4) intraabdominal collateral venous channels indicative of portal hypertension.[20] In all cases, vascular channels are defined in the lesser omentum and gastrohepatic ligament. Gastric varices may also be seen in short gastric veins along the greater curvature aspect of the stomach in the gastrosplenic ligament. These varices are commonly visualized in distal splenic vein obstruction, such as in pancreatic carcinoma.

In this same study only seven of the patients had abnormalities in the upper gastrointestinal series suggestive of gastric varices. The explanation is readily apparent from the CT scan because it is readily seen that only a small percentage of varicosities actually abut the gastric lumen. Varices may be missed when the stomach is not properly distended or when intravenous contrast material is not used. The major differential diagnosis is lymphadenopathy, particularly in the region of the gastrohepatic omentum. This diagnosis can be differentiated by use of intravenous contrast bolus with dynamic scanning.[21] If the equipment used is not adequate to perform dynamic scans, ultrasound may be useful in detecting typical findings of gastric varices.[22]

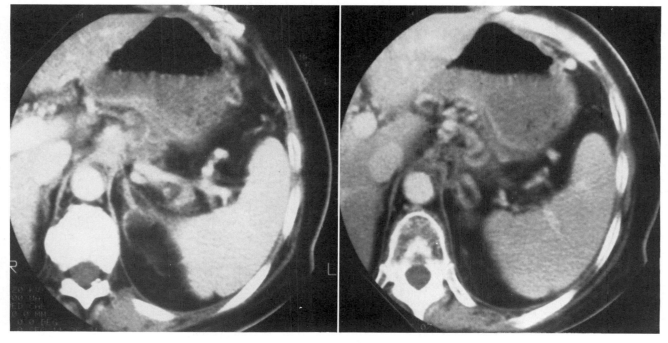

Fig. 3-13. Gastric varices—splenic vein occlusion. **A,** Dynamic scan through the pancreas reveals obstruction of the splenic vein as a result of carcinoma of the tail of the pancreas. Dilated veins in the gastrocolic ligament are seen. **B,** Scan more cephalad reveals multiple varices of short gastric veins in the lesser omentum.

Peptic ulcer disease

The role of CT in evaluating patients with gastric ulcer is to detect complications of the ulcer rather than to further evaluate the appearance of the ulcer. As CT becomes more readily available and as it is used more as a screening examination than special procedure, an appreciation of the appearances and complications of gastric ulcer will be necessary. CT may show walled-off abscess collections in the lesser sac (Figs. 3-14 and 3-15) or in lesser omentum in patients with sealed-off perforations of lesser curve gastric ulcers. Clinical symptomatology is more suggestive of abdominal abscess, leading to CT imaging rather than barium studies.[23,24] Fluid collections in the left anterior subphrenic space should raise the suspicion of a perforated greater curvature ulcer. CT has a little role in differentiation of a benign from malignant gastric ulcer, particularly with the availability of fibroptic endoscopy and biopsy.

Pancreatic disease

Proximity of the stomach to the anterior surface of the pancreas results in direct effects of pancreatic disease on the viscus. Pancreatic masses will displace the stomach anteriorly, and CT will be able to differentiate this displacement from a pancreatic mass versus retrogastric lymphadenopathy.

Brown et al. analyzed the appearance of the gastric wall in patients with pancreatitis. Two thirds of these patients showed wall thickening greater than 1 cm. Findings of thickened wall in association with nonpancreatic fluid collections often indicated that this fluid collection was infected.[25] CT also provides excellent depiction with pancreatic pseudocysts and shows their relation to the stomach, allowing and providing for accurate routes of either surgical or percutaneous cyst gastrostomy[26] (Fig. 3-16).

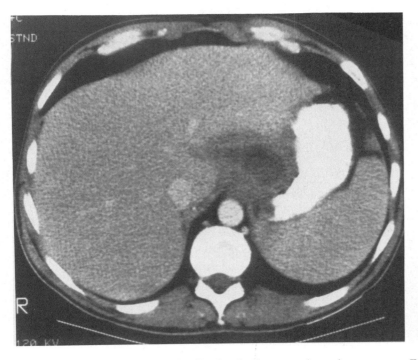

Fig. 3-14. Gastric ulcer. Complex fluid collection in the gastrohepatic omentum. Free air is not seen. The patient was a 26-year-old drug addict evaluated for fever. Subsequent endoscopy revealed a gastric ulcer. Surgery revealed a sealed off perforation. (Courtesy Dr. C.A. Whelan, Mountainside Hospital, Montclair, New Jersey.)

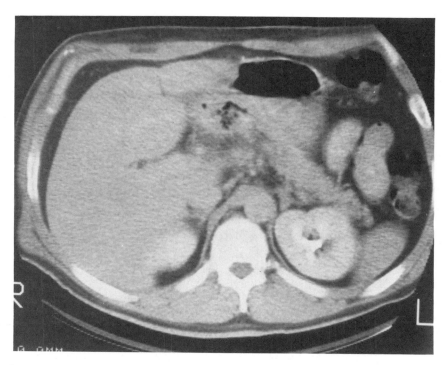

Fig. 3-15. Gastric ulcer with lesser sac abscess. The patient was referred to CT for suspected acute pancreatitis. Scan reveals loculated collection of air in the lesser sac as a result of a perforated, lesser curvature, gastric ulcer. No free air was seen. A small amount of fluid is seen in the subhepatic space (lesser omentum).

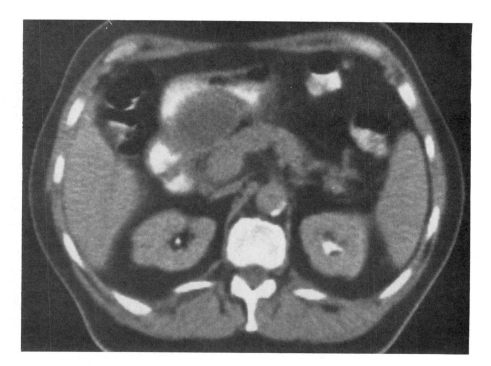

Fig. 3-16. Antral pseudocyst. The precise localization of the cyst in relation to the stomach provides accurate preoperative assessment for subsequent drainage.

GASTRIC NEOPLASMS

CT of the stomach has its greatest application in the evaluation of patients with neoplastic disease. Cross-sectional display of the stomach as well as visualization of the perigastric tissues allows preoperative documentation of the extent and spread of the primary neoplasm. Surgery was averted in 7 of 22 patients in whom Stage III and IV gastric carcinoma was diagnosed by CT.[27] We believe as others that CT should not make the decision as to whether or not to operate on a given patient; however, documentation of more extensive disease than clinically predicted may influence the decision for a palliative resection rather than attempting to perform curative surgery.[28]

Adenocarcinoma

Adenocarcinoma is the most common malignant lesion of the stomach, accounting for 95% of all gastric neoplasms and representing the sixth leading cause of cancer deaths overall. An estimated 24,000 new cases will be diagnosed in 1985 with 14,300 estimated deaths. This neoplasm ranks third behind colo-rectal, and pancreatic cancer in the incidence of gastrointestinal malignancy.[29] Despite the increasing availability of endoscopy and improved operative techniques, the 5-year survival rate in the United States is approximately 18%. Most retrospective surgical series reflect little re-

duction in overall mortality over the past three decades.[30-32] However, some authors note improved survival in radical operations performed for lesions in patients with Stage I and II disease as classified by the TNM system.[33,34] Unfortunately this group of patients is in a distinct minority. Most patients with gastric carcinoma are diagnosed late in the disease on the basis of clinical symptomatology and confirmed with endoscopy or barium radiography. The role of CT in these patients is to document the spread of disease beyond the mucosa of the stomach.

CT findings

The most important finding of gastric carcinoma on CT is focal thickening of the gastric wall. The very fact that thickening can be visualized implies that the tumor has generally extended into the submucosal and probably the serosal layers of the stomach. Therefore it must be emphasized that the *early diagnosis* of gastric carcinoma is *not* to be expected from CT. Gross radiographic appearances can be divided into three groups: (1) polypoid or fungating, (2) ulcerating or penetrating, and (3) infiltrating or scirrhous. These correspond to the well known gross classifications and can be differentiated on CT scanning (Figs. 3-17 to 3-19). It must be stressed that the appearance of the neoplasm itself has no bearing on the prognosis.

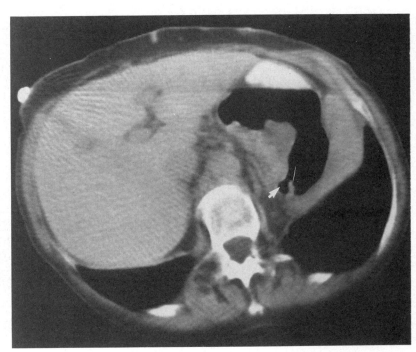

Fig. 3-17. Polypoid gastric carcinoma. A fungating polypoid tumor is seen along the lesser curvature aspect of the proximal stomach. The most posterior portion is ulcerated *(arrow)*. Note that the scan is performed with the patient in the prone position to maximize air distention of the posterior gastric fundus.

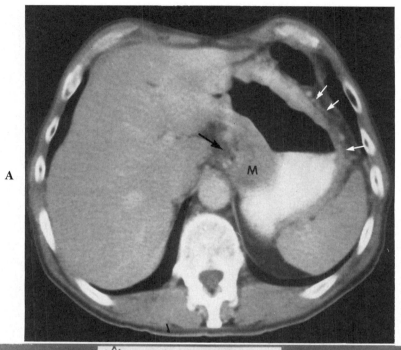

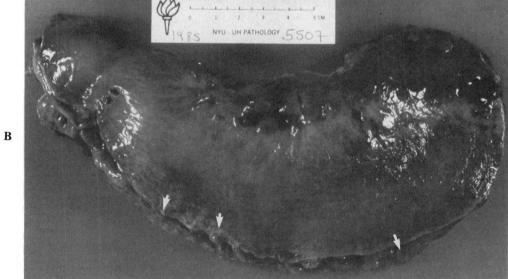

Fig. 3-18. Gastric carcinoma—typical CT findings. **A,** CT scan through the upper abdomen reveals marked thickening of the gastric wall. There is a loss of the normal rugal pattern. The wall shows a variable enhancement. Note the serpiginous, linear densities along the greater curvature of the stomach that represent engorged lymphatic vessels *(small arrows)*. These result from intramural lymphatic obstruction by the neoplasm. Along the lesser curvature aspect a large mass *(M)* extends into the gastrohepatic ligament. Rounded densities adjacent to the mass represent enlarged lymph nodes *(black arrow)*. **B,** Pathologic specimen of *(A)*. Note the nodular, serpiginous structures along the greater curvature. These correspond with dilated lymphatics as discussed above *(arrows)*.

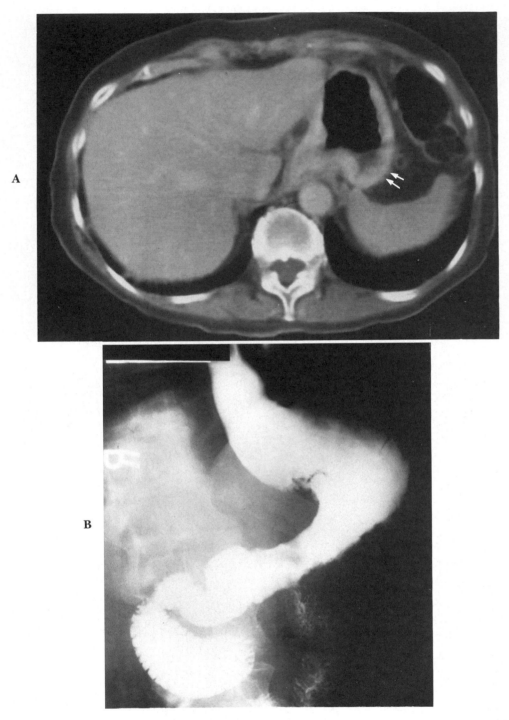

Fig. 3-19. Gastric carcinoma—linitis plastica. **A,** The capacity of the stomach is reduced. The wall is thickened. Note the enhancement of the wall seen during dynamic sequential scanning. Dilated surface lymphatics are seen along the serosa *(arrows)*. **B,** Appearance of typical linitis plastica as seen on gastrointestinal series.

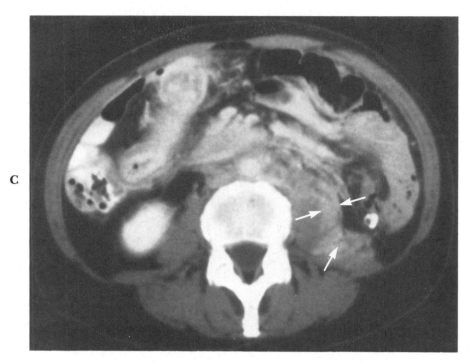

C

Fig. 3-19, cont'd. C, Scan through the retroperitoneum—scans patient as in **A** and **B**. Note the sheetlike regions of bright enhancement in the metastases within the left psoas and paraspinal muscle *(arrows)*. Metastases to the mesentery show a similar appearance.

The luminal surface of the neoplasm is irregular and nodular. The folds are asymmetrically thickened when the wall is infiltrated. The density of the wall may show varying attenuation or may be uniform. The serosal aspect is usually poorly marginated. In advanced cases, there is an increased density in the perigastric fat, and at times small nodules are seen in the serosal aspect of the stomach correlating with the presence of dilated surface lymphatics; a common finding seen in laparotomy resulting from distention of the intramural lymphatic plexi within the stomach (Fig. 3-19). There is a variable tendency for the gastric carcinoma to enhance on a bolus injection of intravenous contrast material. We have seen enhancement of gastric carcinoma exclusively in the linitis plastica or scirrhous forms but not in the polypoid form. The pathologic explanation for this enhancement is not clear. Radiologically it is possible that this may serve as a way of differentiating gastric lymphoma from gastric adenocarcinoma. The enhancement is noted in the metastases from scirrhous carcinoma as well (Fig. 3-19, *C*). One case of calcification within the wall of a mucinous adenocarcinoma has been reported.[35]

Table 3-1. TNM classification of gastric carcinoma

Primary tumor (T)

T_1	Tumor is limited to mucosa or to mucosa and submucosa
T_2	Tumor involves mucosa, submucosa, muscle or serosa, but does not penetrate serosa
T_3	Tumor penetrates through the serosa without invading contiguous structures
T_4	a. Tumor invades adjacent contiguous tissues b. Tumor invades adjacent organs, diaphragm, abdominal wall

Nodal involvement (N)

N_0	No metastases to regional nodes
N_1	Involvement of perigastric nodes within 3 cm of primary tumor along lesser or greater curvature
N_2	Involvement of regional nodes more than 3 cm from primary tumor or along the branches of the celiac axis
N_3	Involvement of other abdominal nodes: para-aorta, hepatoduodenal, retropancreatic, and mesenteric nodes

Distant metastases

M_0	No known distant metastases
M_1	Distant metastases present

Modified from American Joint Committee for Cancer Staging and End Results Reporting. Chicago, 1978, American Joint Committee.

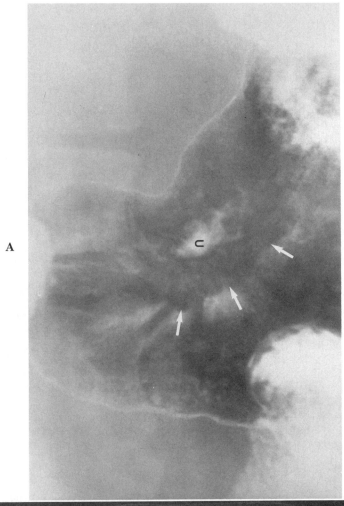

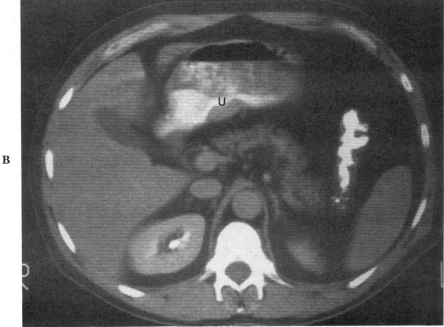

Fig. 3-20. True T$_2$ gastric carcinoma. **A,** Gastrointestinal series—double-contrast film reveals a shallow ulcer crater, *c*, asymmetrically located in a mass. Notice that the radiating folds do not reach the ulcer crater but end at the periphery of the mass *(arrows)*. **B,** CT scan—the ulcer, *u*, is visualized in a soft-tissue mass along the distal, lesser curvature. The lesion did not penetrate to the serosa. No nodes were present at the time of gastrectomy. This is the only gastric carcinoma we have imaged that could be considered less than a T$_3$ lesion.

We have analyzed CT scans in 60 patients with adenocarcinoma of the stomach and attempted to correlate these with the TNM classification when possible (Table 3-1). In 55 of 56 patients a T_3 or T_4 lesion was present. The remaining four patients were seen following surgery. We have seen only one proven T_2 lesion (Fig. 3-20). No T_1 lesions were detected, although we have seen 2 mm, hyperplastic, gastric polyps using the air contrast technique (see Fig. 1-16). Therefore we believe that it is theoretically possible to image small, polypoid, mucosal neoplasms with CT. The thickness of the involved wall measured between 6 and 30 mm (average 14 mm). This measurement is *less* than in other reported series.[1,2] In Komaiko's series the range of abnormal thickening measured between 13 and 45 mm.[36] In the series reported by Balfe, 26 of 28 patients had wall thickening from 12 to 140 mm; however in this series patients with leiomyosarcomas and lymphomas were included in measurements, which probably accounted for the large average size.[2] We believe the reason we could diagnose gastric carcinoma despite less thickening of the wall than has previously been reported is a result of the ability to recognize infiltration of the gastric wall by virtue of loss of a normal fold pattern and the enhancement seen in linitis plastica forms (Fig. 3-21).

We had difficulty in detecting ulcers by CT. There may be several reasons for this phenomenon. First, we had not studied the patients with an empty stomach and therefore were at a disadvantage in analyzing the mucosal surface. Retention of particulate material within the ulcer crater may also obscure its presence, particularly when mixed with the relatively dilute oral contrast material. Since adopting routine air contrast technique, we request scans be performed with an empty stomach. Second, it has been difficult to distinguish an ulcer crater between two mounds of neoplastic tissue from nonulcerated mucosa between heaped-up margins of the neoplasm. However, because CT detects the mass in which the ulcer is present we have found this deficiency to be relatively minor.

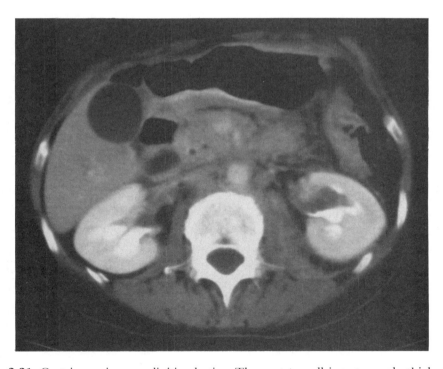

Fig. 3-21. Gastric carcinoma—linitis plastica. The gastric wall is not grossly thickened. This lesion is recognized by the enhanced gastric wall and loss of normal mucosal contours. These findings are appreciable as a result of air contrast techniques. Notice the presence of adenopathy thickening the vessels in a fashion similar to pancreatic carcinoma (T_3N_2).

Carcinoma of the esophagogastric junction

Carcinoma of the esophagogastric junction has risen in frequency from 7% of gastric neoplasms in 1930 to 33% of gastric neoplasms in 1976.[37] Barium radiography remains the procedure of choice in the evaluation of the patient with dysphagia who may have had a carcinoma at the esophagogastric junction, but CT may play a significant role in preoperative staging of this disease. Freeny and Marks found CT to be highly accurate in staging this group of neoplasms and especially in separating resectable from nonresectable lesions. In this series of 21 patients CT predicted nonresectability in 16 cases.[38] In a retrospective study of 19 patients with cardioesophageal carcinoma the intraabdominal esophageal median diameter was 15.6 ± 3.2 mm. Air was seen in the dilated esophageal lumen in 80% of the cases. The median thickness of the adjacent stomach was 10.7 ± 6.2 mm.[39]

We do not routinely measure the thickness of the gastric wall. When the diameter of the esophagus is greater than the immediately posterior aorta and when the lesser curvature aspect of the adjacent cardia is poorly seen as a result of retained secretions, lack of opacification, or suboptimal distention, we believe it necessary to prove that no carcinoma exists in this region. Because the wall thickening may be present in this region as a normal finding, the diagnosis of neoplasm requires additional maneuvers to confirm its presence (Fig. 3-5). When neoplasm is present in the area, the mucosal surface tends to appear lobulated, and in more advanced cases a bulky mass can be seen. Bolus injection of contrast material fails to reveal the enhancement seen in the linitis plastica form of gastric carcinoma (Fig. 3-22). This may best be imaged by giving the patient effervescent granules, then positioning and scanning him in the right-side-down decubitus position (Fig. 3-23). This maximizes distention of the gastric fundus and allows more precise recognition and documentation of the extent of a neoplasm. It is important to include cuts of the lower thorax in the evaluation of these patients. In a series of 101 patients with carcinoma of the esophagogastric junction, the median length of esophageal involvement was 2.8 cm.[34] Esophageal involvement manifests itself as thickening of the wall of the esophagus. This may be difficult to accurately demonstrate because of the relative lack of fat in the periesophageal mediastinal compartment. Decubitus scanning facilitates air distention of the esophagus; however, barium radiography remains the best method of evaluating the length of an esophageal involvement.

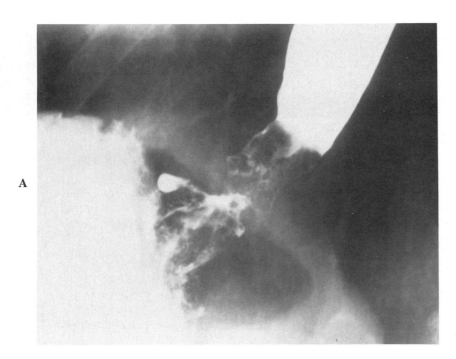

Fig. 3-22. Carcinoma—gastroesophageal junction. **A,** Annular, ulcerated lesion seen in the distal esophagus and proximal stomach.

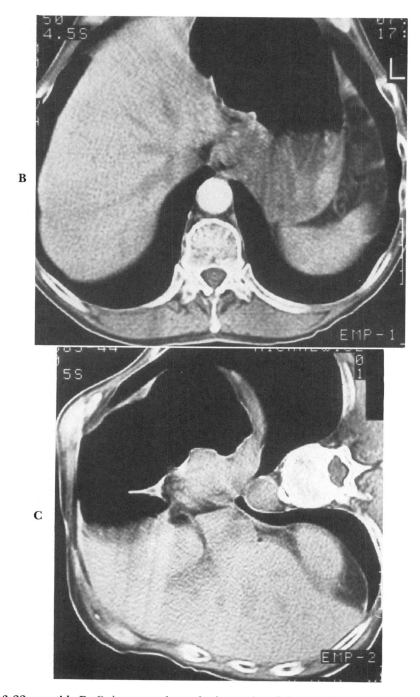

Fig. 3-22, cont'd. B, Bolus scan through the region fails to enhance the tumor mass despite the excellent blood level seen in the aorta. (Compare to Fig. 3-19.) It is difficult to assess the full extent of the tumor with the patient in the supine position. **C,** Scan of the patient in a right-side-down decubitus position shows the true extent of the tumor along the fundus and lesser curvature (same patient as in **B**).

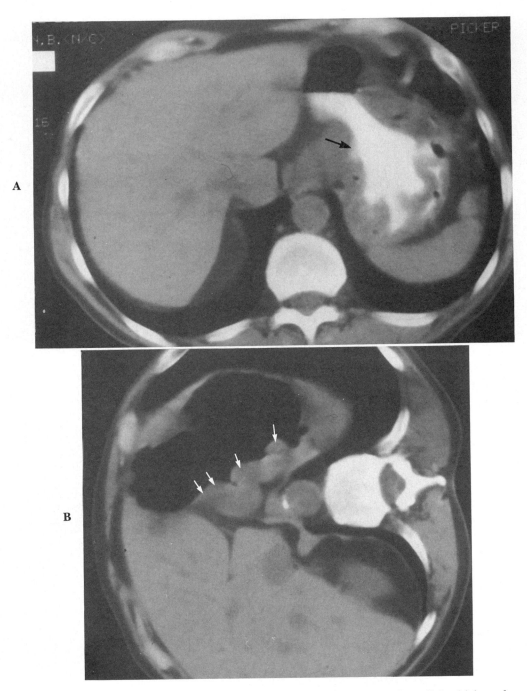

Fig. 3-23. Carcinoma of esophagogastric junction. **A,** The gastric wall is thickened—apparently diffusely. The region of the esophagogastric junction appears bulky. There is an ulcer along the lesser curvature *(arrow)*. **B,** Scan of the patient in a right-side-down decubitus position shows lobulated tumor confined to the lesser curvature aspect *(arrows)*. This position maximizes air distribution in the proximal stomach, providing a more accurate assessment of the walls. The ulcer is not recognized.

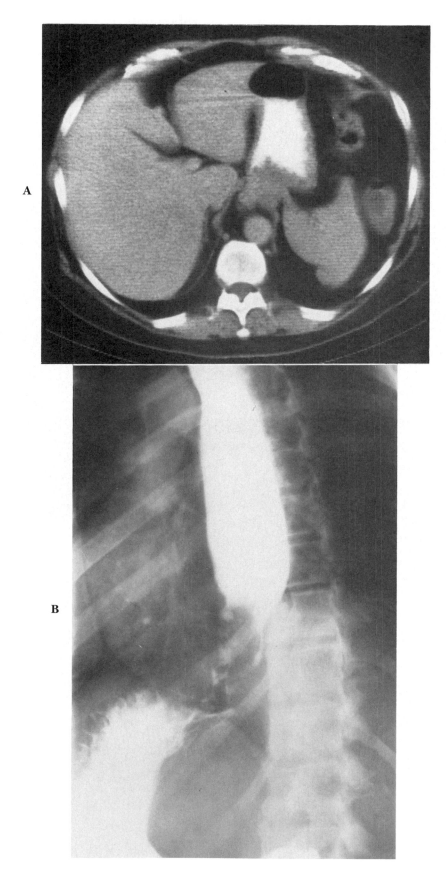

Fig. 3-24. Hiatal hernia or carcinoma? **A,** CT shows bulky mass at esophagogastric junction. The proximal esophagus is dilated on previous scans. **B,** Esophagram shows adenocarcinoma.

Continued.

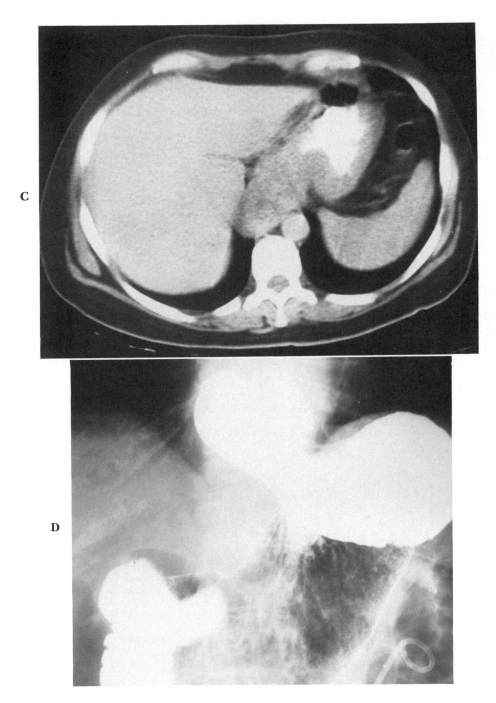

Fig. 3-24, cont'd. C, CT of a different patient showing similar findings. **D,** Esophagogram of patient in **C** with a typical hiatal hernia.

A further differential diagnostic problem in this region is the distinction between a bulky tumor in the esophagogastric junction and a nondistended hiatal hernia (Fig. 3-24). Findings suggestive of a hiatal hernia include a mass in the retrocardiac mediastinum and separation of the crura of the diaphragm (see Chapter Two). In order to evaluate hiatal hernia, additional oral contrast material or effervescent granules should be administered to distend this region of the stomach and ensure that the wall is not thickened or lobulated. Again this may be facilitated by scanning the patient in the decubitus position in order to maximize distention of the herniated portion of the stomach. CT may have a slightly increased sensitivity in the detection of neoplasm within the herniated stomach (Fig. 3-25).

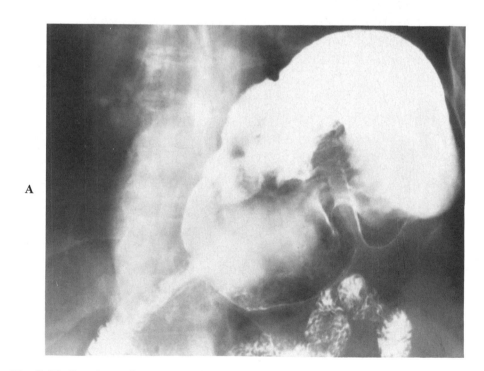

Fig. 3-25. Gastric carcinoma (antral) in a intrathoracic stomach. **A,** Gastrointestinal series shows complex herniation of the stomach into the thorax. This study was interpreted as otherwise normal.   *Continued.*

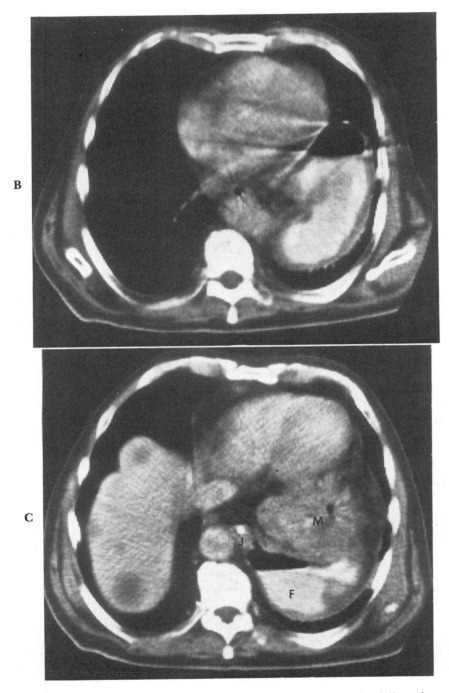

Fig. 3-25, cont'd. B, In the CT scan the posterior fundus can be followed anteriorly toward the greater curvature. **C,** Scan 1 cm caudad shows the esophagogastric juntion (*J*) and the fundus (*F*) to be subdiaphragmatic. A large bulky tumor mass (*M*) occupies the midportion of the stomach. Multiple hepatic metastases are present.

CT manifestations of spread of gastric carcinoma

CT is ideal for imaging the extragastric spread of neoplasm. Spread of gastric carcinoma can occur via a variety of pathways. These included: (1) direct spread along the long axis of the stomach; (2) spread along the peritoneal ligaments toward and ultimately into adjacent viscera; (3) spread to local lymph nodes; (4) hematogenous metastases; and (5) peritoneal metastases.[40] Of 462 patients studied at Charity Hospital, metastatic disease was present in 75% at the time of surgical exploration.[41] These figures are fairly constant in comparison of large surgical series and indicate the frequency of advanced disease in the United States.

Although many staging systems have been proposed, we have adapted the TNM classification where possible (Table 3-2).[42] Use of this system allows for accurate comparison of follow-up scans with the original preoperative study. Furthermore we can often visualize lymph node groups not seen at gastrectomy, particularly the celiac nodes and retroperitoneal nodes (Figs. 3-26 and 3-27). This generally upstages the disease, which will hopefully segregate treatment groups for more precise definition in ongoing oncologic clinical trials. The TNM system addresses the status of the tumor as well as the presence of distant metastases.

Table 3-2. Comparison of staging with TNM system

Staging	TNM
Stage I	$T_1 N_0$, M_0
Stage II	T_2, T_3, N_0, M_0
Stage III	T_1-T_3, N_1, N_2, M_0, T_{4a}, any N_1, M_0
Stage IV	T_1-T_3, N_3, M_0, T_{4b}, any N_1, M_0, any T_1, N_1, M_1

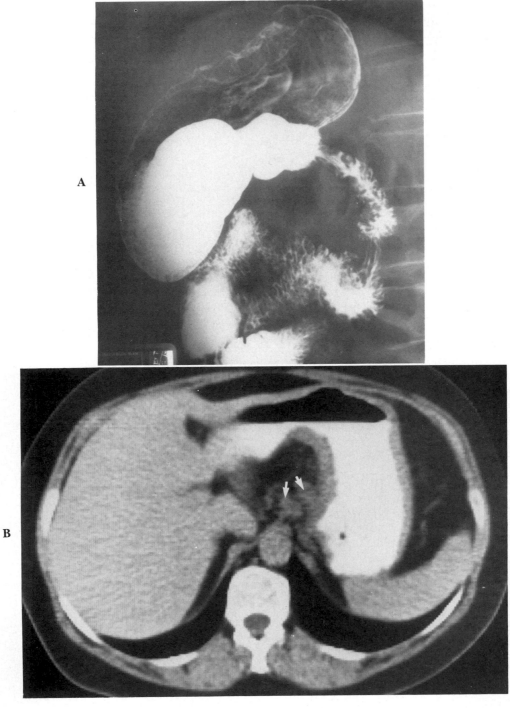

Fig. 3-26. Gastric carcinoma—proximal stomach. **A,** Gastrointestinal series reveals an infiltrating lesion along the greater curvature that extends toward the esophagogastric junction. **B,** CT shows the lesion to be more extensive than predicted by gastrointestinal series. The lesion extends around the gastric fundus and involves a considerable portion of the lesser curvature. Adenopathy is seen in the lesser omentum *(arrows)* (T_3N_1).

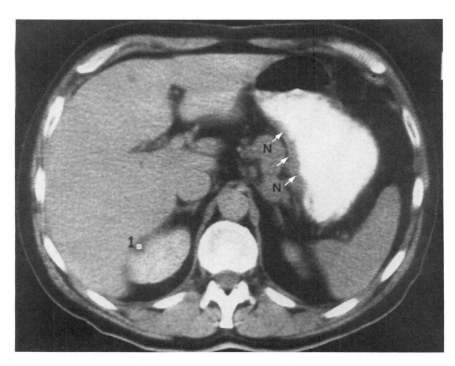

Fig. 3-27. Gastric carcinoma. Minimal thickening is noted, representing the primary neoplasm of the wall along the lesser curvature. Adenopathy is seen in celiac nodes (N). Involvement of these secondary drainage sites indicate a T_3N_2 lesion.

Direct spread along the long axis of the stomach is facilitated by an intricate network of intramural lymphatic plexi in both the submucosal and subserosal layers. This plexus is prominent in the esophagus and may be present in the duodenum in 30% to 40% of patients as well. It is the spread of tumor within these lymphatic plexi that frustrates surgical attempts at obtaining tumor free margins[29] (Fig. 3-28).

Spread to local lymph nodes can occur by way of lymphatic dissemination or direct invasion of local node groups by the primary tumor mass. In our series of 55 preoperative CT scans, 6 of 16 patients considered N_0 had bulky lesions extending across peritoneal surfaces. In these patients it was virtually impossible to determine whether the soft tissue mass was the result of contiguous adenopathy or engulfment of nodes by the tumor. In the series by Freeny and Marks two cases were found where local nodal metastases were misinterpreted as tumor.[38] The difficulty in distinguishing direct extension from lymph node metastases was also noted by Komaki in a recent series of 23 patients studied on fourth generation CT equipment.[43] Our overall accuracy was 93% in detection of the tumor and associated adenopathy. This compares favorably with other reported series.[43a]

The presence of nodal metastases decreases the overall patient survival in any T category[40,42] (Table 3-3). CT is most accurate in detection of adenopathy in the gastrohepatic ligament, celiac nodes, and hepatoduodenal ligament nodes. Nodal metastases in the gastrohepatic ligament are seen as lobulated densities within the fat between the under surface of the liver and lesser curve of the stomach. When using a rapid bolus/rapid infusion technique, nodal metastases can be distinguished from branches of the left gastric artery and coronary vein by virtue of their lack of enhancement. Celiac lymph nodes surround the celiac axis along the lesser curvature of the stomach. Presence of enlargement of these nodes constitutes N_2 lesions even if primary drainage nodes are not seen. Nodes in the hepatoduodenal ligaments surround the pancreatic head and may simulate pancreatic mass. As these nodes enlarge they may obstruct the common bile duct, producing jaundice. Nodes in the subpyloric region and in the gastrosplenic ligament are more difficult to detect. Sunderland shows a rough correlation between the location of the tumor and the nodes involved. This classification of paracardial (I), superior gastric (II), subpyloric (III), inferior gastric (IV), and pancreatic lienal (V) correspond to surgically accessible

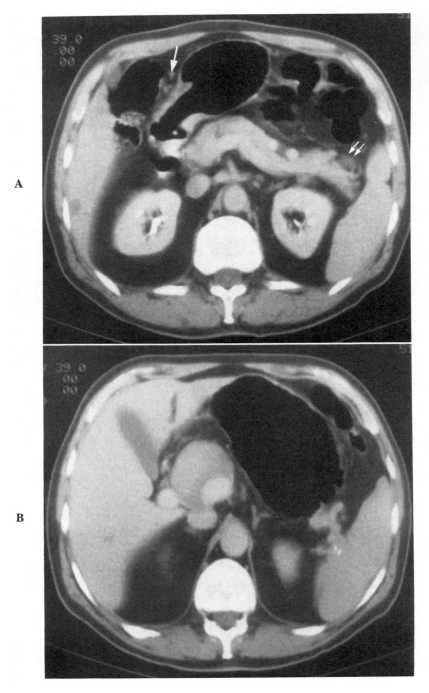

Fig. 3-28. Gastric carcinoma—antrum. **A,** The wall measures approximately 4 mm along the greater curvature aspect. The abrupt transition from normal wall thickness can be seen. Notice nodular densities in the perigastric fat, representing local (greater curvature) nodes *(large arrows).* A low-density node is seen just above the pancreatic tail *(small arrows).* **B,** Same patient as in **A.** Scan slightly more cephalad reveals large lymph node metastases in the hepatoduodenal ligament. Nodes are also seen in the splenic hilum. The lymph node metastases to sites not directly draining the tumor is common in gastric carcinoma and reflects intramural lymphatic communication (T_3N_2).

Table 3-3. Effect of lymph node disease on 5-year survival

TNM stage	5-year survival
T_1	85%
T_2	52%
T_3	47%
$N_1\text{-}N_2$ $\}$ $(T_1\text{-}T_4)$	17%
N_3	5%

Modified from Kennedy, B.J.: TNM classification for stomach cancer, Cancer **26:**971, 1970.

node groups. In 100 cases, an average of 3.75 node groups were involved, with superior gastric nodes (lesser omentum) having the highest occurrence.[12] This corresponds to data from our series in which adenopathy in the lesser omentum was detected in 38 of 40 patients with visualized adenopathy. The presence of the intercommunicating, intramural, gastric lymphatics makes prediction of patterns of lymph node involvement much less reliable for a gastric carcinoma than is apparent for carcinoma of the colon and rectum. Distal gastric lesions may involve splenic hilar lymph nodes in up to 20% of cases.[44] When adenopathy is detected in paraaortic, retropancreatic, and mesenteric nodes, this indicates markedly advanced disease since these node groups cannot be considered regional. Some authors consider nodes in this group as M classification. In 3 of the 60 cases of gastric carcinoma we have seen lymphadenopathy in the retroperitoneum extending below the renal pedicle (Fig. 3-29). In 3 other cases retroperitoneal involvement was manifested by infiltrating sheets of tumor tissue and obscuring retroperitoneal landmarks associated with hydronephrosis. In cases in which linitis plastica forms, carcinomas are present and the retroperitoneal metastases enhance similar to the gastric components (see Fig. 3-19, *C*).

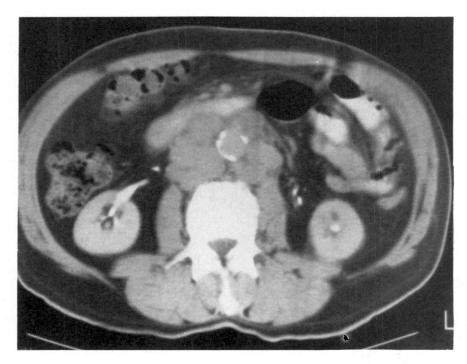

Fig. 3-29. Retroperitoneal adenopathy—gastric carcinoma. Bulky para-aortic, retroperitoneal lymphadenopathy is seen below the level of the renal pedicle. Enlarged retroperitoneal nodes, although uncommon in gastric adenocarcinoma, were seen in 5% of the cases in our series.

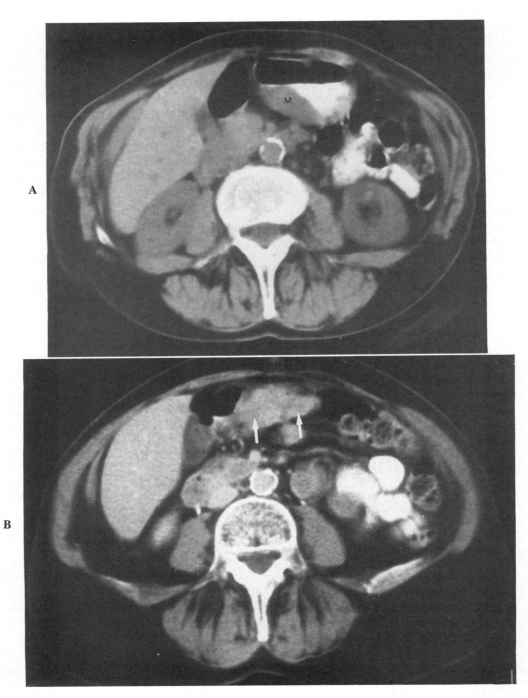

Fig. 3-30. Gastric carcinoma extending across the transverse mesocolon. **A,** CT at mid-stomach showing a gastric neoplasm *(M).* Lobulated densities surrounding the aorta reveal retroperitoneal lymph nodes. **B,** Scan at level of uncinate process of pancreas. Soft-tissue mass is seen abutting the inferior aspect of the transverse colon *(arrows).* Serial scans establish continuously with the primary tumor. The appearance is the result of direct extension along the transverse mesocolon (T_4a).

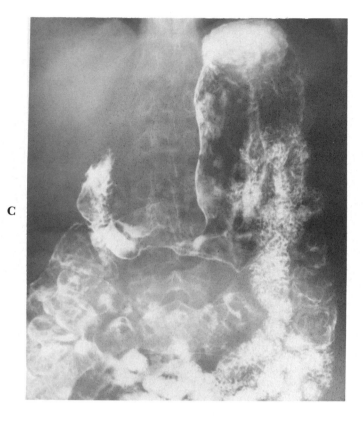

Fig. 3-30, cont'd. C, Corresponding gastrointestinal series.

Radiologic manifestations of spread along the peritoneal ligaments have been documented by Meyers.[45] The peritoneal reflections of the gastrocolic ligament facilitate tumor spread directly along this fascial plane into the transverse colon (Figs. 3-30 and 3-31). The reflections of the transverse mesocolon also allow advanced cases to directly infiltrate into the pancreas. Direct spread can also occur along the lesser omentum into the liver (Fig. 3-32). The submucosal lymphatic plexus facilitate lymphangitic spread of tumor into the esophagus, head of the pancreas, and diaphragm. We have considered patients with direct extension into adjacent viscera as T_4 category (Fig. 3-33).

Peritoneal seeding is a common form of distant metastases and displays a spectrum of findings. Minimal local peritoneal seeding is represented as increased density in the perigastric fat and appears as a finely retriculated latticework of linear densities (Fig. 3-34). More extensive cases reveal loculated fluid collections in the adjacent peritoneal cavity. In more advanced cases loculated fluid deposits within the leaves of the mesentery may be seen accompanied by apparent thickening of the mesenteric vessels. Ultimately, gross ascites is present with omental caking. In female patients, it is important to scan the pelvis to detect ovarian deposits. In gastric carcinoma, ovarian deposits tend to have a homogeneous, soft-tissue density appearance as compared to other lesions that metastasize to the ovary[46] (Fig. 3-35).

Hematogenous metastases may occur to the liver, lungs, adrenal glands, ovaries, and bones.[40] These are all potentially evaluated on CT scanning. The liver is the most commonly affected organ as shown in large series.[47,48] Thoracic and skeletal metastases were seen in 1.8% of 12,061 studied by conventional radiography.[42] In our series 20 patients had metastases that included the peritoneal cavity, gastric ligaments, liver, retroperitoneum, ovary, pancreas, and diaphragm. Hepatic metastases are best detected with a bolus/rapid infusion technique with dynamic, sequential scanning.[49,49a] In most scan sequences, cuts of the lower thorax will be obtained. These should be evaluated at both soft tissue and at "lung" windows to assess the presence of potential lymphangitic metastases within the lung interstitium. Hematogenous metastases are presumably seeded by the portal venous system, and the liver acts as an effective filter in the prevention of further dissemination; thus lung and bone metastases are rare. Balthazar et al. has reported hematogenous metastases to the anal canal from gastric carcinoma[50] (Fig. 3-36).

Text continued on p. 142.

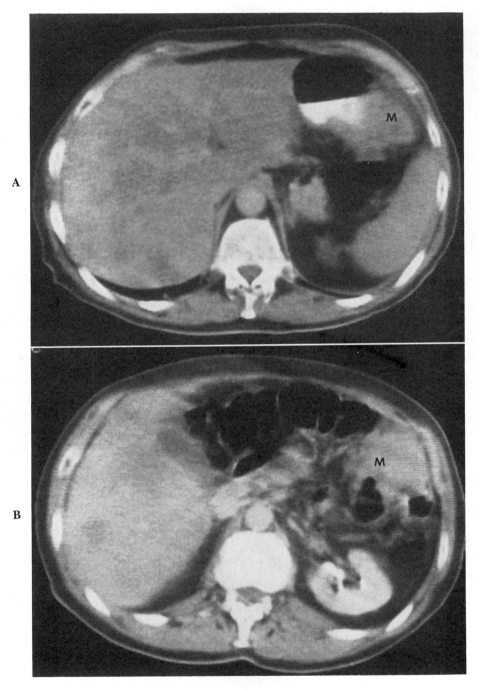

Fig. 3-31. Gastric carcinoma extending across the gastrocolic ligament. **A,** A bulky mass (*M*) is seen extending from the greater curvature aspect of the mid-stomach. Multiple hepatic metastases are seen. **B,** Scan slightly caudad reveals that the mass continues and invades the distal transverse colon. Some proximal distention of the colon is noted. The pathway is along the gastrocolic ligament ($T_4aN_2M_1$).

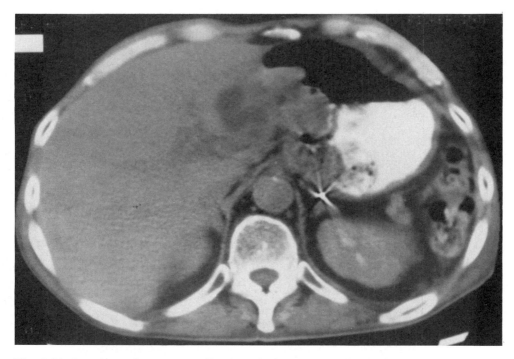

Fig. 3-32. Gastric carcinoma extending into the liver. Scan at level of the esophagogastric junction shows lobulated ulcerated carcinoma of lesser curvature. The low-density region in the liver represents direct extension of tumor rather than metastases. The pathway of spread is across the lesser omentum. It is impossible to determine if the lymph nodes are involved with the tumor or engulfed by the advancing tumor mass (T_4b).

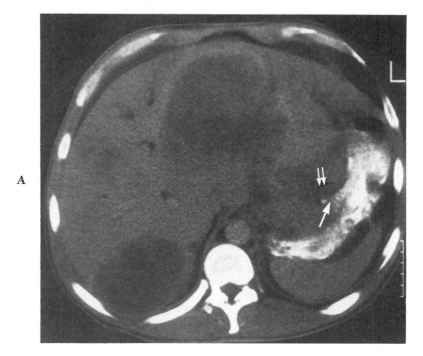

Fig. 3-33. Perforated gastric carcinoma. **A,** CT scan in a 37-year-old patient reveals that the stomach lumen is distorted and displaced to the left. An ulcer is seen *(arrow)*. Note the localized, extraluminal air collection indicating perforation *(small arrows)*. Multiple liver metastases are seen. The lesser omentum is replaced by a huge neoplastic mass.

Continued.

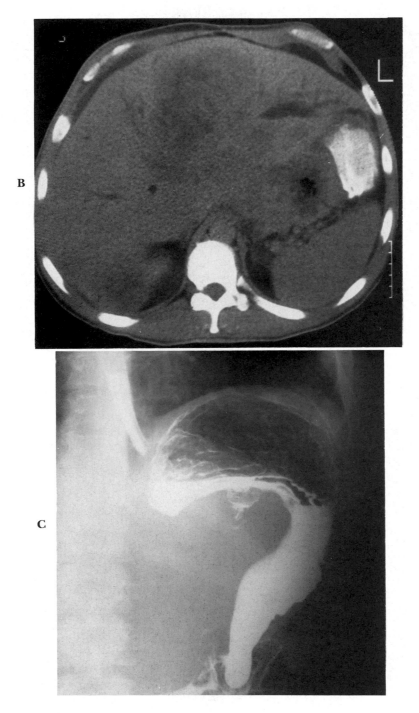

Fig. 3-33, cont'd. B, The low-density region surrounding the air corresponds to the inflammatory component. The remainder of the mass obscures all upper abdominal landmarks, invading the pancreas, diaphragm, and liver. A small amount of ascites is present ($T_4bN_2M_1$). **C,** Corresponding gastrointestinal series. Notice the ulcer with a sinus tract extending into the mass.

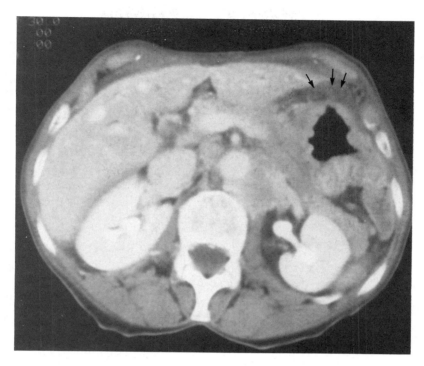

Fig. 3-34. Gastric carcinoma with local peritoneal seeding. The tumor mass thickens the gastric wall, distorts the lumen, and is slightly enhanced (linitis plastica). Reticular densities are seen in the fat anterior to the greater curvature aspect compatible with peritoneal seeding *(arrows)*. Note the retroperitoneal node metastases at the level of the renal pedicle (T_4aN_3).

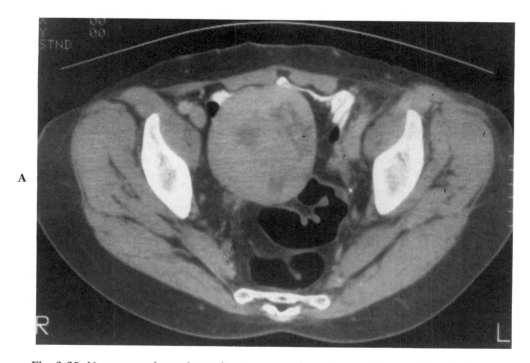

Fig. 3-35. Unsuspected gastric carcinoma presenting with a pelvic mass (Kruckenberg tumor). **A,** Scan of the pelvis reveals a huge, predominantly soft-tissue density mass in the right adnexa. The scan was requested to evaluate the nature of the clinically palpable mass.
Continued.

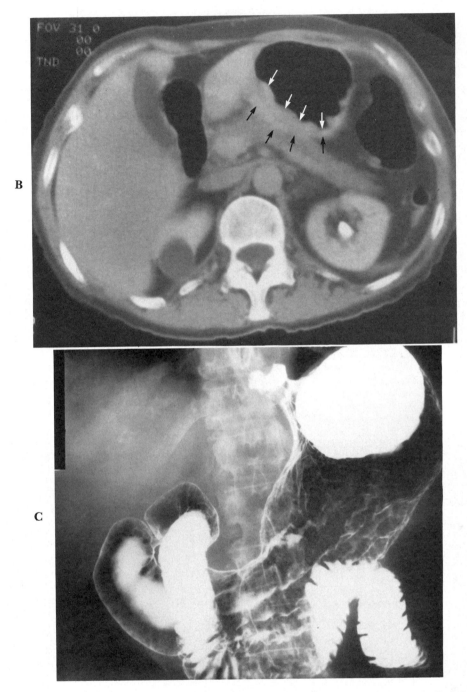

Fig. 3-35, cont'd. B, Routine scanning of the upper abdomen shows a thick-walled, lesser curvature of the stomach *(arrows)*. The diagnosis of gastric carcinoma was suggested by the CT study. **C,** The CT findings led to this gastrointestinal series that shows infiltrated folds in the midstomach compatible with gastric adenocarcinoma. Ovarian metastases from the stomach are true Kruckenberg lesions and have a greater soft-tissue component than metastases from other primaries.

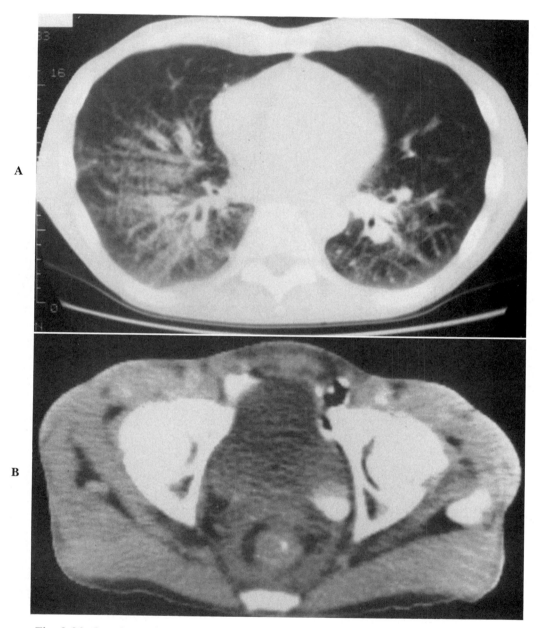

Fig. 3-36. Gastric carcinoma—extra gastric manifestations. **A,** Lymphangitic lung metastases. **B,** Hematogenous metastases to the rectum. The levator ani are thickened, the rectal wall is thick, and the lumen is narrowed. Proximally the colon was obstructed. Because these lesions occur below the peritoneal reflection they are believed to be hematogenously seeded.

Follow-up studies

CT is used extensively as a follow-up examination to assess the status of a patient's response to surgical and chemotherapeutic regimens. We will review the appearance of the postoperative stomach in a subsequent section. This discussion will focus on nodal and extranodal recurrences.

There is little literature, except autopsy data, documenting patterns of regional failure following surgery. In one such series from the University of Minnesota of 107 patients, 80.4% had evidence of recurrent metastatic cancer found at second-look operative procedure. Analysis of the reasons for the failures revealed that the failure rate increased in patients with advanced lesions, increased depth of wall penetration, and the presence of lymph nodes, thereby diminishing the prognosis.[40,47] Failures occur most commonly in the gastric bed in regional nodes.[48]

CT examination in these patients reveals the presence of metastases in a variety of forms. The gastric bed may show increased density in perigastric fat with small lymph nodes present along the serosal aspect of the gastric remnant and reticular densities in the local fat that indicate peritoneal seeding. Masses may be present in the celiac and peripancreatic node groups, particularly in the latter. Masses in this location were seen in all of the five patients that we have studied following gastric resection. In three of these patients, obstructive jaundice was present (Fig. 3-37). In our institution, the surgical procedure performed in gastric carcinoma is subtotal gastrectomy with local lymph node dissection. This surgical exposure does not visualize nodes posterior to the pancreatic head, in the celiac axis, and in the suprapancreatic groups. Thus CT may potentially provide a more accurate TNM assessment than is possible by direct visualization.

Gastric carcinoma remains a lethal disease and the survival rates are unchanged over three decades. There have been some suggestions of statistically significant, improved patient survival with progressive, aggressive, chemotherapeutic regimens and possibly with intraperitoneal chemotherapy. CT will facilitate a more rapid appraisal of these new therapeutic modalities previously available only through second-look surgery. More accurate depiction of lymph node groups will result in a more accurate staging of the disease, allowing better definition of the patient populations that may benefit from aggressive chemotherapy. We do not believe that the role of CT is to deny surgical treatment, rather that it has unique abilities to depict local and distant extent of disease.[43a]

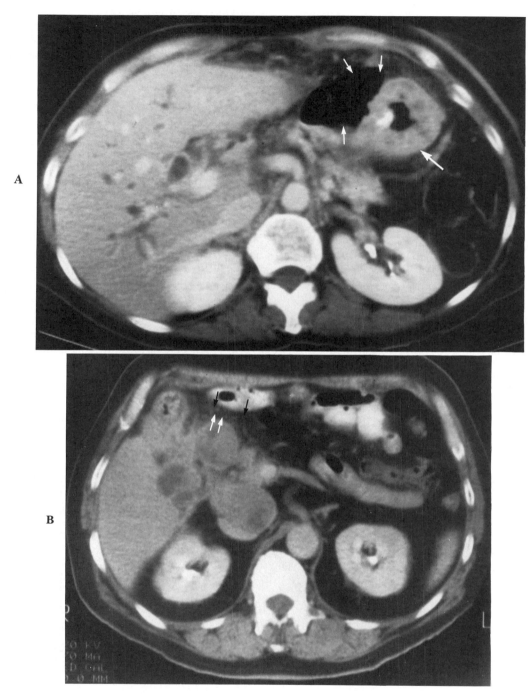

Fig. 3-37. Follow-up CT scan—gastric carcinoma. **A,** Patient was not jaundiced at the time of the CT scan. There are dilated bile ducts obstructed by enlarged peripancreatic lymph nodes seen on more caudad images. Note the appearance of the fat in the lesser omentum and gastrocolic ligament compatible with peritoneal seeding. The patient has undergone gastrojejunostomy. Note the gastric remnant *(arrow)* is markedly thickened. The jejunal portion has a normal wall *(small arrows)*. **B,** Scan in another patient reveals massive adenopathy surrounding the pancreatic head (pancreatico-duodenal nodes). Local stippling in the fat of the free margin of the transverse mesocolon is also seen *(arrows)*. The patient underwent total gastrectomy approximately 10 months previously—failures in the peripancreatic nodes are common. These nodes are not routinely visualized at laparotomy.

OTHER GASTRIC NEOPLASMS
Gastric lymphoma

The stomach is the portion of the gastrointestinal tract most commonly affected by lymphoma. Lymphoma accounts for 2% to 5% of all gastric malignancies and for 25% of extranodal lymphoma. Most patients will have non-Hodgkins lymphoma with hystiocytic cell-type being the most common variety.[51]

The importance of the recognition of lymphomatous involvement of any portion of the gastrointestinal tract is apparent when the clinical consequences of its presence are considered. It has been shown that the presence of gastrointestinal lymphoma may require alterations and proposed therapy. These lesions tend to perforate and/or bleed during treatment, especially with rapid resolution during chemotherapy.[52] This complication can lead to premature cessation of therapy with less than optimal results. In a patient with known gastrointestinal lymphoma, it is important to determine if the lesion is isolated to the gastrointestinal tract or if the bowel is involved as part of the disseminated disease.[53] Lewin showed that previous survival rates in patients with isolated bowel lymphoma range from 71% to 82% as compared with patients with Stage IV disease, leading to a 0% 2-year survival rate.[54]

We reviewed the CT scans of 275 patients with positive CT findings of abdominal lymphoma. Twenty-six patients (9.5%) had bowel involvement. Only 13 of these had symptoms directly referable to the gastrointestinal tract. Seventeen of these patients had gastric involvement.[55] Three CT appearances were encountered. The most common finding was a diffuse involvement in which more than 50% of the length of the stomach was involved (Fig. 3-38). In four patients segmental involvement of the wall was seen, and in two patients ulcerated masses were detected. The average thickness of the wall was 5 cm. Segmental forms seem to have a predilection for the proximal portions of the stomach, although more recent experience tends to suggest that this distribution is random (Fig. 3-39).

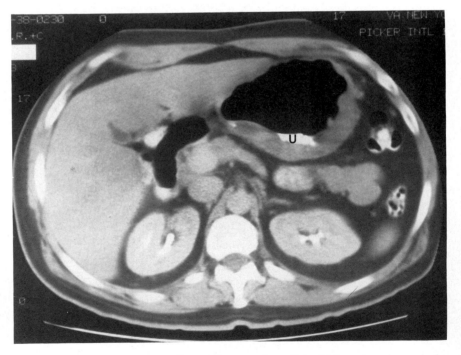

Fig. 3-38. Gastric lymphoma—diffuse. The gastric wall is thicker than in typical carcinoma cases. Residual barium is seen in an ulcer crater *(U)* that is difficult to recognize on the basis of the CT scan.

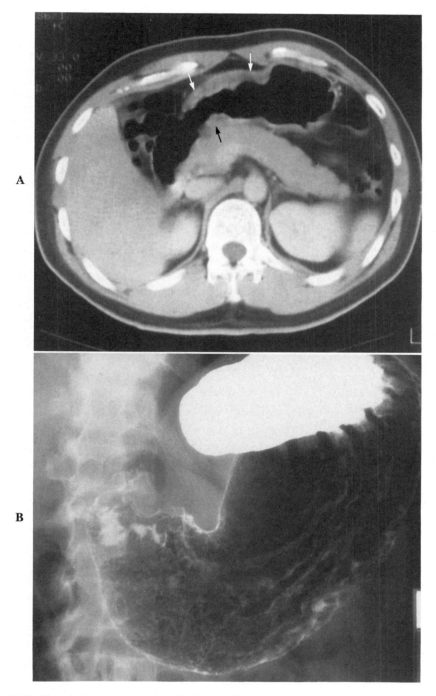

Fig. 3-39. Gastric lymphoma—localized. **A,** The patient was studied because of epigastric pain. There is focal wall thickening seen along the antrum. The inner surface has an undulating quality. The perigastric fat is not involved, and the serosal margin is sharply defined. The fat planes between the mass and the pancreatic body are preserved *(arrows)*. **B,** Gastrointestinal series. The lobulation is best seen along the lesser curvature aspect of the antrum. The greater curvature folds are effaced typical of a "soft" gastric lesion. No adenopathy was seen elsewhere. Histiocytic lymphoma localized to the stomach without serosal penetration was found at surgery.

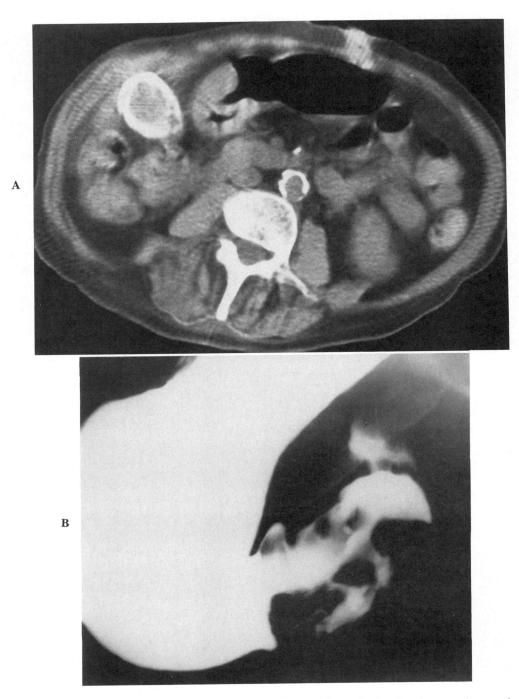

Fig. 3-40. Localized antral lymphoma. **A,** CT scan through the distal stomach reveals abrupt transition to a thick-walled lesion in the antrum. Air collection within the mass represents an ulcer. A porcelain gallbladder is present. **B,** Spot film from gastrointestinal series reveals a stenotic lesion of the antrum with a large linear ulcer within the substance of the mass.

The thickened wall has a homogeneous, uniform density (Fig. 3-40). Although bolus injections were not performed in the evaluation of the lesions in the original series, subsequent bolus work has been performed. There is significantly less enhancement of gastric lymphoma when compared to linitis plastica, usually approximately 10 to 20 H units. However, in one patient a rapid bolus injection produced an enhancement of 45 H units; further case experience must be accumulated. The average thickness of the wall in all cases was approximately 5 cm. This is significantly thicker than in patients with gastric carcinoma. Buy and Moss reviewed the scans of 12 patients with gastric lymphoma. Standard barium studies were positive in 9 of the 12 cases. CT findings included irregularity of the lumen in 66%, hyperogosity in 58%, and wall thickening in 100%. In their series the average thickness was 4 cm.[56] They observed that lymphoma less frequently invaded perigastric fat and adjacent organs. Furthermore they found that lymphomatous involvement occurred over greater portions of the stomach in comparison to gastric carcinoma. In patients with disseminated disease they found that the distribution of lymphadenopathy may be helpful in suggesting lymphoma.[56] Lymphadenopathy below the level of the renal pedicle in gastric carcinoma occurred in 3% of the patients in our series; however it is significantly more common in lymphoma (Fig. 3-39). Pillari et al. called attention to the club-like digitations that the thickened folds assume more often in gastric lymphoma than in gastric carcinoma.[57]

False-negative studies were obtained in patients with "bulls-eye" lesions of the gastrointestinal tract. Both of these patients had clinical evidence of gastrointestinal bleeding, and a subsequently performed gastrointestinal series revealed the lesions. The reason for this difficulty may be in the small size of the lesions, the lack of associated mass, and the difficulty in recognizing the ulcer mound from thickened or normal, nondistended adjacent folds (Fig. 3-41).

When the thickening of the wall in a patient with gastric lymphoma appears nonhomogeneous, particularly when fluid density is present within the wall, the possibility of perforation or sinus tract should be ruled out. These may often occur without clinical symptomatology. Perforations have been reported in from 9% to 40% of patients.[58] Thirteen percent of perforations may be clinically silent during the life of the patient.[59] Careful monitoring of the appearance of the gastric wall on CT during chemotherapy is a useful way of detecting this complication, often before clinical symptomatology becomes apparent (Fig. 3-42).

CT is highly sensitive to the presence of gastric lymphoma. The appearance should be recognized on CT scanning because many patients with lymphoma elsewhere will undergo CT as their initial diagnostic procedure. In symptomatic patients in whom the CT scan is negative, barium radiography is recommended to rule out the presence of small ulcerating lesions.

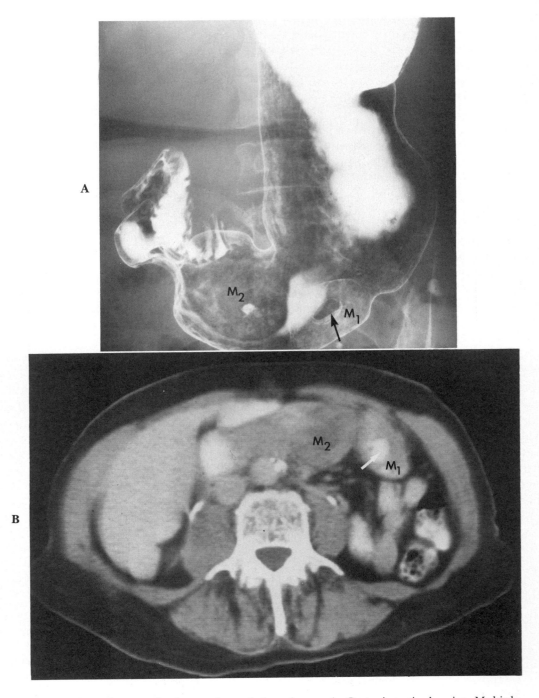

Fig. 3-41. Submucosal, ulcerated gastric lymphoma. **A,** Gastrointestinal series. Multiple submucosal masses ($m_1 m_2$) are seen. Note the air within the ulcer crater along the greater curvature *(arrow).* **B,** CT scan through greater curvature of stomach. The plane of the section is tangent to the ulcerated mass making it difficult to realize that the mass is gastric in location. Adjacent is the larger, greater curvature mass (m_2). Ulcerated masses are difficult to visualize on CT scanning.

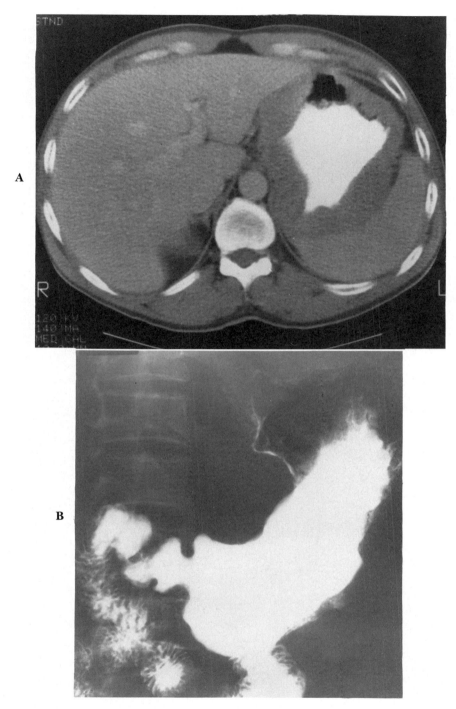

Fig. 3-42. Gastric lymphoma—complication of therapy. **A,** CT reveals a thickened gastric wall with an irregular luminal surface (effacement of the rugal pattern). The density is less than hepatic parenchyma and is only minimally enhanced. The appearance is homogenous with sharply outlained perigastric fat. Endoscopic biopsy was inconclusive; surgical biopsy was histiocytic lymphoma. **B,** Corresponding gastrointestinal series.

Continued.

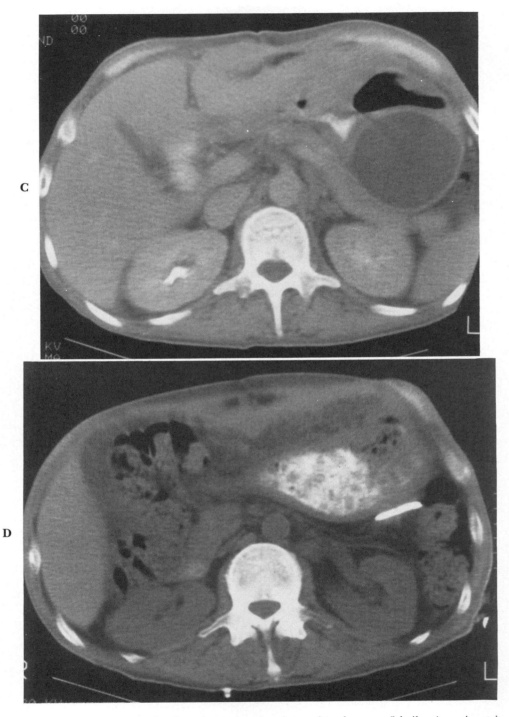

Fig. 3-42, cont'd. C, Following chemotherapy the patient became febrile. A perigastric fluid collection along the greater curvature was noted. Fluid collections should be considered the result of occult perforations, which have an increased incidence during this phase of rapid tumor lysis. **D,** CT provides a guide for successful percutaneous drainage. (Courtesy C.A. Whelan, M.D., Montclair, New Jersey.)

Mesenchymal tumors

Mesenchymal tumors of the stomach account for less than 5% of gastric neoplasms.[60] They vary in size from small nodules found incidentally at autopsy to huge necrotic masses that may occupy the entire abdomen. The most common lesions are leiomyomas, which account for anywhere from 30% to 60% of benign, submucosal, gastric neoplasms. Other lesions in this category include neurogenic neoplasms, lipomas, fibromas, carcinoid tumors, glomus tumors, duplication cysts, and pancreatic rests. Each of these tumors may have a malignant counterpart. CT can definitively diagnose lipomas because of its exclusive sensitivity to fat. A lipoma examined by CT will have an attenuation value of approximately −70 to −90 H units because of its fat content. This is diagnostic of the lesion.[61,62] Benign lipomas are homogeneous mass-es (Fig. 3-43). Internal septations of soft tissue within the lipoma should suggest the presence of malignant liposarcoma.

Gastric duplication cysts account for 3.8% of all gastrointestinal duplications, and although most are diagnosed in infancy, some may appear in adult life. CT scanning reveals a low-density, nonenhancing mass smoothly marginated by the stomach and located along the greater curvature. Radiographic differentiation from pancreatic pseudocysts may be impossible. These lesions may ulcerate into the stomach in 15% of cases. Extension through the crus of the diaphragm into the thorax has been reported.[63] In one reported case, aspiration of cyst fluid yielded clear serous fluid with an amylase value of 9000 International units. The lesion was associated with a pulmonary sequestration (Fig. 3-44).[64]

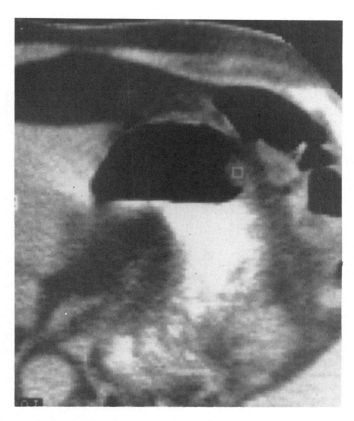

Fig. 3-43. Gastric lipoma. The tiny lesion along the greater curvature measured −75H units. This is compatible with fat and diagnostic of a lipoma.

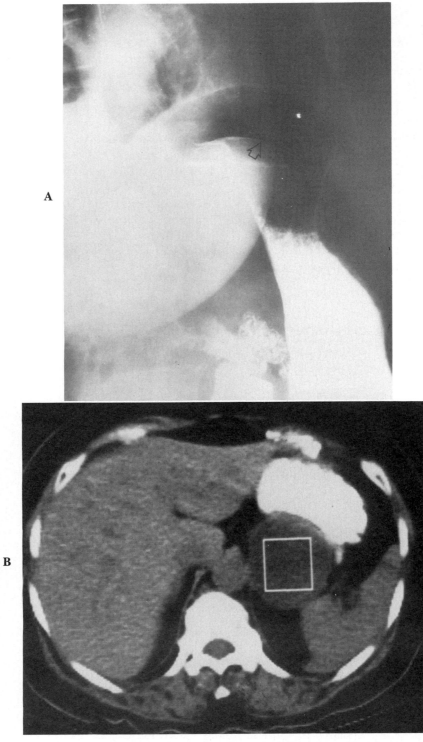

Fig. 3-44. Gastric duplication cyst. **A,** Smooth, extrinsic pressure effect is seen along the lesser curvature of the greater fundus *(open arrow).* **B,** CT scan shows a 9H unit (water-density) mass slightly below the esophagogastric junction. Surgery revealed a duplication cyst of the stomach. Differentiation from a pancreatic pseudocyst or leiomyoblastoma may be impossible. (Courtesy Dr. H. Morehouse, Albert Einstein College of Medicine, Bronx, New York.)

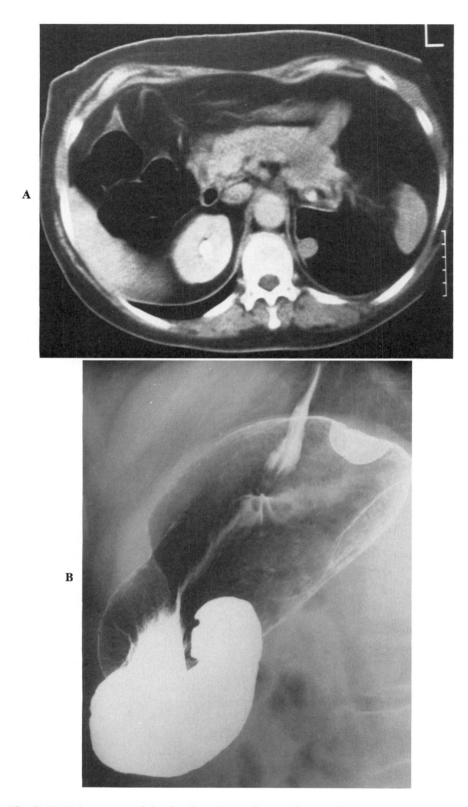

Fig. 3-45. Leiomyoma of the fundus. **A,** Small, round, smooth homogenous mass seen in the fundus. The right angle interface with the gastric wall suggests a mural origin. **B,** Gastrointestinal series corresponding to **A.** Features are typical of leiomyoma.

We have reviewed the CT appearance of 29 patients with mesenchymal nonepithelial tumors of the gastrointestinal tract.[65] There were 9 leiomyomas, 5 leiomyoblastomas, and 15 leiomyosarcomas studied. In this group 18 gastric lesions were seen. CT was useful in showing the extent of these typically exophytic tumors. The benign and malignant lesions had a considerably different CT appearance. The average size of the benign lesions was 4.8 cm as compared to the 12 cm average size of the malignant lesions. The benign lesions displayed homogeneous appearance with densities ranging between 40 to 60 H units and were enhanced diffusely and symmetrically (Fig. 3-45). The malignant lesions had a nonhomogeneous appearance and a complex enhancement pattern.

The outer soft-tissue density rim enhanced significantly as compared to the unenhancing center, which approaches water density (Figs. 3-46 and 3-47). This ability of CT to depict a gross appearance of the lesion makes it useful in helping distinguish benign from malignant lesions.[66] This difference in gross appearance, particularly size and homogeneity are well known pathologic criteria for distinguishing benign from malignant lesions, perhaps more reliably than histology.[67] We have seen two cases thought to be histologically benign based on biopsy material. In both cases CT revealed nonhomogeneous, nonlocalized, lobulated tumor masses. In one case liver metastases were present. Another recent series of 6 patients with gastric leiomyosarcoma also described similar gross CT appearance.[68]

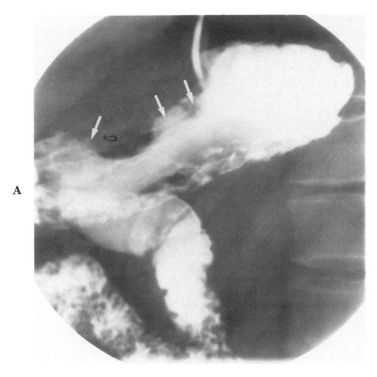

Fig. 3-46. Leiomyosarcoma. **A,** Gastrointestinal series. An ulcerated mass is seen along the lesser curvature aspect of the body of the stomach *(arrows).*

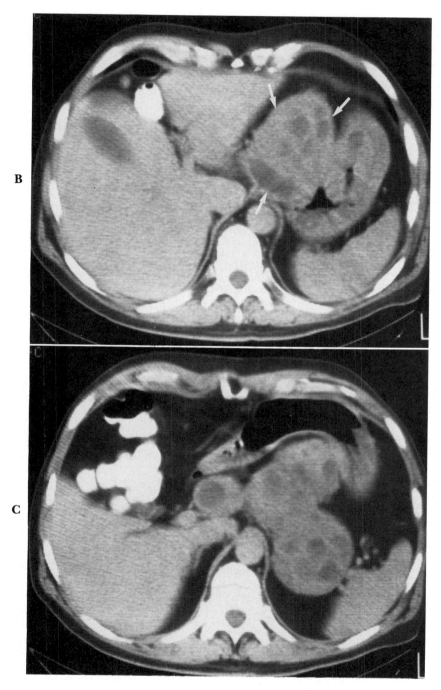

Fig. 3-46, cont'd. B, CT scan reveals nonhomogeneous, rounded tumor mass. The appearance is that of leiomyosarcoma *(arrows)*. **C,** Scan slightly caudal to **B** reveals that the tumor is more extensive than predicted by the gastrointestinal series.

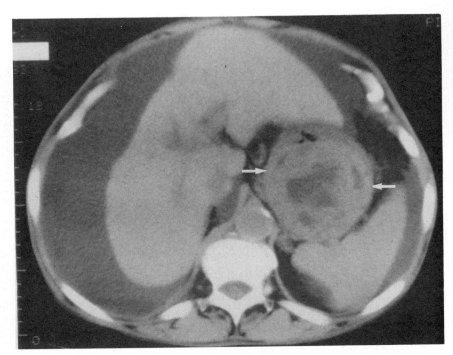

Fig. 3-47. Leiomyosarcoma. The stomach is collapsed. A nonhomogeneous, round mass is seen along the posterior aspect of the fundus *(arrows)*. The patient is cirrhotic (ascites and scarred liver). Needle biopsy was compatible with leiomyosarcoma.

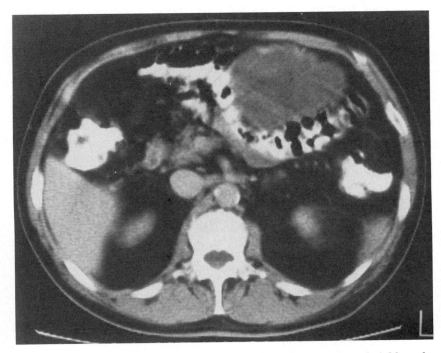

Fig. 3-48. Leiomyoblastoma. This large, exophytic lesion has a rim of viable enhancing tissue and a low-density center. The point of attachment could not be seen on the scan. However, the transverse colon is displaced both inferiorly and posteriorly, suggesting that the lesion is growing across the gastrocolic ligament. The CT appearance suggests leiomyosarcoma or cystic leiomyoblastoma. (Courtesy Dr. S. Gross, Muhlenberg, New Jersey.)

Leiomyoblastoma is classified as a benign tumor, although lymphatic and hepatic metastases have been reported.[69] These lesions have also been termed cellular epithelioid leiomyoma. We have studied six patients with leiomyoblastomas. The CT appearance ranges from well-defined, rounded masses with small fluid collections to large excavated masses undistinguishable from leiomyosarcoma by CT criteria. The cystic appearance of leiomyoblastoma has previously been reported both by CT and ultrasound.[70] Pathologically, the low-density material may be the result of hemorrhage within the lesion (Fig. 3-48).[71]

CT is accurate in depicting the origin of these masses from the wall of the stomach. No matter how large the exophytic component is in comparison to the point of attachment, careful scanning should visualize the portion of the thickened gastric wall representing the point of attachment (Fig. 3-49). At times however the masses become so large that it may be impossible to predict the organ of origin of a given mass in the upper abdomen, and selective angiography will be necessary to demonstrate the predominant blood supply of the lesion.

The differential diagnosis of these lesions includes other gastric neoplasms and extragastric, left, upper, abdominal masses. Gastric carcinoma rarely appears as a large exophytic mass, although we have seen three cases presented at local conferences of bulky exophytic adenocarcinomas of the stomach. In all three cases, the preoperative diagnosis on CT scan barium studies and angiography was that of leiomyosarcoma. In our institution, we have not seen this form of adenocarcinoma of the stomach, but the reader should be aware that this morphologic form does occur, although rarely. Lymphoma may appear as a bulky mass with an exophytic component, however there is usually a greater component of gastric wall involvement in lymphoma. The enhancement pattern of lymphoma has been described previously. In the absence of perforation, abscess or sinus tract lymphoma should enhance in a homogeneous pattern quite different from large bulky leiomyosarcomas. Histologic differentiation between other soft-tissue neoplasms may also be impossible (Fig. 3-50). Differentiation from cystic lesions of the tail of the pancreas, particularly cystadenocarcinoma and complicated pancreatic pseudocysts, may be impossible. In many cystic pancreatic lesions we have been able to detect splaying of the pancreatic parenchyma around the neoplasm (Fig. 3-51). In thin patients in whom the pancreas is poorly visualized, a selective angiography may be necessary to determine the predominant blood supply and enhance the organ origin.

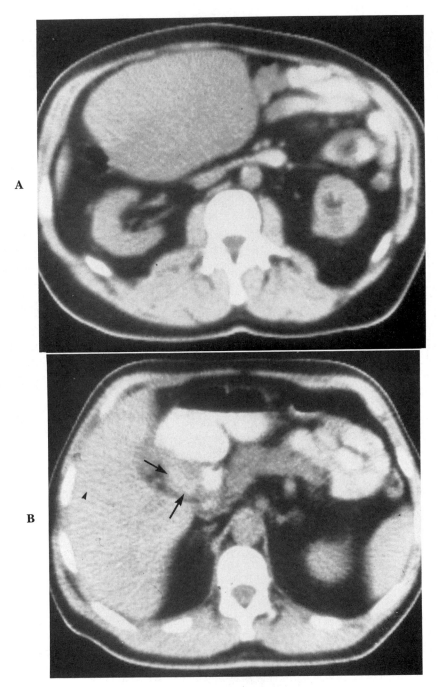

Fig. 3-49. Exophytic leiomyoma. **A,** Large mass is seen in the right upper quadrant. **B,** Thickening of the pyloric region allows identification of the point of origin of the mass. Occasionally, the exophytic myomatous tumors have a small pedicle-like attachment *(arrow)*. In these cases, angiography may be necessary to determine the organ of origin. Despite the size, the mass is homogeneous, suggesting a benign rather than malignant histology.

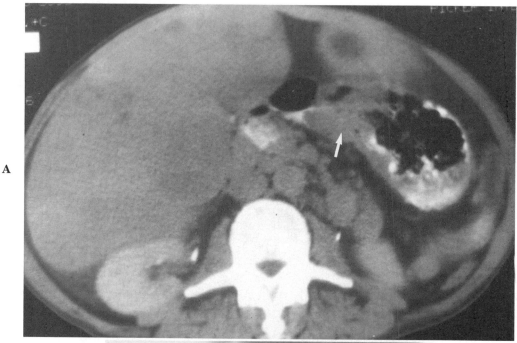

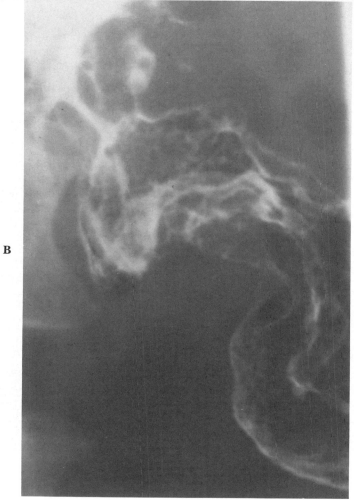

Fig. 3-50. Gastric carcinoid. **A,** Focal region of wall thickening is seen along the inferior portion of the antrum *(arrow).* There is massive hepatomegaly with low-attenuating metastases. **B,** Gastrointestinal series. Spot film reveals submucosal mass along greater curvature. Biopsy of lesion reveals carcinoid tumor.

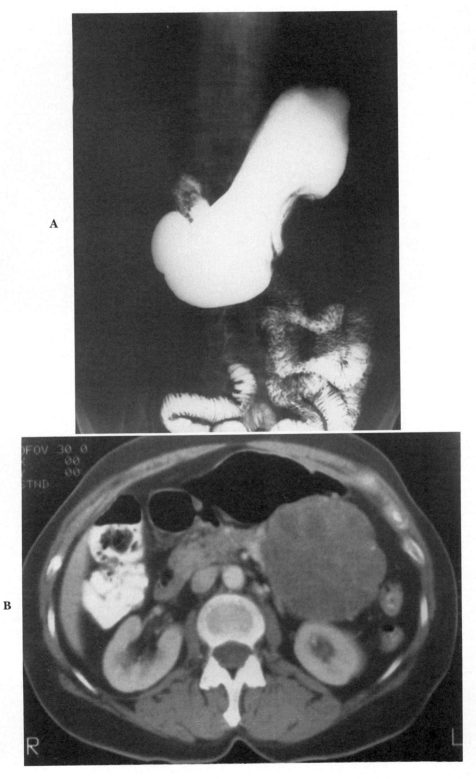

Fig. 3-51. Cystadenoma pancreas. **A,** Gastrointestinal series shows left upper quadrant mass with an apparent point of origin from the greater curvature of the stomach. **B,** CT scan through midportion of mass. The pancreatic parenchyma is splayed around a septated wall marginated mass arising from the pancreatic tail. Despite the lack of central calcification, this mass proved to be a microcystic, serous cystadenoma.

Metastases to the stomach

Metastases to the stomach may occur by way of direct extension of a contiguous neoplasm, lymphatic dissemination, or hematogenous spread. Direct extension from the pancreas is probably the most common form of metastases to the stomach.[72] On CT scanning it may be impossible to differentiate pancreatic carcinoma invading the stomach from gastric carcinoma invading the pancreas. In patients with carcinoma of the gallbladder, the antrum may be involved by the large pericholecystic mass (Fig. 3-52). Carcinoma of the breast metastasizes frequently to the gastric antrum, presumably by way of lymphatic dissemination, and radiographically it may simulate linitis plastica (Fig. 3-53). Some authors state that in any woman with a picture of linitis plastica, carcinoma of the breast should be the primary consideration in the differential diagnosis of each patient.[73] Hematogenous metastases may also appear as focal bulls-eye lesions. This occurs most frequently in melanoma and occasionally in patients with lung, kidney, and bladder carcinomas. We have studied several patients with Kaposi's sarcoma complicating AIDS and failed to detect the small submucosal lesions present in the stomach.

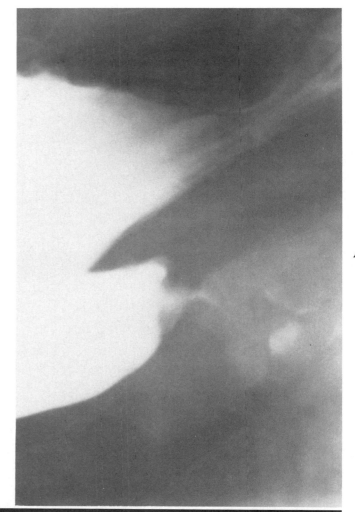

A

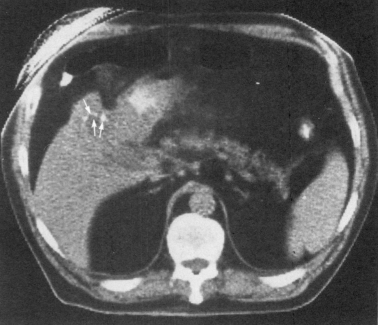

B

Fig. 3-52. Metastases to the stomach—gallbladder cancer (direct extention). **A,** Gastrointestinal series in patient with gastric outlet obstruction. The pyloroduodenal region is narrowed. **B,** CT scan shows a mass in the gallbladder bed extending across the lesser omentum into the antrum of the stomach. Note the calcification within the gallbladder *(arrows).*

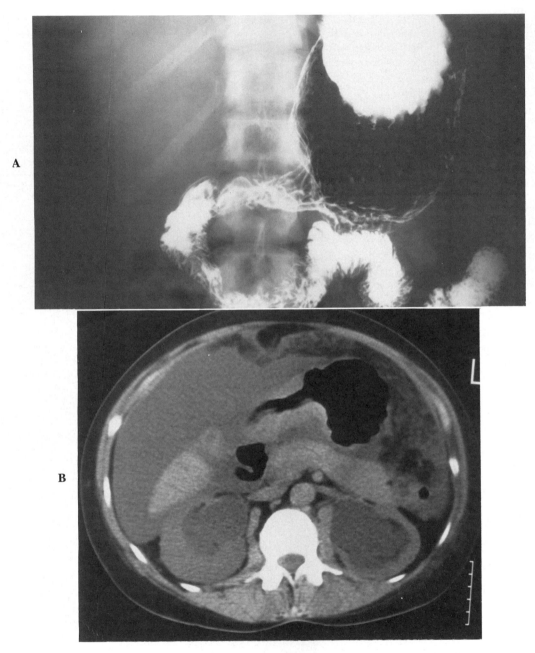

Fig. 3-53. Breast carcinoma metastases to the antrum. **A,** Gastrointestinal series. Narrowing of the antrum with relative preservation of the mucosa is seen. This suggests a lesion infiltrating the submucosal layers rather than a mucosal-based lesion. Multiple blastic bone lesions are seen in the lower thoracic spine. **B,** Air contrast CT. There is thickening of the antral wall. The duodenal bulb is spared. Bilateral hydronephrosis is seen. Massive ascites and peritoneal seeding is noted. The findings are identical to primary gastric carcinoma.

THE POSTOPERATIVE STOMACH

The postoperative stomach, especially following the Billroth II gastrojejunostomy, may be encountered as an incidental finding on CT examination of the abdomen, or the patient may be referred for scanning to evaluate complications related to the previous surgery. Barium radiography remains the procedure of choice for the radiologic evaluation of early and late postoperative complications in these patients. However, CT is emerging in an increasingly important role in evaluating early postoperative complications as well as the detection of carcinoma developing within the gastric remnant.

Anatomy

The classic Billroth II gastrojejunostomy will result in alteration of the normal relationships of the left upper quadrant, obviously as the result of the mobilization of the bowel during the formation of the gastric jejunal anastomosis. Most surgeons agree that the procedure of choice for placement of the anastomosis is antecolic, with the afferent loop applied to the lesser curvature aspect of the stomach and with the efferent loop along the greater curvature aspect of the stomach. This results in the gastrojejunostomy being located anteriorly, along the lesser curvature side of the gastric remnant.[74] Therefore in studying these patients, the anastomosis may best be visualized by the use of air within the gastric remnant delivered either by effervescent granules or nasogastric tube. Air contrast in immediate postoperative patients has a further safety factor since it is less desirable to give the patient oral contrast material (Fig. 3-54). The detail possible with air contrast allows recognition of changes of gastritis (Fig. 3-55) or suture granuloma (Fig. 3-56).

CT has been useful in our practice in detecting the following complications of gastrojejunostomy: postoperative abscesses, duodenal stump blowout, postoperative stomal obstruction, postoperative intraabdominal hemorrhages, postoperative pancreatitis and pseudocyst formation, anastomic leak, de novo carcinoma arising in the gastric remnant, and recurrent and metastatic carcinoma following gastric surgery from malignancy.

Text continued on p. 168.

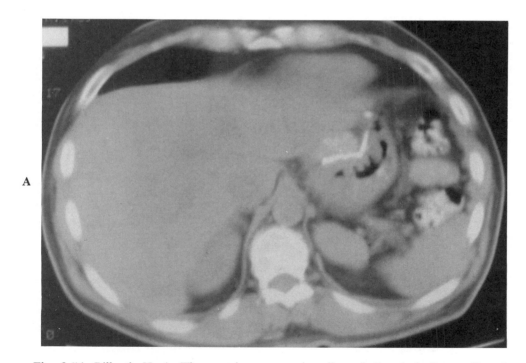

A

Fig. 3-54. Billroth II. **A,** The gastric remnant is collapsed. Surgical clips outline the margin of resection. *Continued.*

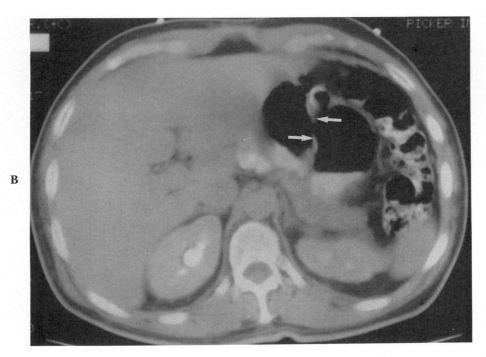

Fig. 3-54, cont'd. B, Following administration of effervescent granules, the remnant is distended. Note air rising into the anastomosis, which is placed along the greater curvature of the stomach *(arrows)*.

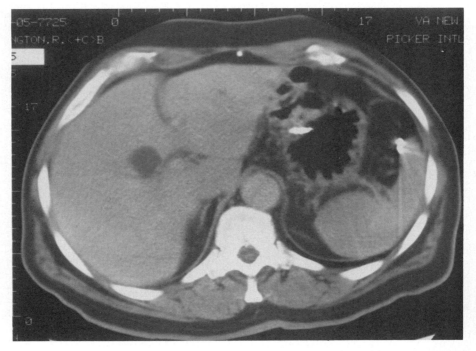

Fig. 3-55. Billroth II—bile reflux gastritis. Surgical clips are seen at the anastomosis. The folds of the anastomosis are thickened. The rugal folds in the remnant are thickened but contain their symmetric circumferential orientation. Endoscopically these findings were found to be caused by bile reflux gastritis.

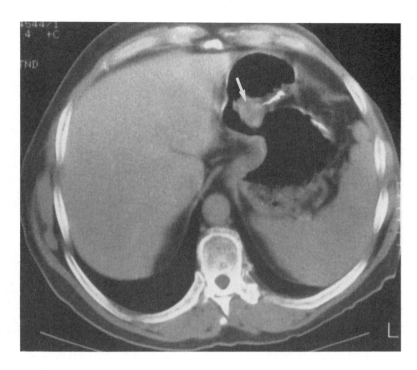

Fig. 3-56. Suture granuloma. Surgical clips are seen at an anastomotic region following a Billroth II. The greater curvature portion of the anastomosis is thickened *(arrow)*. Suture granuloma was found endoscopically.

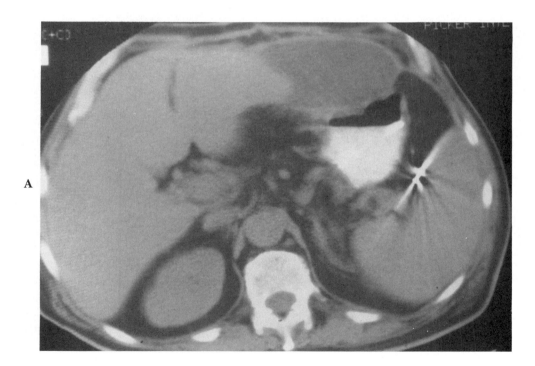

Fig. 3-57. Postoperative abscess. **A,** CT scan in a febrile patient approximately 10 days following gastrojejunostomy. A fluid collection is seen in the left anterior subphrenic space.   *Continued.*

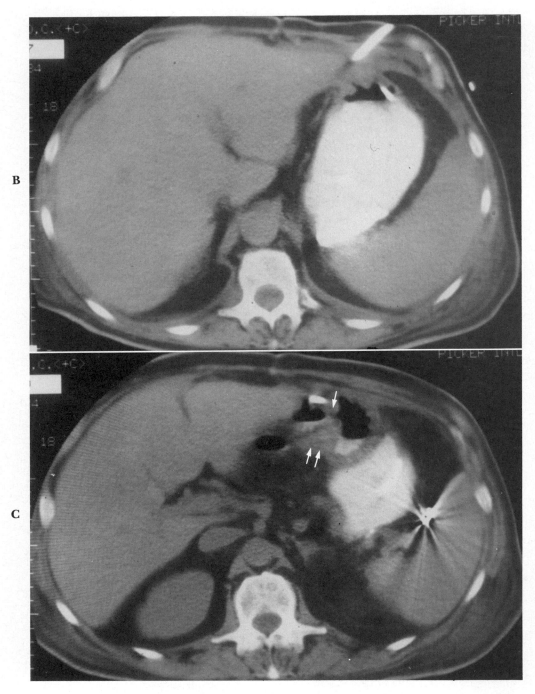

Fig. 3-57, cont'd. B, Diagnostic aspiration yielded pus, and percutaneous drainage was performed. CT confirms that the drainage catheter is in the cavity. **C,** Follow-up scan revealing the abscess to have been successfully drained. The anastomosis is edematous *(arrows)*, but no residual pus is seen.

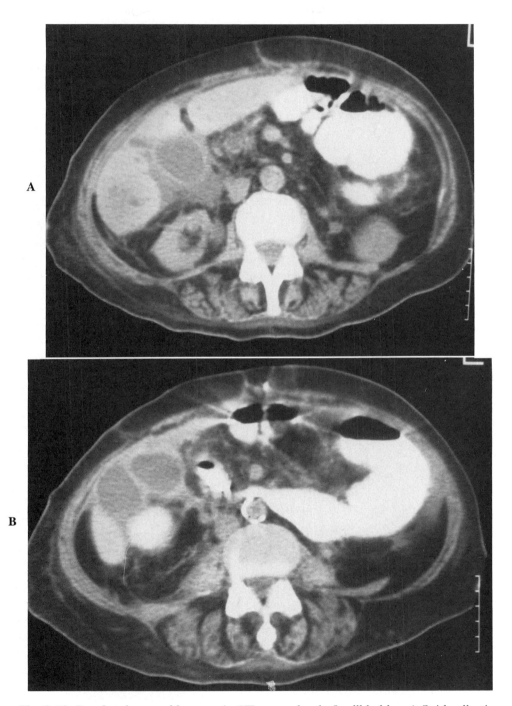

Fig. 3-58. Duodenal stump blowout. **A,** CT scan at level of gallbladder. A fluid collection surrounds the gallbladder. A contrast-filled gastrojejunostomy is seen in the left upper quadrant. **B,** Scan slightly caudad shows contrast in a dilated afferent loop. The proximal end is narrowed with thickening of local tissues. The patient had a benign course, was managed with conservative therapy and was monitored with CT scans for changes in the size and location of the fluid collections.

Postoperative abscesses may occur as a result of anastomic leaks, intraoperative contamination, or inadequate lavage of the peritoneal cavity during the operative procedure. These abscesses manifest as loculated fluid collections (Fig. 3-57). Only a small percentage of these abscesses contain air, and if air is seen within the abscesses, the possibility of communication to the bowel should be considered. Halvorsen et al. has noted the frequency of abscesses in the left anterior subphrenic space when a gastric source is present.[75]

Duodenal stump blowout will result in a fluid collection in the subhepatic space related to the lesser omentum. This is because the stump of the duodenal segment has been mobilized from the hepatoduodenal portion of the lesser omentum and thus fluid collections will track along this fascial plane. This complication has a high mortality.[76] CT is useful in helping establish the location of abscess collection, allowing accurate mapping and leading to more adequate surgical drainage following re-exploration (Fig. 3-58).

Stomal obstruction

In patients who have a slow return to normal gastric emptying following surgery, CT may be requested to rule out the possibility of abscess collections surrounding the gastric jejunal anastomosis. Stomal obstruction can be divided clinically into a temporary reversible obstruction versus late-appearing, mechanical closure of the anastomosis. Early obstruction is probably the result of edema at the suture line and possibly the result of abscess or hematomas of the suture line with localized peritonitis. Metabolic factors, including potassium deficiency resulting from prolonged postoperative vomiting or inadequate electrolyte replacement, hypoproteinemia, and postoperative hyperacidity, have been implicated as factors that may lead to this reversible form of stomal obstruction.[62] CT can obviously rule out the presence of structural or inflammatory complications that produce early, postoperative, stomal obstruction (Fig. 3-59). In late obstruction, 75% of cases are presumably the result of ulcer disease in the stoma. Therefore barium radiography should be considered the procedure of choice in the evaluation of these patients.

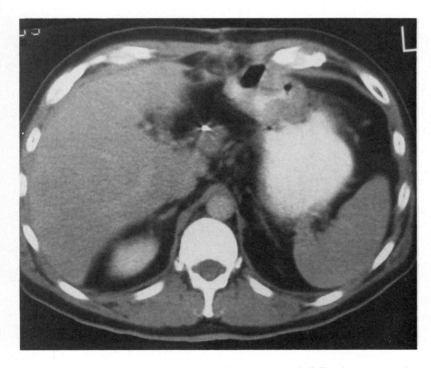

Fig. 3-59. Postoperative stomal obstruction. CT scan 1 week following gastrojejunostomy in a patient with high nasogastric output. The region of the anastomosis is markedly thickened and edematous. This finding is compatible with reversible stomal obstruction and not with abscess or other emergent surgical conditions.

Afferent loop obstruction

The afferent loop syndrome is a symptom complex that is caused by inflammatory disease, neoplasm, mechanical factors (e.g., intussuception, adhesions, linking), or ideopathic motor dysfunction and that results in partial intermittent obstruction of the afferent loop. The loop becomes overdistended with digestive juices and is relieved by bilious vomiting. Failure of these pancreatic and biliary secretions to mix may cause malabsorption, anemia, and vitamin B_{12} deficiency.[77] Prior to CT, the diagnosis was suggested by clinical symptomatology and confined by testing for shown low levels of vitamin B_{12} or intubation of efferent loop with continued aspiration of contents and timing of the appearance of the afferent loop content. Nuclear medicine studies using ^{99m}Tc-IDA agents may also be of value.[78] On barium studies in patients following Billroth II gastrojejunostomies we routinely attempt to fill the afferent loop and get a delayed film in one half hour to assure that the loop empties normally.

Etiologic factors in afferent loop obstruction include: adhesions, kinking of a redundant loop, and neoplastic infiltration of the local mesentery or anastomosis. The CT appearance of afferent loop obstruction has been described by Gale et al. One sees rounded, fluid-filled masses adjacent to the head and tail of the pancreas, which on sequential sections can be traced contiguously to conform to the U-shaped afferent loop.[79] Because of the obstruction, contrast material administered orally may not enter the loop accounting for the water density appearances. When severe, there may be an increased pressure at the ampulla with resulting distention of the biliary tree (Fig. 3-60).

Pancreatitis can occur as a complication of gastric surgery. This is presumably the result of trauma at the time of surgery. In cases when inadvertent splenic injury occurs during the gastrectomy resulting in a splenectomy, the distal duct of Santorini may be embedded in the splenic hilum, and the possibility of a postoperative pseudocyst in he left upper quadrant may occur.[80] CT has been universally accepted as a method of choice in evaluating the presence and extent of acute pancreatitis.[81]

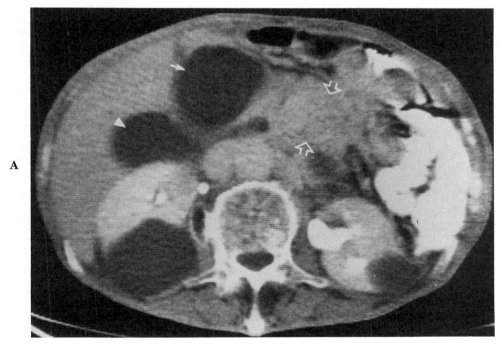

Fig. 3-60. Afferent loop obstruction. **A,** Several fluid collections are seen. The most superior fluid collection represents the proximal afferent loop *(small arrow);* just below this is a dilated gallbladder *(arrowhead).* *Open arrows* point to a mesenteric mass representing recurrent gastric carcinoma.   *Continued.*

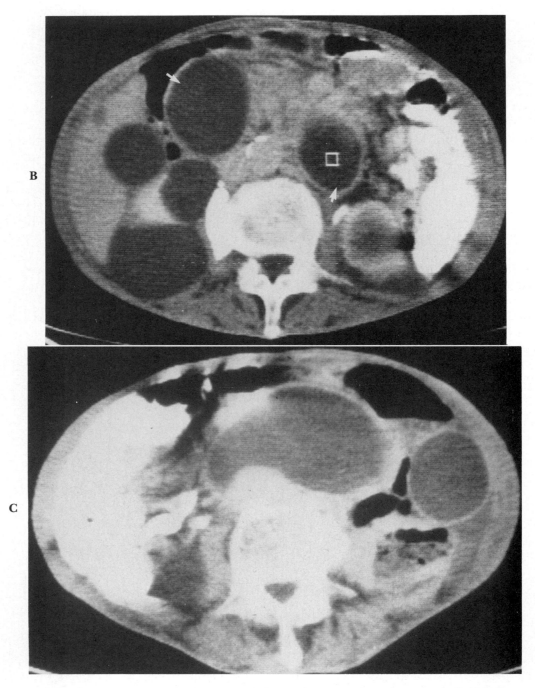

Fig. 3-60, cont'd. B, Scan slightly caudad reveals apparent peripancreatic fluid collections. These actually represent the limbs of the afferent loop. **C,** The dilated afferent loop can be followed caudally to continuity.

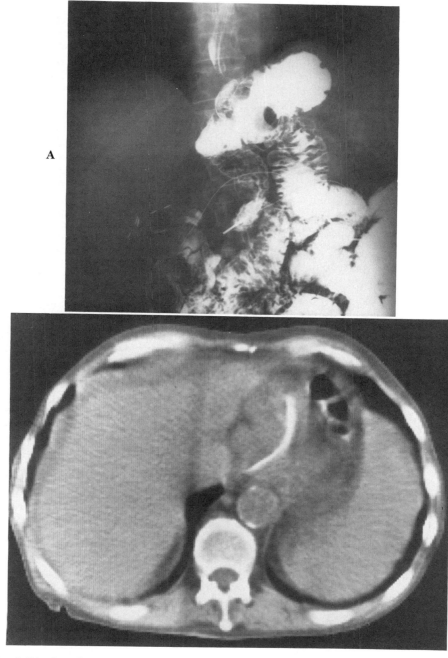

Fig. 3-61. Gastric carcinoma arising in remnant. **A.** Gastrointestinal series. Patient 20 years following gastrojejunostomy for ulcer disease, who is now experiencing weight loss. **B,** CT scan. The collapsed lumen is marked by the nasogastric tube. The fat along the greater curvature is infiltrated. Lobulated densities in the lesser omentum represent lymph nodes. A small amount of ascitic fluid can be seen. Multiple endoscopic biopsies failed to reveal neoplasm. At jejunostomy adenocarcinoma entirely submucosal in location was found.

Carcinoma may arise de novo in the gastric remnant following ulcer surgery or may recur following partial resection for advanced cases. As in carcinoma of the preoperative stomach, the CT findings include a thickened wall, peritoneal infiltration, and the presence of nodal or hepatic metastases. Because of the diminished gastric reserve in any patient with gastrojejunostomy, it may be difficult to achieve adequate distention of the stomach during an examination and therefore a false-positive examination may occur. Therefore we recommend studying all patients with gastrojejunostomies with air contrast technique for maximal distention of the gastric remnant as well as the relatively anterior anastomosis. If the gastric remnant is collapsed and if the wall is suspected of being thickened as a result of neoplasm, a repeat examination over the area should be obtained following ingestion of effervescent granules to ensure that the wall is truly thickened. As in patients with carcinoma arising in the preoperative stomach, care must be taken in inspection of the perigastric fat and local lymph node as well as distantly for evidence of distant metastasis (Fig. 3-61). Lymph node metastases in the peripancreatic and hepatoduodenal nodes is common.[82] CT aids in documenting the extent of the disease and in mapping for possible radiotherapy.

REFERENCES

1. Lee, K.R., Levine, E., Moffat, E.R., et al.: Computed tomographic staging of malignant gastric neoplasm, Radiology **133:**151-155, 1979.
2. Balfe, D.M., Koehler, R.E., Karstedt, N., et al.: Computed tomography of gastric neoplasms, Radiology **140:**431-436, 1981.
3. Komaki, S.: Normal or benign gastric wall thickening demonstrated by computed tomography, J. Comput. Assist. Tomogr. **6:**1103-1107, 1982.
4. Griffith, C.A.: Anatomy. In Harkins, H.N., and Nyhus, L.M., editors: Surgery of the stomach and duodenum, Boston, 1969, Little, Brown and Co., Inc.
5. Arey, L.B.: Developmental anatomy, Philadelphia, 1954, W.B. Saunders Co.
6. Berliner, L., Bosniak, M.A., and Megibow, A.J.: Adrenal pseudotumors on computed tomography, J. Comput. Assist. Tomogr. **6:**281-285, 1982.
7. Kaye, M.D., Young, S.W., Hayward, R., et al.: Gastric pseudotumor on CT scanning, AJR **135:**190-193, 1980.
8. Marks, W., Callen, P.W., and Moss, A.A.: Gastroesophageal region: a source of confusion on CT, AJR **140:**359-362, 1981.
9. Balfe, D.M., Mauro, M.A., Koehler, R.E., et al.: Gastrohepatic ligament: normal and pathologic CT anatomy, Radiology **150:**485-490, 1984.
10. Olipant, M., and Berne, A.S.: Computed tomography of the subperitoneal space: demonstration of direct spread of intraabdominal disease, J. Comput. Assist. Tomogr. **6:**1127-1137, 1982.
11. Coller, F.N., Kay, E.B., McIntyre, R.S.: Regional lymphatic metastases of carcinoma of the stomach, Arch. Surg. **43:**748-761, 1941.
12. Sunderland, D.A.: Lymphatic spread of gastric carcinoma. In McNeer, G., and Pack, G.T., editors: Neoplasms of the stomach, Philadelphia, 1967, J.B. Lippincott and Company.
13. Jeffries, G.I., Schlessinger, M., and Fordtran, J., editors: Gastrointestinal disease, ed. 2, Philadelphia, 1978, W.B. Saunders Co.
14. Fishman, E.K., Magid, D., Jones, B., et al.: Ménétrièr disease: case report, J. Comput. Assist. Tomogr. **7:**143-145, 1983.
15. Williams, S.M., Harned, R.K., and Settles, R.H.: Adenocarcinoma of the stomach in association with Ménétrièr's disease, Gastrointest. Radiol. **3:**387-390, 1978.
16. Nelson, S.W.: Small interesting manifestations of Crohn's disease (regional enteritis) of the stomach, duodenum and small intestine, AJR **107:**86-101, 1969.
17. Farman, J., Faegenberg, D., Dollinard, S., et al.: Crohn's disease of the stomach: the "rams-horn" sign, AJR **123:**242-251, 1985.
18. Anderson, M.F., and Diminich, N.R.: Pseudotumor caused by gastric varices, Dig. Dis. Sci.: **22:**929-932, 1977.
19. Cho, J.K., and Martel, W.H.: Recognition of splenic vein occlusion, AJR **131:**439-444, 1978.
20. Balthazar, E.J., Megibow, A.J., Naidich, D.P., et al.: Computed tomographic recognition of gastric varices, AJR **142:**1121-1125, 1984.
21. McCain, A.H., Bernardino, M.E., Somes, P.J., et al.: Varices from portal hypertension: correlation of CT and angiography, Radiology **154:**63-71, 1985.
22. Subramanyam, B.R., Balthazar, E.J., Raghavendra, B.N., et al.: Sonographic evaluation of patients with portal hypertension, Am. J. Gastroenterol. **78:**369-373, 1983.
23. Jeffrey, R.B., Federle, M.P., and Wall, S.: Value of computed tomography in detecting occult gastrointestinal perforation, J. Comput. Assist. Tomogr. **7:**825-827, 1983.
24. Lee, H., Vibharkar, S., and Ballon, E.: Gastroduodenal perforation: early diagnosis by computed tomography, J. Comput. Assist. Tomogr. **7:**226-229, 1983.
25. Brown, B.M., Federle, M.P., and Jeffrey, R.B.: Gastric wall thickening and extragastric inflammatory processes: a retrospective CT study, J. Comput. Assist. Tomogr. **6:**762-765, 1982.
26. Ho, C.S., and Taylor, B.: Percutaneous transgastric drainage for pancreatic pseudocysts, AJR **143:**623-625, 1984.
27. Moss, A.A., Schnyder, P., Marks, W., et al.: Gastric adenocarcinoma: a comparison of the accuracy and economics of staging by computed tomography and surgery, Gastroenterology **80:**45-50, 1981.
28. McFee, A.S., and Aust, J.B.: Gastric carcinoma and the CAT scan, Gastroenterology **80:**196-198, 1981.
29. Silverberg, E.: Cancer statistics, 1985, CA **35:**19-35, 1985.
30. Weed, T.E., Nuessie, W., and Ochsner, A.: Carcinoma of the stomach: why we are failing to improve survival. Ann. Surg. **193:**407-413, 1981.
31. Diehl, J.T., Hermann, R.E., Cooperman, A.M., et al.: Gastric carcinoma: a ten year review, Ann. Surg. **198:**9-12, 1983.
32. Hoerr, S.O.: Prognosis for carcinoma of the stomach, Surg. Gynecol. Obstet. **137:**205-209, 1973.
33. Shiu, M.H., Papachristou, D.N., Kosloff, C., et al.: Selection of operative procedure for adenocarcinoma of the mid stomach, Ann. Surg. **192:**730-737, 1980.

34. Papachristou, D.N., and Fortner, J.G.: Adenocarcinoma of the gastric cardia: the choice of gastrectomy, Ann. Surg. **193:**58-64, 1980.

35. Nishimura, K., Togashi, K., Tohdo, G., et al.: Computed tomography of calcified gastric carcinoma, J. Comput. Assist. Tomogr. **5:**1010-1011, 1984.

36. Komaiko, M.S.: Gastric neoplasm: ultrasound and CT evaluation, Gastrointest. Radiol. **4:**131-137, 1979.

37. Antonioli, D.A., and Goldman, H.: Changes in the location and type of gastric adenocarcinoma, Cancer **50:**775-781, 1982.

38. Freeny, P.C., and Marks, W.M.: Adenocarcinoma of the gastroesophageal junction: barium and CT examination, AJR **138:**1077-1084, 1982.

39. Schneeckloth, G., Terrier, F., and Fuchs, W.A.: Computed tomography in carcinoma of the esophagus and cardia, Gastrointest. Radiol. **8:**193-206, 1983.

40. Gunderson, L.L., and Sosin, H.: Adenocarcinoma of the stomach: areas of failure in a reoperation series (second or symptomatic look)—Clinicopathologic correlations and implications for adjuvant therapy, Int. J. Radiat. Oncol. Biol. Phys. **8:**1-11, 1982.

41. Dupont, J.B., Lee, J.R., Burton, G.R., et al.: Adenocarcinoma of the stomach: review of 1497 cases, Cancer **41:**941-947, 1978.

42. Kennedy, B.J.: TNM classification for stomach cancer, Cancer **26:**971-983, 1970.

43. Komaki, S., and Toyoshima, S.: Computed tomography's capabilty in detecting advanced gastric cancer, Gastrointest. Radiol. **8:**307-313, 1983.

43a. Dehn, T.C.B., Rezneck, R.H., Nockler, I.B., et al.: The preoperative assessment of advanced gastric cancer by computed tomography, Br. J. Surg. **71:**413-417, 1984.

44. Fly, O.A., Waugh, J.M., and Dockerty, M.B.: Spleen hilar nodal involvement in carcinoma of the distal part of the stomach, Cancer **9:**459-462, 1956.

45. Meyers, M.A.: Dynamic radiology of the abdomen, New York, 1976, Springer-Verlag New York, Inc.

46. Megibow, A.J., Hulnick, D.H., Bosniak, M.A., et al.: Ovarian metastases: computed tomographic appearances, Radiology **156:**151-164, 1985.

47. Clarke, J.S., Cruze, K., ElFarra, S., et al.: The natural history and results of surgical therapy for carcinoma of the stomach: an analysis of 250 cases, Am. J. Surg. **102:**143-152, 1961.

48. MacDonald, J.S., Cohn, I., and Gunderson, L.L.: Cancer of the stomach. In DeVita, V.T., Hellman, S., and Rosenberg, S.A., editors: Cancer: principles and practice of oncology, ed. 2, Philadelphia, 1985, J.B. Lippincott Co.

49. Foley, W.D., Berland, L.L., Lawson, T.L., et al.: Contrast enhancement techniques for dynamic hepatic computed tomographic scanning, Radiology **147:**797-803, 1983.

49a. Alpern, M.B., Lawson, T.L., Foley, W.D., et al.: Focal hepatic masses and fatty infiltration detected by enhanced dynamic CT, Radiology **158:**45-49, 1986.

50. Balthazar, E.J., and Rosenberg, H.D.: Primary and metastatic scirrhous carcinoma of the rectum, AJR **132:**711-715, 1979.

51. Gray, G.M., Rosenberg, S.A., Cooper, A.D., et al.: Lymphoma involving the gastrointestinal tract, Gastroenterology **82:**143-152, 1982.

52. Hande, K.R., Fischer, R.I., DeVita, V.T., et al.: Diffuse histiocytic lymphoma involving the gastrointestinal tract, Cancer 1984-1989, 1978.

53. Weingrad, D.N., DeCosse, J.J., Sherlock, P., et al.: Primary gastrointestinal lymphoma: a 30 year review, Cancer **49:**1258-1265, 1982.

54. Lewin, K.J., Ranchod, M., and Dorfman, R.E.: Lymphoma of the gastrointestinal tract, Cancer **42:**693-707, 1978.

55. Megibow, A.J., Balthazar, E.J., Naidich, D.P., et al.: Computed tomography of gastrointestinal lymphoma, AJR **141:**541-543, 1983.

56. Buy, J.N., and Moss, A.A.: Computed tomography of gastric lymphoma, AJR **138:**859-865, 1982.

57. Pillari, G., Weinreb, J., Vernace, F., et al.: CT of gastric masses: image patterns and a note on potential pitfalls, Gastrointest. Radiol. **8:**11-17, 1983.

58. Hertzer, N.R., and Hoerr, S.O.: An interpretive review of lymphoma of the stomach, Surg. Gynecol. Obstet. **143:**113-124, 1976.

59. Friedman, A.F.: Primary lymphosarcoma of the stomach: a clinical study of 75 cases, Am. J. Med. **26:**783-796, 1958.

60. Chatterjee, D., and Powell, A.: Mesenchymal tumors of the stomach: report of cases, review of the literature and analysis of leiomyosarcomas, Br. J. Clin. Radiol. **36:**26-33, 1982.

61. Megibow, A.J., Redmond, P.E., Bosniak, M.A., et al.: CT diagnosis of gastrointestinal lipomas, AJR **133:**743-745, 1979.

62. Heiken, J.P., Forde, K.A., and Gold, R.P.: Computed tomography as a definitive method for diagnosing gastrointestinal lipomas, Radiology **142:**408-413, 1982.

63. Lo, J., Sage, M.R., Paterson, H.S., et al.: Gastric duplication in an adult, J. Comput. Assist. Tomogr. **7:**328-330, 1983.

64. Thornhill, B.A., Cho, K.C., and Morehouse, H.T.: Gastric duplication associated with pulmonary sequestration: CT manifestations, AJR **138:**1168-1171, 1982.

65. Megibow, A.J., Hulnick, D.H., Balthazar, E.J., et al.: CT of leiomyomas and leiomyosarcomas, AJR **144:**727-733, 1985.

66. Salmela, H.: Smooth muscle tumors of the stomach: a clinical study of 112 cases, Acta Chir. Scand. **134:**384-391, 1968.

67. Appelman, H.D., and Helwig, E.B.: Sarcomas of the stomach in 49 patients, Am. J. Clin. Pathol. **67:**2-10, 1977.

68. Scatarige, J.C., Fishman, E.K., Jones, B., et al.: Gastric leiomyosarcoma: CT observations, J. Comput. Assist. Tomogr. **9:**320-327, 1985.

69. Cathcart, P.M., Cathcart, R.S., and Yarbrough, D.R.: Tumors of gastric smooth muscle, South. Med. J. **73:**18-20, 1980.

70. Slasky, B.S., Denese, L., and Skocnice, M.L.: Exogastric leiomyoblastoma: diagnosis by CT and ultrasonography, South. Med. J. **75:**1275-1277, 1982.

71. Faegenberg, D., Farman, J., Dallemond, S., et al.: Leiomyoblastoma of the stomach, Radiology **117:**247-302, 1975.

72. Marshak, R.H., Lindner, A.E., and Maklansky, D.: Carcinoma of the stomach. In Marshak, R.H., Linder, A.E., Marklansry, D., editors: Radiology of the stomach, Philadelphia, 1983.

73. Cormier, J., Jeffrey, T., and Welch, J.: Linitis plastica caused by metastatic lobulated carcinoma of the breast, Mayo Clinic Proc. **55:**747-753, 1980.

74. Tanner, N.C.: Gastric resection: Billroth II. In Harkins, H.N., and Nyhus, C.M., editors: Surgery of the stomach and duodenum, ed. 2, Boston, 1969, Little, Brown & Co., Inc.

75. Halvorsen, R.A., Jones, M.A., Rice, P., et al.: Anterior left subphrenic abscess: characteristic plain film and CT appearance, AJR **139:**283-289, 1982.

76. Moore, H.C.: Complications of gastric surgery. In Harkus, H.N., and Nyhus, L.M., editors: Surgery of the stomach and duodenum, Boston, 1969, Little, Brown & Co., Inc.

77. Meyer, J.H.: Chronic morbidity after ulcer surgery. In Schlesinger, M.H., and Fordtran, J.S., editors: Gastrointestinal disease, ed. 2, Philadelphia, 1978.

78. Thomas, J.L., Cowan, R.J., Maynard, D., et al.: Radionuclide demonstration of small bowel anatomy in afferent loop syndrome: case report, J. Nucl. Med. **18**:897-898, 1977.

79. Gale, M.E., Gerzof, S.C., Kiser, L.C., et al.: CT appearance of afferent loop obstruction, AJR **138**:105-108, 1982.

80. Balthazar, E.J., Megibow, A.J., Rothberg, M., et al.: CT evaluation of pancreatic injury following splenectomy, Gastrointest. Radiol. **10**:139-144, 1985.

81. Freeny, P.C., and Lawson, T.L.: Radiology of the pancreas, New York, 1982, Springer-Verlag New York, Inc.

82. Mullin, D., and Shirkhoda, A.: CT after gastrectomy for gastric carcinoma, J. Comput. Assist. Tomogr. **9**:30-33, 1985.

Chapter Four

DUODENUM

Alec J. Megibow

In comparison to its use with the stomach and colon, CT has relatively little to offer in terms of improving diagnosis and assessment of duodenal lesions. However, because the duodenum has important anatomic relations with vital structures in the upper abdomen, the most intimate being the relation between the duodenum and the pancreas, successful examination of the upper abdomen is dependent on reliable opacification and identification of the duodenum. CT techniques of duodenal opacification are discussed in Chapter One. This chapter concerns CT diagnosis of the disease processes directly involving the duodenum and attempts to highlight those instances where CT may aid in differential diagnosis of duodenal pathology.

ANATOMY AND RELATIONSHIPS

The duodenum begins just distal to the pyloric channel and extends to the ligament of Treitz—the duodenal jejunal (DJ) junction. This portion of the alimentary tube becomes retroperitoneal in location immediately beyond the hepatoduodenal ligament, the right border (free margin) of the lesser omentum. As it sweeps posteriorly, the medial aspect of the second portion of the duodenum or C-loop is adjacent to the right margin of the pancreatic head separated from the parenchyma by variable amounts of fat. In patients with sufficient fat the gastroduodenal and pancreaticoduodenal vessels may be seen in this space. The origin of the transverse mesocolon reflects from the anterior aspect of the second portion of the duodenum.[1] The mesocolon can be recognized by fibrofatty vascular tissue extending toward the colon. The lateral aspect of the second portion of the duodenum is adjacent to the anterior portion of the inferior surface of the caudate lobe and gallbladder. The genu of the duodenum is related medially to the lateral inferior border of the pancreatic head, inferiorly to the inferior vena cava and right renal vein, and posterolaterally to the right kidney. The latter is separated from the duodenum by the perirenal fascia, which separates the right perirenal space from the right anterior pararenal space in which the duodenum lies. It is this portion of the duodenum that, when filled with fluid, may simulate a peripancreatic mass or a retroperitoneal mass, particularly in thin patients. On more caudal sections, the transverse duodenum is consistently seen traversing the inferior vena cava and aorta. Just superior to the transverse duodenum, the superior mesenteric artery and vein are seen. The fourth portion is recognized on more cephalad sections than the horizontal segments as it ascends to meet the ligament of Treitz (Fig. 4-1).

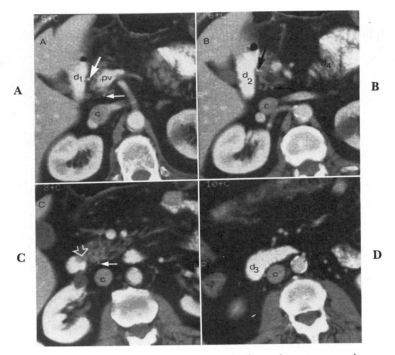

Fig. 4-1. Normal duodenum. Sequential CT images show the course and appearance of the normal duodenum filled with positive contrast material. **A** and **B,** Note the gastroduodenal artery *(arrow)* in the fat between the lumen (d_1) and the neck of the pancreas. **A** through **C,** The *small arrow* points to pancreaticoduodenal arterial branches. **B,** The fourth portion of the duodenum (d_4) is seen at the level of the duodenal bulb. **C,** The soft-tissue density of the papilla of Vater *(open arrow)* may be recognized along the medial duodenal wall. Normal nodes are not seen (*c,* inferior vena cava). The junction of the second and third portion *(d_3)* is seen in **D.** This is a useful landmark in establishing that the entire pancreas has been scanned.

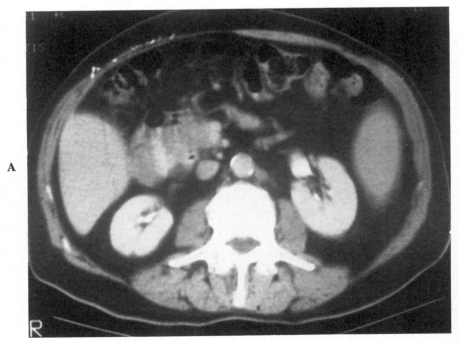

Fig. 4-2. Duodenal nonrotation. **A,** Scan at the level of the uncinate process of the pancreas. There is a suggestion of mass surrounding the duodenum.

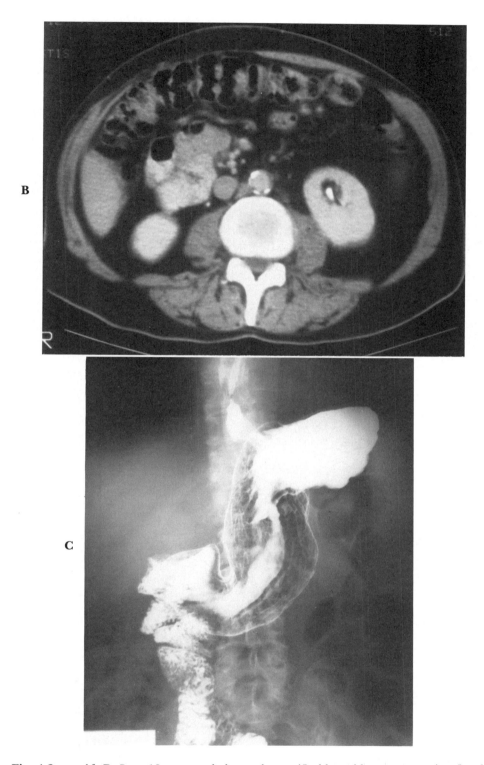

Fig. 4-2, cont'd. B, Scan 10 mm caudad reveals opacified bowel loops accounting for the mass. Notice the mesenteric vessels to the right of the aorta *(arrows)*. No duodenal segments were visualized crossing the spine. **C,** Film from gastrointestinal series. Notice the lack of duodenal and jejunal loops in the left upper quadrant.

The horizontal portion is not visualized in patients with rotational abnormalities. In these patients, on analysis of contiguous sections, one can follow the duodenum into the jejunum on the right side of the abdomen. An ancillary finding indicative of rotational abnormality is a reversal in the axis of the mesenteric vessels (Fig. 4-2). This redundant noncrossing duodenum may be confused with a peripancreatic mass.[2]

The duodenum is also bordered by multiple lymph node groups. The anterior and posterior pancreaticoduodenal lymph nodes, which are located in the groove between the pancreatic parenchyma and duodenum, are the most frequently visualized. When enlarged these nodes may displace and engulf the duodenum.[3] These nodes may enlarge in a variety of conditions, which shall be discussed subsequently. Normal lymph nodes may be seen in up to 77% of patients with no upper abdominal adenopathy.[4]

The normal duodenal wall is thinner than the gastric wall, measuring approximately 1 mm in thickness. The papilla is infrequently seen on routine scans. It is occasionally recognized as a soft-tissue nodule along the medial aspect of the second portion of the duodenum (see Fig. 4-1). The papilla is more often recognized on air contrast CT scans performed with thin sections and hypotonia induced by glucagon as described in Chapter One.

Duodenal diverticula rarely cause clinical symptoms and most commonly occur along the medial border of the descending duodenum. They are acquired lesions. They are usually seen in air collection insinuated between the inferolateral aspect of the pancreatic head and the junction of the second and third duodenal segments (Fig. 4-3). Occasionally they may become obstructed leading to duodenal diverticulitis. The major concern of the CT radiologist is in those patients being studied for choledocholithiasis in whom a diverticulum filled with contrast material may be potentially confused with a distal common duct stone. Some authors have recommended not administering oral contrast material in patients with suspected choledocholithiasis to avoid mistaking a partially-filled diverticulum for a common duct stone.

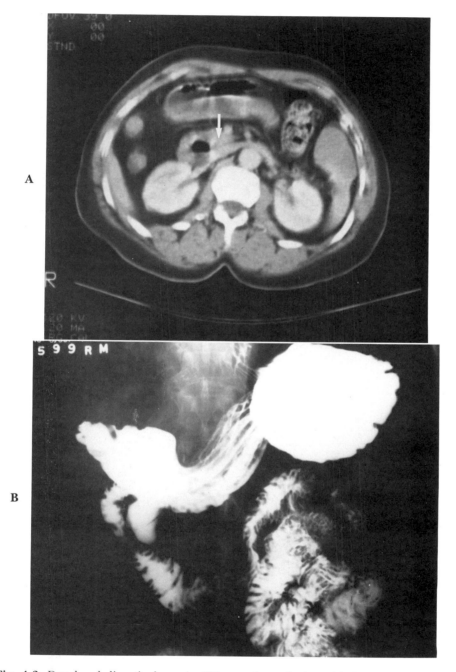

Fig. 4-3. Duodenal diverticulum. **A,** CT scan through the mid-abdomen reveals an air fluid level just lateral to the uncinate process of the pancreas *(arrow)*. **B,** Gastrointestinal series in the same patient shows typical duodenal diverticulum. (Case courtesy Dr. S. Toder, Hospital Center at Orange, Orange, New Jersey.)

INFLAMMATORY DISEASE
Duodenitis

Intrinsic inflammatory disease of the duodenum is diagnosed by history and double-contrast duodenography. Endoscopy may be warranted occasionally. Therefore peptic duodenitis is rarely diagnosed by CT scanning. Severe cases may reveal a diffusely thickened, slightly low-density, duodenal wall. The lumen is compressed centrally, and there is little differential diagnostic difficulty in distinguishing symmetric inflammatory wall thickening from neoplastic wall thickening. Reactive changes along contiguous fascial planes (Gerota's fascia) signal more severe inflammation (Fig. 4-4).

The more common situation in which we detect duodenitis is as a secondary manifestation of acute pancreatitis. The direct proximity of the pancreas and medial wall of the duodenum provide anatomic correlation for this direct effect of the inflammatory exudate on the duodenum.[5] Duodenal paresis, edematous folds, widening of the C-loop, and edema of the duodenal papilla are classic signs on barium studies and may be present in from 70% to 80% of patients.

Two complications of acute pancreatitis deserve special mention. First, duodenal obstruction may occur as a result of the presence of a fulminant inflammatory exudate in the root of the mesentery compressing the third portion of the duodenum.[6] The obstruction occurs at this point because the inflammatory mass leads to narrowing of the angle between the aorta and superior mesenteric artery constricting the duodenal lumen[7] (Fig. 4-5).

Second pseudocyst of the pancreas may surround and obstruct the descending duodenum.[7a] CT provides accurate depiction of the mass and its relation to the duodenal lumen providing guidance for surgical therapy (Fig. 4-6). One should remember that duodenal atony with the resultant dilation and secretion may result in an image in which a dilated duodenum may be mistaken for a pseudocyst. Air insufflation of the duodenum and scanning the patient in a left-side-down lateral decubitus position should differentiate the dilated, fluid-filled atonic C-loop from an actual pancreatic pseudocyst (see Fig. 1-15).

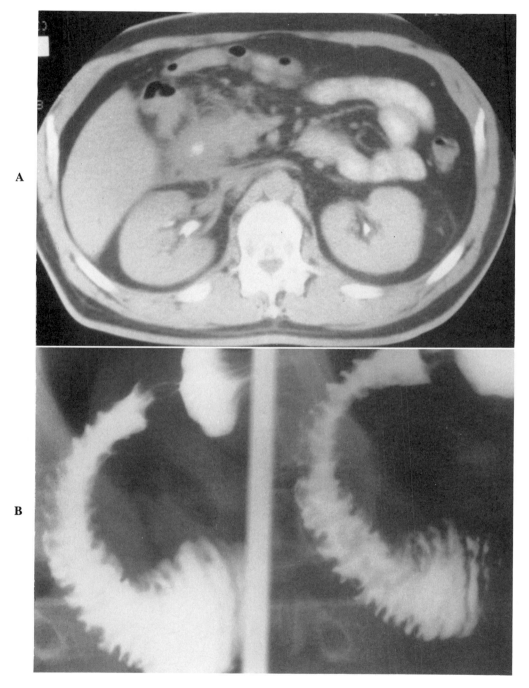

Fig. 4-4. Doudenitis. **A,** CT scan through the head of the pancreas. The duodenal wall is thickened and has a relatively low density. Increased density in the fat reflects reaction to the diffuse inflammatory process. The pancreatic head is not enlarged. Serum amylase was normal. **B,** Spot film from gastrointestinal series reveals changes of submucosal edema with mild narrowing of the lumen.

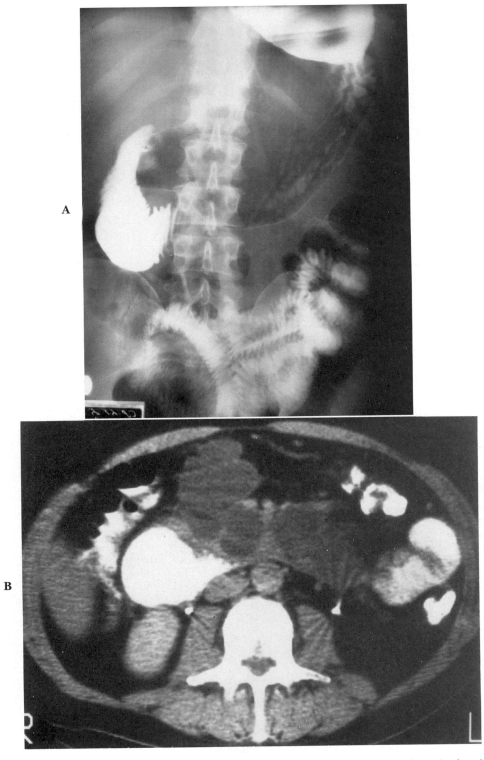

Fig. 4-5. Acute pancreatitis—duodenal obstruction. **A,** Films from gastrointestinal series. There is narrowing of the duodenum at the level of the root of the mesentery. The air-filled, transverse colon is inferiorly displaced. The opacified small bowel loops are edematous. **B,** CT scan through the transverse duodenum reveals extrinsic narrowing by pancreatic phlegmon at the aortomesenteric angle that results in partial duodenal obstruction.

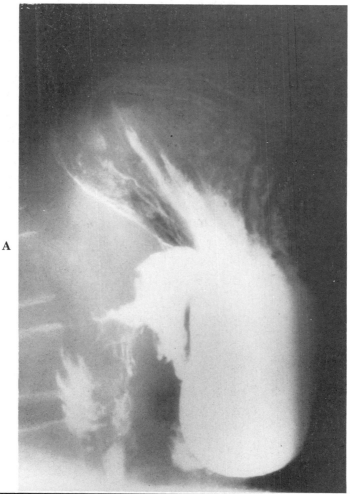

A

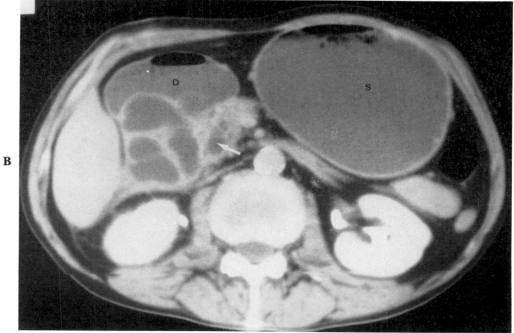

B

Fig. 4-6. Pancreatic pseudocyst with duodenal obstruction. **A,** Oblique film from gastrointestinal series shows a long segment of narrowing in the second portion of the duodenum. A large amount of secretion is present in the stomach. **B,** CT scan in same patient. The stomach *(S)* is dilated and filled with fluid. A similar appearance is seen in the duodenal bulb *(D)*. A multiseptated mass is seen immediately below the dilated duodenal bulb. Notice the dilated pancreatic duct in the uncinate process of the pancreas *(arrow)*. Surgery confirmed a multiloculated pseudocyst.

TRAUMA

Duodenal and pancreatic injury occurs as a result of blunt abdominal trauma most often associated with steering wheel injuries. Early recognition is important because unrecognized duodenal perforation has a 65% mortality rate as opposed to a 5% mortality rate when injury is recognized and operated on within the first 24 hours of the traumatic event.[8] Plain films are insensitive to retroperitoneal duodenal rupture, approximating at 33% sensitivity.[9]

Two small series have been reported in which CT shows the presence of gas and fluid in the right anterior pararenal space.[10,11] These findings are highly suspicious for duodenal retroperitoneal perforation in the appropriate clinical setting.

Walsh has described two false-positive cases based on these signs; one case resulted from dissection of gas posterior to the transverse duodenum from a pneumothorax and a second from migration of fluid from a retroperitoneal rupture of the bladder into the anterior pararenal space.[12] Pancreatic trauma occurs in 3% to 12% of abdominal injuries. Manifestations may include acute pancreatitis, pseudocyst, contusion, laceration or complete fracture.[13] A peripancreatic hematoma may impress and narrow the duodenal lumen, and patients may have symptoms of upper gastrointestinal obstruction. CT, when performed within 3 days of the event, will show the increased blood density in the peripancreatic hematoma (Fig. 4-7).

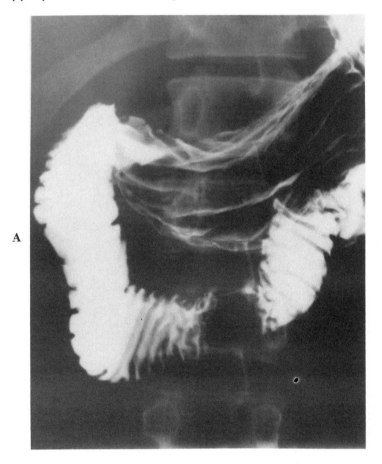

Fig. 4-7. Peripancreatic hematoma. **A,** Gastrointestinal series in a 31-year-old patient who sustained blunt abdominal trauma in a motor vehicle accident. Persistent vomiting lead to the study. A persistent area of narrowing was detected with focal, proximal, submucosal edema.

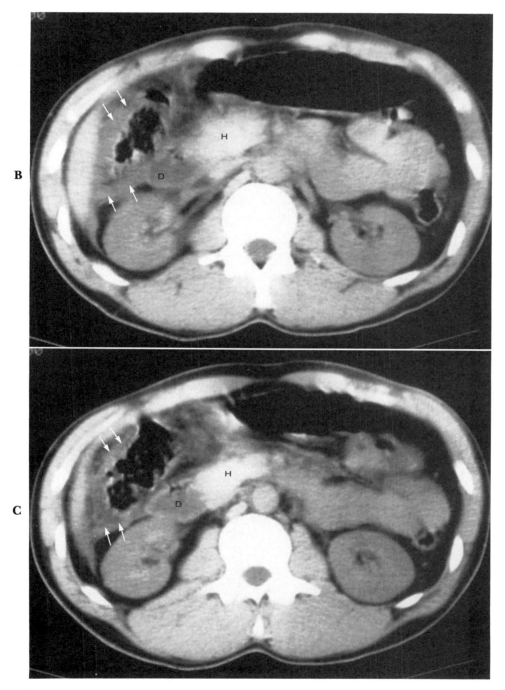

Fig. 4-7, cont'd. B and **C,** CT through the transverse duodenum reveals an area of increased density compatible with a periduodenal hematoma *(H).* The high density of blood is accentuated by not using oral or intravenous contrast material. Notice the fluid-filled duodenal lumen associated with mild dilation. Fluid in the anterior pararenal space results from mild pancreatic injury *(arrows).* (Case courtesy Dr. S. Toder, Hospital Center at Orange, Orange, New Jersey.)

PEPTIC ULCER DISEASE

CT has no primary role in the diagnosis of peptic ulcer disease. Occasionally patients with chronic peptic ulcer disease develop sealed off perforations in the hepatoduodenal ligament lesser sac or pancreatic head and may be referred for CT for a suspected abscess. Madrazo and associates[14] have reported CT findings in 4 patients with peptic ulcer disease who were referred for CT as a result of back pain. Findings included visualization of the ulcer, a sinus tract between the ulcer and head of the pancreas, pancreatic head enlargement, and edema at the site of the ulcer crater. They stress the fact that these cases may be confused with pancreatic masses unless the ulcer itself is visualized (Fig. 4-8).

Occasionally, giant duodenal ulcers may appear as regions of edema surrounding the duodenal bulb. This complication of ulcer disease is rarely seen because of the advent of improved drug therapy for ulcer disease. However, we still see giant ulcers in patients treated with large doses of corticosteroid therapy (Fig. 4-9).

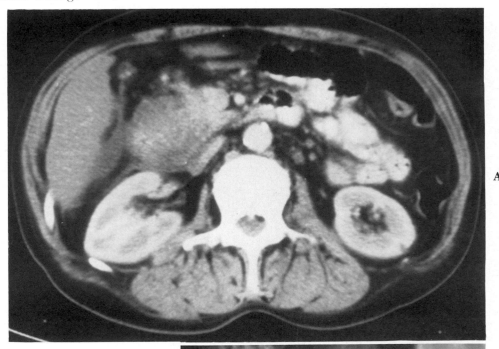

A

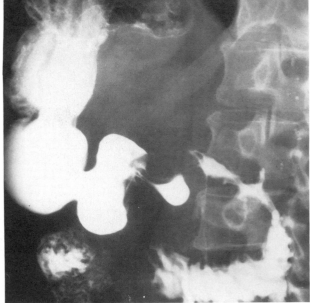

B

Fig. 4-8. Penetrating post-bulbar peptic ulcer. **A,** CT through mid-kidneys shows an apparent mass in the head of the pancreas. Fluid collections are noted in the right anterior pararenal space. **B,** Gastrointestinal series shows a post-bulbar ulcer resulting in periduodenal sinus tracts. The "mass" in the pancreatic head resulted from penetration of the ulcer into the head of the pancreas, which produced a localized pancreatitis. (Case courtesy Dr. R. Meisell, M.D., Booth Memorial Hospital, Flushing, New York.)

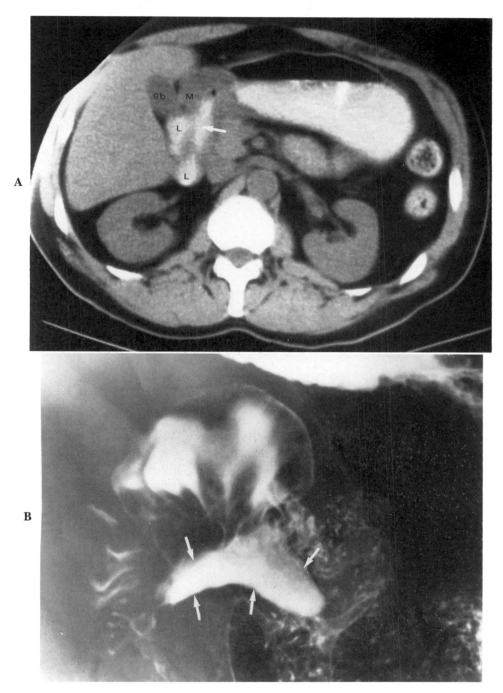

Fig. 4-9. Peptic ulcer disease. **A,** Non-contrast CT through gallbladder fossa. An irregular mass *(M)* surrounds the duodenal bulb. The density is similar to the gallbladder *(gb)*. No air is noted in the mass. The duodenal lumen *(L)* is narrowed. A second collection of barium parallels the lumen medially *(arrow)*. **B,** Spot film from upper gastrointestinal series shows a large ulcer along the inferior margin of the bulb *(arrows)*. The superior portion of the bulb is a large pseudodiverticulum. This patient had a giant duodenal ulcer at surgery.

Fistulous lesions of the duodenum

Crohn's disease may exist isolated to the duodenum but is almost always associated with gastric involvement. In a clinical study of 300 patients with Crohn's disease, duodenal involvement was documented in 4%.[15] CT scanning is of value in assessing the extramucosal complications of the disease, specifically the extent and location of fistulous tracts and the presence of abscesses. The duodenum appears thick-walled and may enhance following administration of intravenous contrast material. Extraluminal, linear air collections may be seen in the sinus tracts within the hepatoduodenal ligament, transverse mesocolon, peripancreatic fat, or gastrocolic omentum. The diagnosis on CT is suggested by the combination of these changes with more typical changes in the small bowel (Fig. 4-10).

Other fistulous lesions may occur from the gallbladder, right kidney, colon, and aorta. They are generally recognized on barium studies or cholangiography. We have reported one case of fistula from the common bile duct to the duodenum diagnosed by CT.[16] Soft-tissue, linear densities demarcating the fistulous tract are seen in association with air within the common bile duct in a patient without a surgical history.

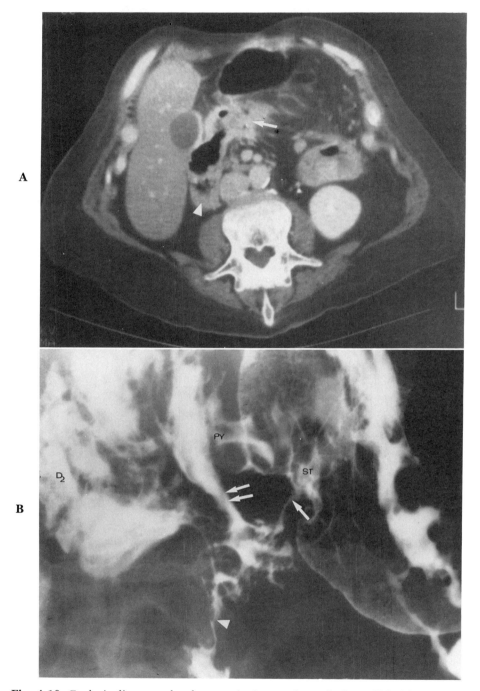

Fig. 4-10. Crohn's disease—duodenum. **A,** A scan through the gallbladder fossa reveals thickening of the duodenal wall. Marked stranding is seen in the peripancreatic fat. Extraluminal gas bubbles are seen in the fistulous tract *(arrow)*. A gas/fluid collection is present below the duodenal lumen *(arrowhead)*. **B,** Spot film from gastrointestinal series shows gastroduodenal *(arrow)* and duodenoduodenal fistulas *(double arrows)*. A blind sinus tract is also noted filling the fluid collection seen on the CT scan *(arrowhead)*. (*ST,* stomach; *PH,* pyloric channel; *D₂,* duodenal sweep.)

Aortoduodenal relationships

The third portion of the duodenum crosses over the abdominal aorta at the L3 level. Anteriorly the root of the mesentery, with the mesenteric artery and vein, encloses the duodenum in a narrow angle between those vessels and the vertebral body. Occasionally in patients with aortic aneurysm the duodenum may become obstructed where it crosses the aorta (Fig. 4-11). Aortic aneurysms may be considered a cause of the superior mesenteric artery syndrome because it results in a narrowing of the aortomesenteric angle trapping the duodenum. Uncomplicated aneurysm rarely produces obstruction.[17,18]

We have used CT to image patients recently postoperative from abdominal aortic aneurysm surgery.[19] In these patients, inflammatory thickening in the root of the mesentery that results from traction of the duodenum during surgical proce-dure may lead to transient partial obstruction at this level. CT will show a spectrum of findings from induration of local fat to fluid collections adjacent to the duodenum. Postoperative fluid may result from trauma to adjacent structures with persistent seroma or localized pancreatitis. High-density fluid collections in this region may represent hematomas signifying anastomotic or perigraft leakages (Fig. 4-12).

Aortoduodenal fistula is a serious complication of aortic reconstructive surgery best studied by angiography. CT has no clear role in the evaluation of this complication.[20] If there is a suspicion of aortoduodenal fistula, angiography should be performed immediately. Aortoduodenal erosion is seen directly with endoscopy. We have studied one patient with an aortoduodenal erosion in which *no* CT finding was present to suggest the presence of erosion of the graft into the duodenal lumen.

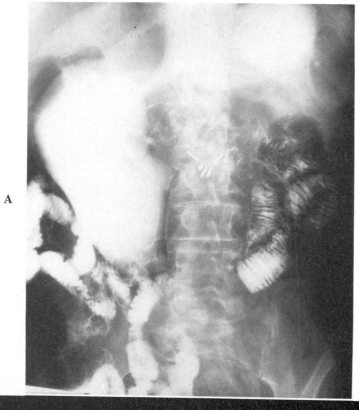

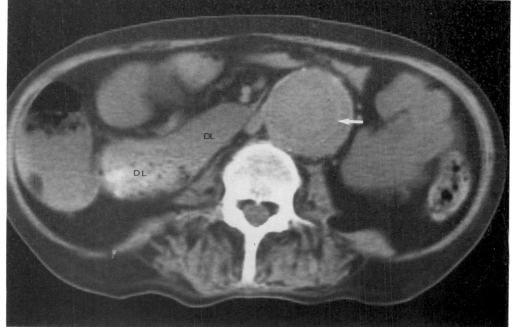

Fig. 4-11. Duodenal obstruction—aortic aneurysm. **A,** Gastrointestinal series shows massively distended, featureless, descending duodenum. Note the surgical clips at the level of the lumbar spine. **B,** CT reveals dilated, fluid-filled duodenum *(DL)* with marked narrowing of the lumen adjacent to an abdominal aortic graft site. The graft wall is seen within the shell of the aneurysm *(arrow)*. Transient duodenal obstruction occurs in the perioperative period in patients undergoing aneurysm surgery. Chronic obstruction is rarely seen.

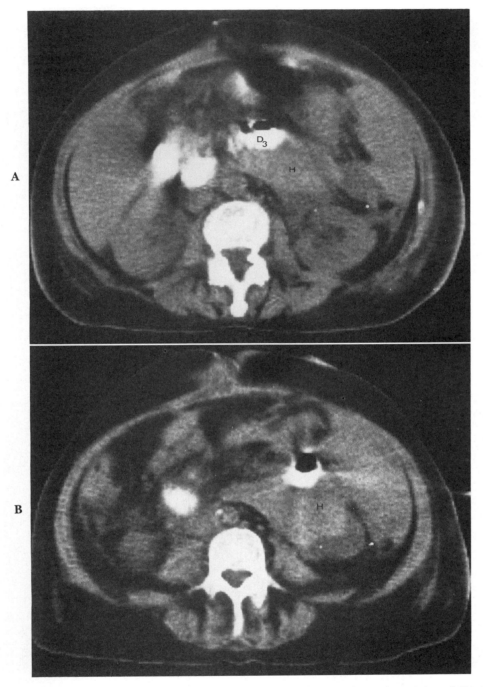

Fig. 4-12. Retroduodenal hematomas. **A** and **B,** Two scans of a patient 4 days following superior mesenteric artery embolectomy. The patient experienced a rapid drop in hematocrit. CT was performed as an emergency. The scans reveal a high-density fluid collection in the retroduodenal region elevating the transverse duodenum from the aorta *(H)*. The increased CT number suggested the acute hemorrhage found at surgery. The hemorrhage was a result of the rupture of a traumatic pseudoaneurysm at the origin of the superior mesenteric artery. Fluid collections from postsurgical pancreatitis frequently accumulate in this space. CT is invaluable in discriminating the nature of these fluid collections in extremely ill patients following aortic surgery. (D_3, third portion of the duodenum.)

DUODENAL NEOPLASMS

Duodenal tumors account for a small number of alimentary tract neoplasms.[21] They may produce a variety of symptoms including bleeding, jaundice, and intermittent obstruction. CT is useful in characterization of benign lesions and in determining the extent of malignant neoplasms. CT has unique applicability in two instances (1) in evaluation of periampullary neoplasms and (2) in determining intrinsic versus extrinsic etiologies of neoplastic duodenal lesions.

Benign neoplasms

The common benign neoplasms involving the duodenum include Brunner gland adenomas, adenomatous polyps, lipoma, leiomyoma, angioma, and hamartoma. The diagnosis is made by barium radiography and endoscopy. CT has the ability to evaluate intramural lesions. The fat density of lipoma is easily recognized confirming their diagnosis. Even small lipomas may be detected when careful technique using proper positioning and air distention of the duodenum is used (Fig. 4-13). Benign leiomyoma has a soft-tissue density and appears as a round homogeneous mass usually less than 3 cm (Fig. 4-14). Other neoplasms may be visualized but CT adds no further diagnostic specificity.

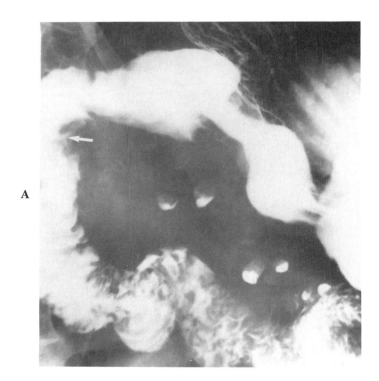

A

Fig. 4-13. Benign intramural mass—duodenal sweep. **A,** Film from the upper gastrointestinal series reveals a smoothly marginated defect along the medial wall of duodenal sweep *(arrow)*.   *Continued.*

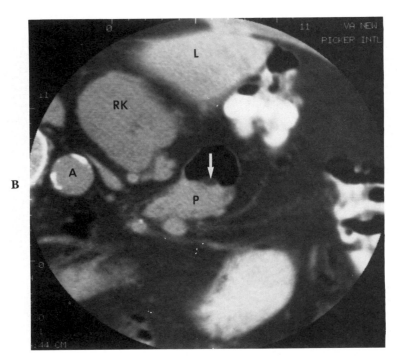

Fig. 4-13, cont'd. B, CT scan performed with the patient in a left-side-down decubitus position reveals a portion of the mass. The attenuation was −70 H units, allowing definitive diagnosis of a lipoma *(arrow)*. (Compare to the papilla seen in Fig. 4-1.) (*P*, pancreas; *RK*, right kidney; *L*, liver; *A*, aorta.)

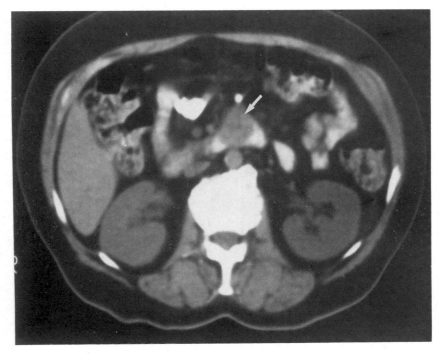

Fig. 4-14. Benign duodenal leiomyoma. Smoothly marginated soft-tissue density mass is seen along the medial margin of the third portion of the contrast-filled duodenum *(arrow)*. The homogeneous density and relatively small size (approximately 3.5 cm) compatible with a benign soft-tissue neoplasm. (Case courtesy Dr. R. Pochachevsky, Long Island Jewish Medical Center, New York, New York.)

MALIGNANT TUMORS
Adenocarcinoma

The duodenum is the most common site of small bowel adenocarcinoma with approximately 40% of lesions occurring in this segment, particularly in the second and third portions.[22] The gross appearance is that of alimentary adenocarcinoma elsewhere, and therefore stenotic or polypoid forms may be encountered. In CT scanning they are recognized as focal areas of wall thickening extending over several centimeters. Large lymph nodes are generally not seen adjacent to the neoplasm (Fig. 4-15).

Ochsner and Kleckner have classified periampullary duodenal neoplasms based on the relationship of the tumor to the papilla.[23] Group I or suprapapillary tumors cause intestinal obstruction and bleeding (Fig. 4-16). Group II periampullary tumors cause extrahepatic jaundice (Fig. 4-17), and Group III intrapapillary lesions are generally associated with gastrointestinal bleeding. In a patient with extrahepatic biliary obstruction we have found CT to be useful in distinguishing periampullary tumors from pancreatic masses. This requires careful scanning of the pancreas and distal common bile duct using 5 mm thick sections (Fig. 4-18). Air contrast techniques and scanning the patient in the left lateral decubitus position may be necessary to distend the duodenum with air and visualize the papilla. We have studied three patients with intrapapillary and periampullary tumors. In all of these patients the pancreatic duct as well as the common bile duct was dilated to the level of the ampulla. No mass was seen in the pancreatic head using the closely spaced 5 mm thin cut. In one case of an intrapapillary neoplasm, air distention allowed visualization of an irregularly thickened ulcerated papilla (Fig. 4-19). In other cases of periampullary tumors, the duodenum has a thick wall with an irregular inner surface signaling the presence of a neoplasm. If no masses are demonstrated by thin section CT scanning, ERCP must be obtained to evaluate the ampulla and attempt biopsy. We have seen one patient with an impacted stone in the ampulla causing marked swelling of the papilla with a resultant pseudotumor appearance. Interestingly in this patient, the pancreatic duct was not dilated as in those with periampullary neoplasms. However, the pseudotumor appearance of the enlarged papilla may cause significant differential diagnostic difficulties (Fig. 4-20). *Text continued on p. 203.*

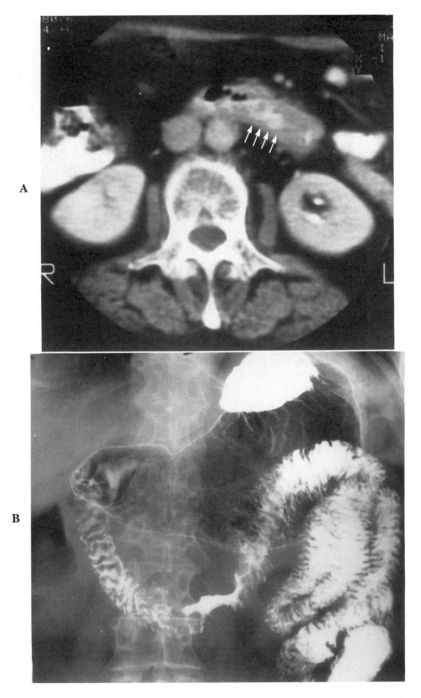

Fig. 4-15. Adenocarcinoma—duodenum. **A,** CT scan through the transverse duodenum. The duodenal wall is thickened and the mucosa (outlined by barium) is irregular (arrows). The appearance is similar to primary annular adenocarcinoma throughout the gastrointestinal tract. **B,** Film from the gastrointestinal series. The neoplasm appears as an ulcerated lesion with overhanging edges.

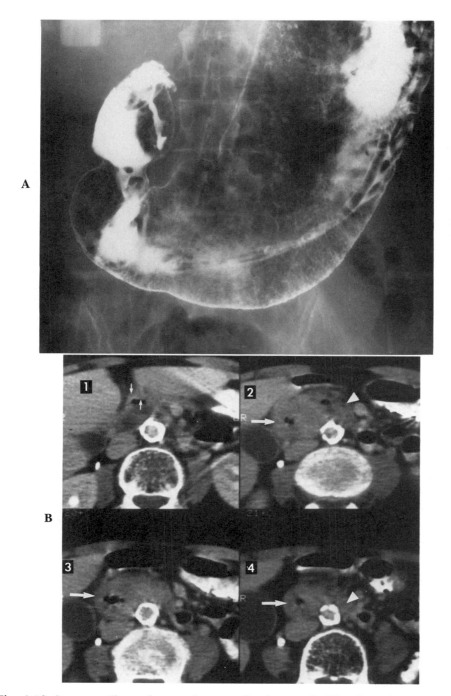

Fig. 4-16. Suprapapillary adenocarcinoma—duodenum. **A,** Film from the gastrointestinal series reveals a high-grade stenotic lesion in the second portion of the duodenum. The radiographic picture is compatible with neoplasm, although endoscopic biopsies failed to obtain a positive result for tumor. **B,** Sequential films from CT examination. The first image (1) shows a dilated, fluid-filled duodenal bulb. Note the normal thickness of the duodenal wall. A markedly thickened wall with a lobulated inner contour is revealed (2-4) *(arrows).* The mass is easily separated from the "acinerized" appearance of the pancreatic head *(arrowhead).*

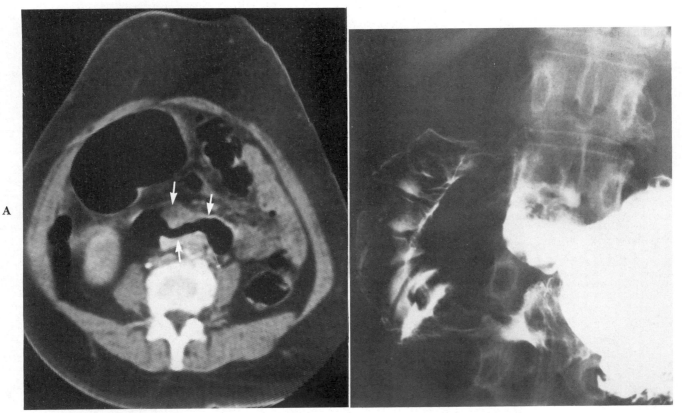

Fig. 4-17. Periampullary duodenal neoplasm. **A,** CT through the third duodenal segment reveals a lobulated, annular, constricting lesion in the third portion of the duodenum (*arrows*). The lumen is outlined with air; the patient was positioned on the left side. This patient was studied for obstructive jaundice. Cephalad scans revealed dilated intrahepatic bile ducts and a dilated common bile duct. No pancreatic mass was present. **B,** Film from the gastrointestinal series shows an annular, ulcerated lesion in the third duodenal segment. The lesion had infiltrated the papilla, leading to biliary obstruction.

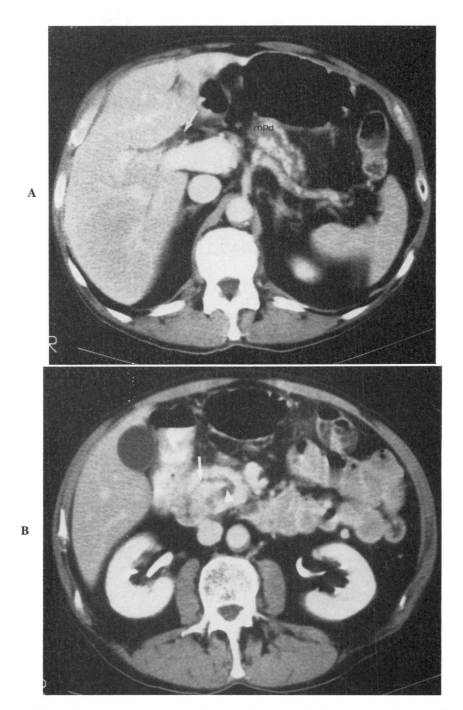

Fig. 4-18. Periampullary duodenal adenocarcinoma. **A,** CT scan through porta hepatis reveals minimally dilated, intrahepatic bile ducts *(arrow)*. The main pancreatic duct (mpd) is dilated as well. **B,** Scan through the level of the ampulla shows dilation of the accessory pancreatic duct *(arrow)* and common bile duct *(arrowhead)*. No mass is identified.

Continued.

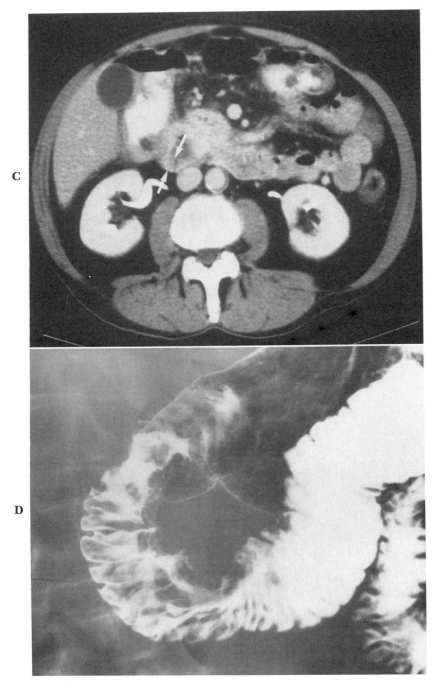

Fig. 4-18, cont'd. C, Scan approximately 10 mm caudad reveals a thickened duodenal wall. The lumen is filled with fluid and the mucosal surface appears nodular. These findings localize the obstructive process to the duodenum. **D,** Film from the gastrointestinal series. The papilla is enlarged and the mucosa is effaced. Adenocarcinoma of duodenal origin was resected. CT is of inestimable value in distinguishing between primary duodenal neoplasms and adjacent malignant processes.

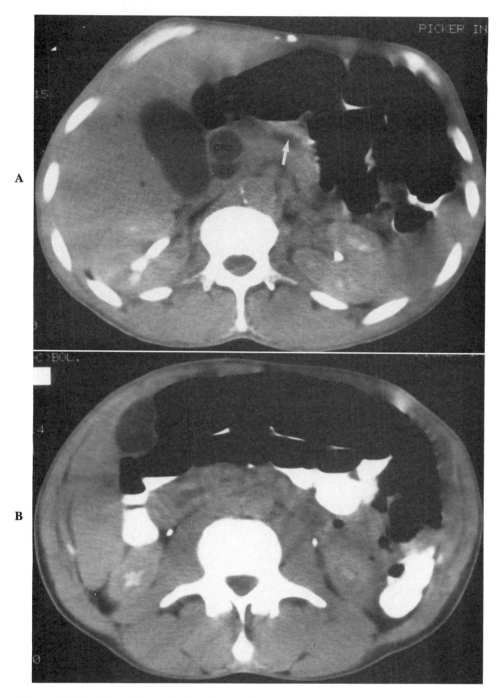

Fig. 4-19. Small papillary duodenal neoplasm. **A,** Air contrast CT scan in a jaundiced patient reveals a dilated gallbladder, cystic duct *(CD)*, common bile duct *(CBD)*, and main pancreatic duct *(arrow)*. **B,** Scan at level of papilla reveals dilated common duct without a visible mass, despite good, positive contrast opacification.   *Continued.*

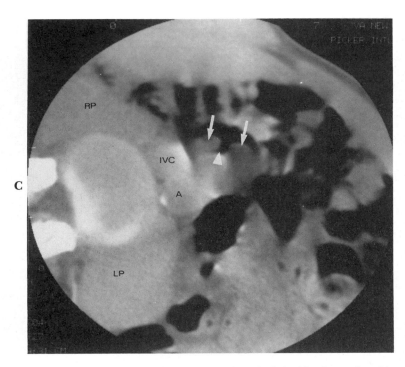

Fig. 4-19, cont'd. C, Air contrast scan with patient in left-side-down decubitus position. The duodenal lumen is now filled with air. The neoplasm is visualized as a bilobed mass *(arrows)* with a central depression *(arrowhead)*. The contour of the papilla is enlarged, lobulated, and distorted compared with a normal papilla. *(A, aorta; P, psoas; IVC, inferior vena cava.)*

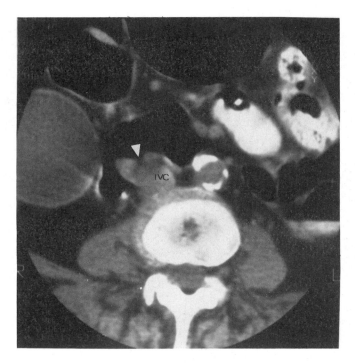

Fig. 4-20. Enlarged papilla from impacted common duct stone. Scan through the papilla in a jaundiced patient reveals an enlarged papilla *(arrowhead)*. The inferior vena cava *(IVC)* is immediately posterior. The patient was clinically jaundiced and this scan was interpreted as being consistent with a periampullary neoplasm. Surgery revealed a markedly swollen papilla resulting from an impacted common duct stone.

SARCOMAS

Leiomyosarcoma appears as a large, ulcerated, exophytic mass. On barium studies these tumors may elevate the transverse colon and produce ulceration along the third portion of the duodenum[24] (Fig. 4-21). As in the remainder of the alimentary tract, CT is useful in distinguishing malignant from benign, soft-tissue neoplasms.[25]

Lymphoma rarely affects the duodenum. When it does, it causes marked wall thickening and bulky periduodenal lymphadenopathy[26] (Fig. 4-22). We have seen one patient who had Hodgkin's disease of the duodenum in which the adenopathy could not be recognized; however, duodenal involvement is extraordinarily rare in Hodgkin's disease.[27] Therefore the CT appearance of this rather unique duodenal lesion may be an exception rather than a rule (Fig. 4-23). In cases of duodenal lymphoma, because the surrounding nodes are so large, it may be difficult to predict actual duodenal involvement versus extrinsic distortion by bulky extrinsic adenopathy. Barium radiography is necessary to distinguish these possibilities.

A

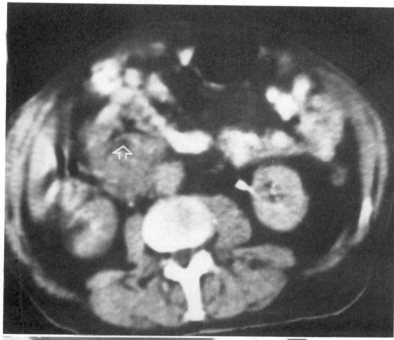

B

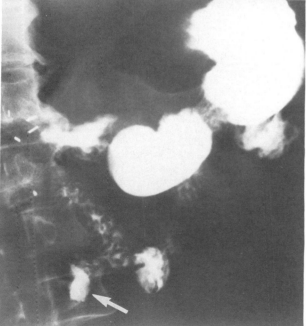

Fig. 4-21. Leiomyosarcoma—duodenum. **A,** CT through the mid-kidneys. The contrast-filled duodenum is elevated and medially displaced (*arrows*) by a large exophytic mass. Air is seen within the mass representing an ulcer crater (*open arrow*). CT was the first examination in this patient who was complaining of ill-defined epigastric pain. **B,** Film from water-soluble gastrointestinal series shows preserved mucosa along the second portion of the duodenum. The sweep is displaced medially. Contrast material fills the ulcer crater (*arrow*) (compare to Fig. 4-13). Leiomyosarcomas are differentiated by their size, inhomogeneity, and tendency toward ulceration.

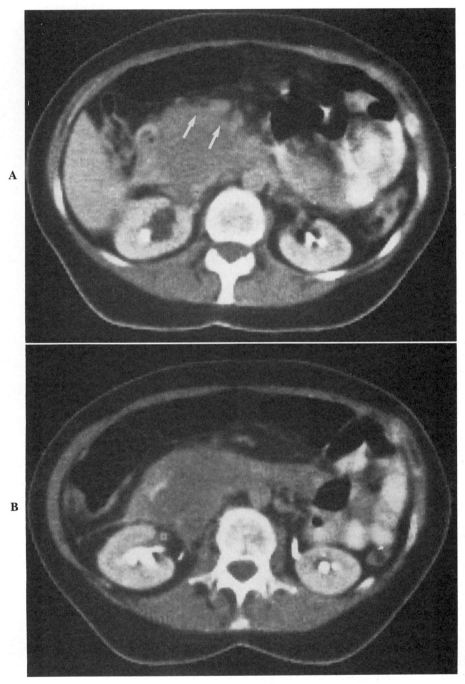

Fig. 4-22. Histiocytic lymphoma—duodenum. **A** and **B,** CT scans reveal a poorly defined soft-tissue mass within the right anterior pararenal space. Notice the anteromedial displacement of the pancreatic head *(arrows)*. The presence of duodenal involvement is impossible to predict on the basis of CT alone.

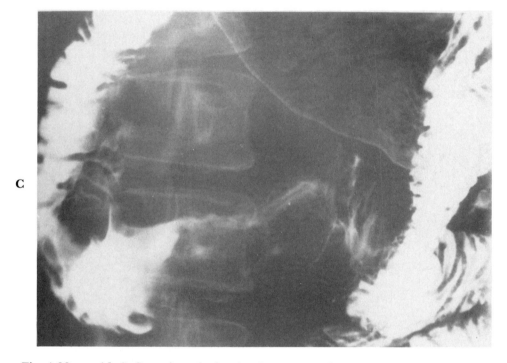

C

Fig. 4-22, cont'd. C, Gastrointestinal series shows narrowing of the lumen and infiltration of the folds of the third portion of the duodenum. Surgery revealed histiocytic lymphoma.

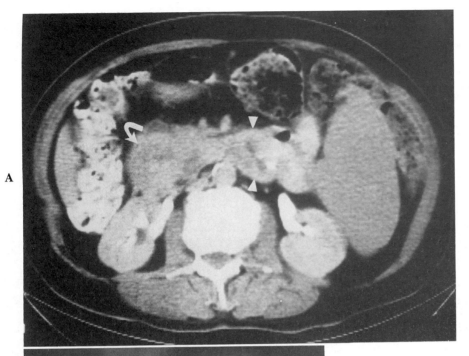

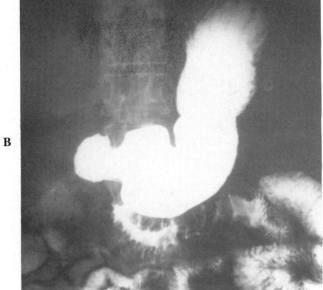

Fig. 4-23. Hodgkin's disease—duodenum. **A,** CT through the transverse duodenum reveals a diffusely thickened duodenal wall in both the junction of second and third portions *(curved arrow)* and third and fourth portions *(arrowheads).* No adenopathy is seen. The abnormality is restricted to the duodenal wall. **B,** Film from the gastrointestinal series shows marked submucosal infiltration of the transverse duodenum without mucosal destruction. Biopsy revealed Hodgkin's disease. (Case courtesy Dr. K.Y. Cho, Albert Einstein College of Medicine, Bronx, New York.)

SECONDARY INVOLVEMENT OF THE DUODENUM BY MALIGNANT DISEASE

Because the duodenum interfaces with a variety of retroperitoneal structures, neoplasms in any of these structures may directly invade the duodenum, giving the appearance of a mucosal based lesion.

Pancreas

Carcinoma of the pancreas may directly invade the medial wall of the duodenum causing ulceration and obstruction. We have seen 5 cases with duodenal obstruction in over 200 patients with pancreatic carcinoma. Infiltration of the duodenal mucosa, which produces the classic "barium findings" of spiculation and focal tethering of mucosal folds, are more difficult to detect (Fig. 4-24). We do not recognize duodenal mucosal changes in from 76% to 84% with pancreatic cancer studied by CT as compared to reports of hypotonic duodenography.[28] However, the advantages of directly imaging the pancreatic mass and assessing the status of peripancreatic vessels and the liver has supplanted hypotonic duodenography in the diagnostic evaluation of pancreatic carcinoma. CT is also useful in predicting those patients in whom duodenal obstruction is imminent and thus in selecting patients for palliative gastrojejunostomies.

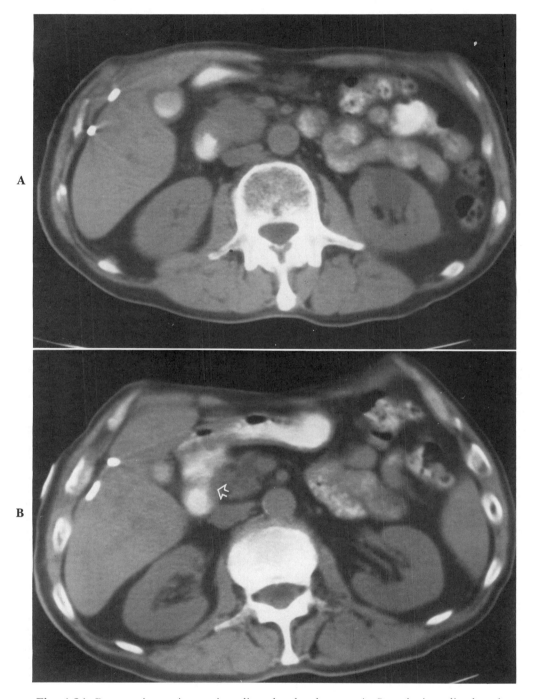

Fig. 4-24. Pancreatic carcinoma invading the duodenum. **A,** Scan in jaundiced patient reveals a mass in the head of the pancreas. The superior mesenteric vessels are free of the mass. **B,** Scan slightly cephalad reveals an irregular appearance to the medial wall of the proximal duodenum. Compare to the lateral wall *(open arrow)*. At surgery the duodenum was infiltrated.

Peripancreatic nodal metastases

Neoplasia in peripancreatic nodes may invade the duodenum. These patients will have signs of upper intestinal obstruction and vomiting. CT reveals bulky masses surrounding the pancreatic head and encasing the duodenum. Lymphoma, lung, and breast primaries are the most likely neoplasms to produce neoplastic invasion or encasement of the duodenum from adjacent nodal metastases (Fig. 4-25).

Retroperitoneal nodal metastases may invade the transverse portion of the duodenum. We have seen three cases of metastatic retroperitoneal lymph nodes (seminoma, endometrial carcinoma, and bladder carcinoma) eroding the duodenal mucosa. Gastrointestinal series suggest intrinsic duo-

denal pathology. The CT scan shows a retroperitoneal mass of lymphadenopathy and may show air or contrast material within the mass indicating direct fistulization into the duodenum (Fig. 4-26). Hulnick et al. have reported peripancreatic tuberculous lymph nodes invading the duodenum and producing large ulcerations within the duodenal lumen. Needle biopsy is necessary in these patients to prove the diagnosis of tuberculosis and to differentiate it from lymphoma. This possibility should be considered in any patient who is immunocompromised or has a history of intravenous drug abuse.[29] Skinny needle biopsy may be performed and specimens should be cultured for *Mycobacterium tuberculosis* or atypical forms of tuberculosis in any of the above situations (Fig. 4-27).[30]

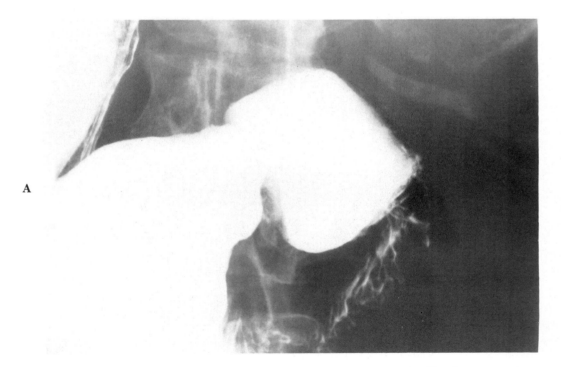

Fig. 4-25. Peripancreatic adenopathy obstructing the duodenum. **A,** Film from gastrointestinal series in a patient with known breast carcinoma and gastric outlet obstruction. There is abrupt narrowing of the lumen just distal to the apex of the duodenal bulb. This is the point at which the duodenal bulb becomes the retroperitoneal.

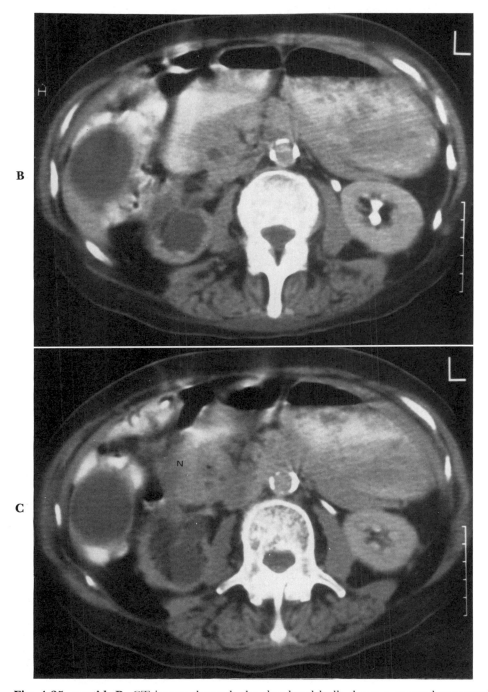

Fig. 4-25, cont'd. B, CT image through the duodenal bulb shows a normal pancreatic neck; the intrapancreatic common bile duct is dilated. There is evidence of right hydronephrosis. **C,** CT scan slightly caudad reveals enlarged peripancreatic lymph nodes surrounding the duodenum with obliteration of fat planes around the inferior vena cava. Needle biopsy confirmed metastatic breast carcinoma. (*N,* nodes.)

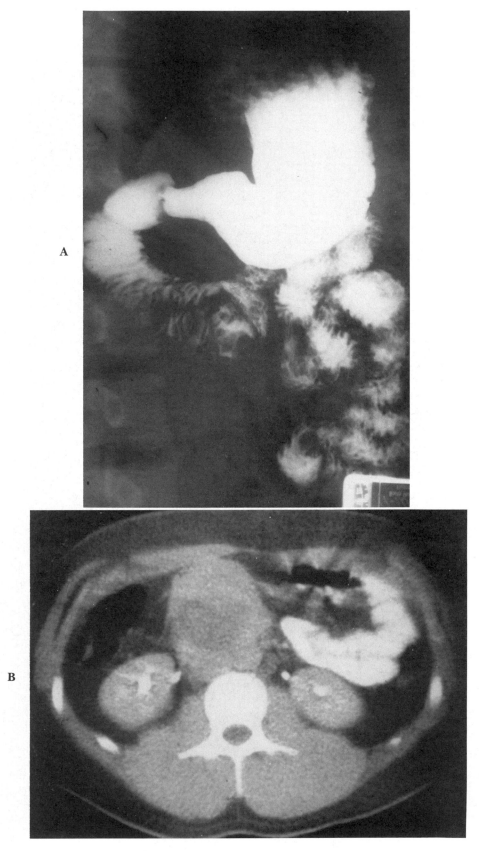

Fig. 4-26. For legend see opposite page.

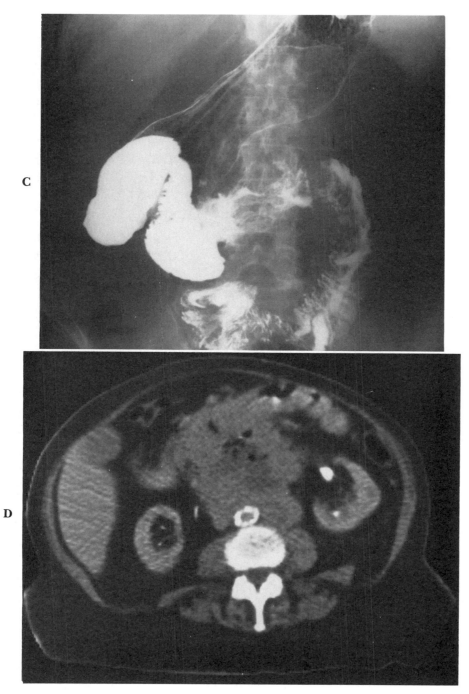

Fig. 4-26. Retroperitoneal metastases invading the duodenum. **A,** Film from gastrointestinal series. An ulcerated lesion is noted along the inferior aspect of the transverse duodenum. The findings are compatible with a primary duodenal neoplasm. **B,** CT through the transverse duodenum shows a large retroperitoneal mass engulfing the duodenal lumen. Surgery revealed a retroperitoneal seminoma. **C,** Gastrointestinal series in another patient revealing a distended lesion along the transverse duodenum. A mass impression is seen along the proximal small bowel. **D,** CT scan shows a large retroperitoneal mass invading the third portion of the duodenum. The presence of air results from fistulization into the duodenal lumen. This had a known endometrial carcinoma; the retroperitoneal mass represented metastatic disease. (**A** and **B** courtesy Drs. B. Held and R. Meisell, Booth Memorial Hospital, Flushing, New York.)

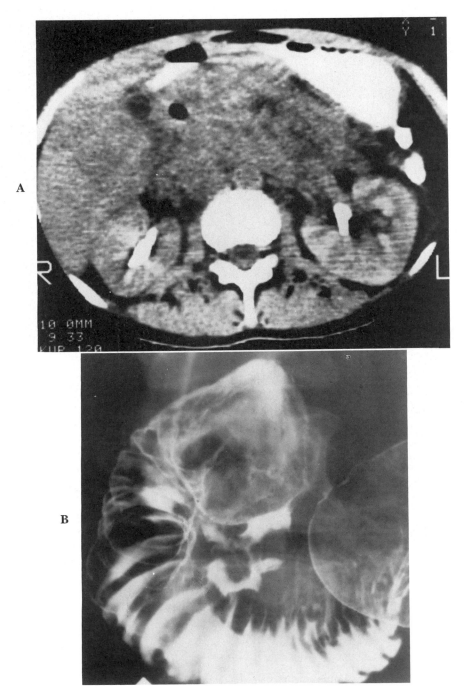

Fig. 4-27. Peripancreatic nodes with fistulization into the duodenum. **A,** A CT scan through the pancreas reveals a poorly defined mass elevating the duodenal bulb and obliterating normal anatomy. An air collection is noted within the mass. **B,** A spot film from the gastrointestinal series reveals spiculation of the mucosal folds along the medial aspect of the duodenum. A large cavity fills with barium. Needle biopsy reveals *Mycobacterium avium-intracellulare* in a patient with AIDS. (Courtesy Dr. K.Y. Cho, Bronx, New York.)

Direct extension from adjacent viscera

Carcinoma of the gallbladder extends into the colon and duodenum. We have seen one case of pyloroduodenal obstruction from infiltrating gallbladder carcinoma into the proximal duodenum (see Fig. 3-42). Carcinoma of the hepatic flexure may extend across the transverse mesocolon into the second portion of the duodenum. These changes may lead to symptoms suggestive of upper gastrointestinal pathology (Fig. 4-28). CT provides a single imaging modality to assess the primary tumor and its extension into adjacent bowel loops.[31]

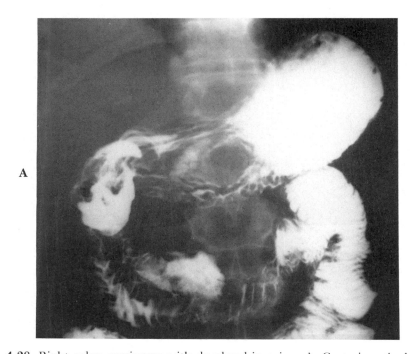

A

Fig. 4-28. Right colon carcinoma with duodenal invasion. **A,** Gastrointestinal series reveals infiltration and ulceration in the duodenal sweep. *Continued.*

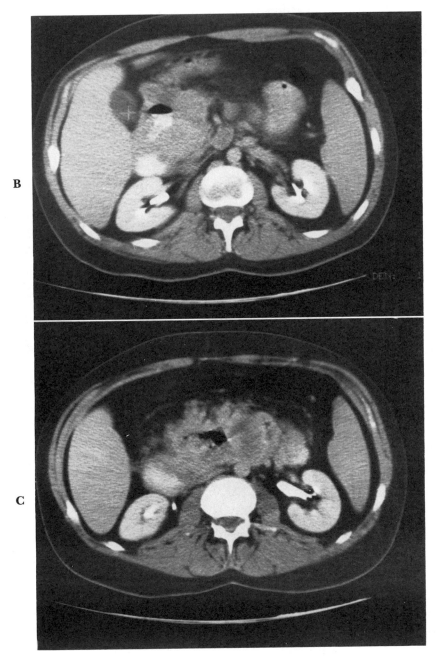

Fig. 4-28, cont'd. B and **C,** CT scans at adjacent levels reveal the presence of a large soft-tissue mass surrounding the duodenum. The irregular air collection seen in **C** signifies the presence of ulceration. The patient was treated for right colon carcinoma 2 years previous. Needle biopsy confirms recurrent tumor invading the duodenum.

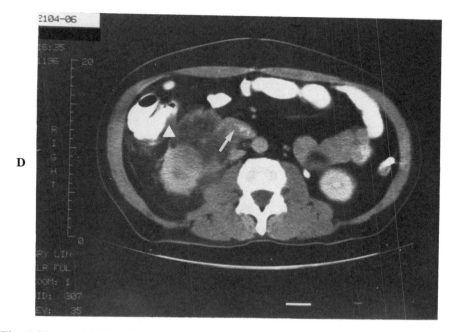

Fig. 4-28, cont'd. D, A CT scan in another patient reveals a low-density mass infiltrating the lateral aspect of the third portion of the duodenum *(arrow)* and the right kidney. A small zone of attachment can be appreciated along the medial border of the ascending colon at the level of a previous ileo transverse colon anastomosis *(arrowhead)*. Needle biopsy confirmed recurrent mucin producing carcinoma of the colon. (Cases courtesy Dr. R. Surapeneni, Brooklyn Veterans Administration Hospital, Brooklyn, New York.)

REFERENCES

1. Meyers, M.A.: Dynamic radiology of the abdomen, New York, 1976, Springer-Verlag New York Inc.
2. Lieberman, J.M., and Haaga, J.A.: Duodenal malrotation, J. Comput. Assist. Tomogr. **6:**1019-1920, 1982.
3. Zeman, R.K., Schiebler, M., Clark, L.R., et al.: The clinical and imaging spectrum of pancreatico-duodenal lymph node enlargement. AJR **144:**1223-1227, 1985.
4. Zirinsky, K., Auh, Y., Rubenstein, W.A., et al.: The porta caval space: CT with MR correlation, Radiology **156:**453-460, 1985.
5. Schultz, E.H.: Aids to diagnosis of acute pancreatitis by Roentgen study, AJR **89:**825-836, 1963.
6. Jeffrey, R.B., Federle, M.P., and Laing, F.C.: Computed tomography of mesenteric involvement in fulminant pancreatitis, Radiology **147:**185-188, 1983.
7. Simon, M., and Lerner, M.A.: Duodenal compression by mesenteric root in acute pancreatitis, Radiology **79:**75-80, 1962.
7a. McGowan, M.J., and Federle, M.P.: Computed tomography of pancreatic pseudocysts of the duodenum, Am. J. Roentgenot. **145:**1003-1009, 1985.
8. Roman, E., Silva, Y., and Lucas, C.: Management of blunt duodenal injury, Surg. Gynecol. Obstet. **132:**7-14, 1971.
9. Toxopeus, M.D., Lucas, C.E., and Krabbenhoft, K.L.: Roentgenographic diagnosis in blunt retroperitoneal duodenal rupture, Radiology **115:**281-288, 1972.
10. Glazer, G.M., Buy, J.N., Moss, A.A., et al.: CT detection of duodenal perforation, AJR **137:**333-336, 1981.

11. Karnaze, G.C., Sheedy, P.F., Stephens, D.H., et al.: Computed tomography in duodenal rupture due to blunt abdominal trauma, J. Comput. Assist. Tomogr. **5:**267-269, 1981.
12. Cook, D.E., Walsh, J.W., Vick, C.W., et al.: Upper abdominal trauma; pitfalls in CT diagnosis, Radiology **159:**65-69, 1986.
13. Jeffrey, R.B., Federle, M.P., and Crass, P.A.: Computed tomography of pancreatic trauma, Radiology **147:**491-494, 1983.
14. Madrazo, B.L., Halpert, R.D., Sandler, M.A., et al.: Computed tomographic findings in penetrating peptic ulcer, Radiology **153:**751-754, 1984.
15. Fielding, J.F., Toye, D.K.M., Beton, D.C., et al.: Crohn's disease of the stomach and duodenum, Gut **11:**1001-1006, 1970.
16. Harkavy, L.A., Balthazar, E.J., and Naidich, D.P.: CT diagnosis of cholecysto duodenal fistula, Am. J. Gastroenterol. Am. J. Gastroenterol. **80:**569-571, 1985.
17. Edwards, K.C., and Katzen, B.T.: Superior mesenteric artery syndrome due to large dissecting aortic aneurysm, Am. J. Gastroenterol. **79:**72-75, 1974.
18. Reasbeck, P.G.: Vascular compression of the duodenum following resection of an abdominal aortic aneurysm, NZ Med. J. **92:**198-199, 1980.
19. Hilton, S., Megibow, A.J., Naidich, D.P., et al.: Computed tomography of the postoperative abdominal aorta, Radiology **145:**403-407, 1982.

20. Pelz, D.M., and Roetgen, R.M.: Alternate bleeding sites in suspected graft enteric fistula, AJR **136**:707-709, 1981.

21. Qizilbash, A.H.: Epithelial neoplasms of the duodenum and periampullary region. In Appelman, H.D., editor: Pathology of the esophagus, stomach, and duodenum, New York, 1984, Churchill Livingstone Inc.

22. Wilson, J.M., Mubrin, D.P., Gray, G.F., et al.: Primary malignancies of the small bowel: a report of 96 cases and review of the literature, Ann. Surg. **180**:175-179, 1974.

23. Ochsner, S., and Kleckner, M.S.: Primary malignant neoplasms of the duodenum, JAMA **163**:413-417, 1957.

24. Meyers, M.A.: Leiomyosarcoma of the duodenum: radiographic and arteriographic appearances, Clin. Radiol. **22**:257-260, 1971.

25. Megibow, A.J., Balthazar, E.J., Hulnick, D.H., et al.: CT evaluation of leiomyomas and leiomyosarcomas, AJR **144**:727-733, 1985.

26. Balthazar, E.J.: Hodgkins disease of the duodenum. Am. J. Gastroenterol. **68**:306-311, 1977.

27. Megibow, A.J., Balthazar, E.J., Naidich, D.P., et al.: CT of gastrointestinal lymphoma, AJR **141**:541-548, 1983.

28. Bilbao, M.E., Rosch, J., Frische, L.H., et al.: Hypotonic duodenography in the diagnosis of pancreatic disease, Semin. Roentgenol. **3**:280-287, 1968.

29. Willis, R.A.: Secondary tumors of the stomach, pancreas, and gallbladder. In The spread of tumors in the human body, Baltimore, 1952, Butterworth Publishers.

30. Hulnick, D.H., Megibow, A.J., Naidich, D.P., et al.: Abdominal tuberculosis evaluated by computed tomography, Radiology **157**:199-205, 1985.

31. Meyers, M.A. and Whalen, J.P.: Roentgen significance of duodeno-colic relationships: anatomic approach, AJR **117**:263-274, 1973.

Chapter Five

SMALL INTESTINE

Donald H. Hulnick

Signs and symptoms of disease in the small intestine are often nonspecific, and clinical attention is usually focused on more common conditions involving the upper gastrointestinal tract, biliary system, or colon. Beyond the reach of the endoscope, the small bowel lumen and its mucosal surface are best evaluated by barium studies. However, even when performed to high standards, these examinations provide only indirect signs of extramucosal disease. Intramural, serosal, mesenteric, or peritoneal disease are imaged only indirectly by their effects on the bowel lumen. It is particularly in relation to these extramucosal manifestations of small bowel disease that CT becomes most important.

The indications for CT evaluation of the small intestine are multiple and still growing in number. Following abnormal results from barium studies, CT may provide important correlative and additional information about the extraluminal component of bowel disease, the relationship of adjacent organs and tissues, and ancillary intra-abdominal findings. Patients may also be referred for evaluation of unusual or nonspecific abdominal complaints, unexplained bleeding, or clinical suspicion of disease undetected by barium studies or endoscopy. Not being organ-specific, CT is evolving as a survey or screening modality, and in many instances, CT may be the first diagnostic examination performed. Therefore it behooves the radiologist to optimize CT techniques that delineate the small bowel, recognize and categorize the site and nature of small bowel disease, and direct further diagnostic or therapeutic management.

TECHNIQUES

CT evaluation of the abdomen and pelvis in general, and of the small intestine in particular, requires optimal opacification of the bowel lumen. Positive contrast opacification is achieved by orally administering a dilute barium suspension (1.5% to 3% W/W) or water-soluble iodinated solution (e.g. 10 to 12 ml Gastrografin to 400 ml water), if there is a question of bowel perforation or complete small bowel obstruction. In order to delineate the entire small bowel in most patients, the contrast material must be given beginning at least 45 minutes before scanning. Apart from patient tolerance, there is no maximum dose, and in general, the more contrast material given the more reliable the bowel opacification. A minimum of 750 ml should be given with approximately 250 ml being given within 15 minutes of scanning. If an interpretive problem arises in distinguishing unopacified fluid-filled or collapsed bowel loops from pathologic mass, administration of more oral contrast material or a change in patient position may be necessary (see Chapter One).

These traditional techniques for positive opacification of the bowel lumen have proved quite reliable. Negative contrast techniques using air or gas to outline the bowel lumen are of enormous value in evaluation of those portions of the alimentary tube that can easily be reached by orally administered effervescent granules or insufflation of air through a rectal tube. However, these techniques are less easily applied to the jejunum and ileum because of their less accessible location and less predictable position. Although orally administered enteric-coated time release effervescent tablets have shown promising preliminary results in outlining the small bowel lumen with negative contrast,[1] positive opacification remains the method of choice.

NORMAL ANATOMY

Several features of normal mesenteric small bowel anatomy are particularly relevant for CT analysis. On CT, as on barium studies, jejunal loops with their feathery mucosal pattern and valvulae conniventes are usually seen in the left upper abdomen (Fig. 5-1, *A*). Ileal loops, with a less featured mucosal pattern, tend to lie in the right lower abdomen and pelvis (Fig. 5-1, *B*). The ileocecal valve appears as a fat density, intraluminal mass in the cecum and is useful in orienting pathology in the right lower quadrant (Fig. 5-2).

In general, the normal luminal diameter of the small intestine does not exceed 3 cm. Normal intestinal wall thickness is less than 3 to 4 mm and valvulae conniventes or mucosal folds are barely apparent, although increasing use of higher resolution scanners reveals mucosal detail in a greater percentage of cases (Fig. 5-1). However, the bowel wall or mucosal folds may spuriously appear thickened if the lumen is not physiologically distended. Furthermore, bowel wall thickness can accurately be measured only when the lumen is clearly defined, well-contrasted by either intraluminal gas or densely opacified fluid.

The peritoneal folds that form the small bowel mesentery itself are usually not directly visible by CT, but the neurovascular bundles they carry can easily be identified between the mesenteric leaves. The superior mesenteric artery and vein are always recognized in their retropancreatic position. Inferior mesenteric trunks, being considerably smaller, are less routinely visualized.[2] Depending primarily on the relative amount of intra-abdominal body fat, portions of branch vessels feeding the bowel from jejunum to rectum can usually be identified.

Mesenteric lymph nodes are normally not identified or are seen only as small, less than 5 mm linear or nodular soft tissue densities.[3] Adenopathy may be manifest as enlargement greater than 15 mm of a few nodes or as an increased number of small nodes. The greater omentum extends from the transverse colon inferiorly, draping over the ventral aspect of the mesentery and small bowel loops. Differentiation of mesenteric or other peritoneal surfaces from the greater omentum may not always be possible in thin patients with insufficient abdominal fat.

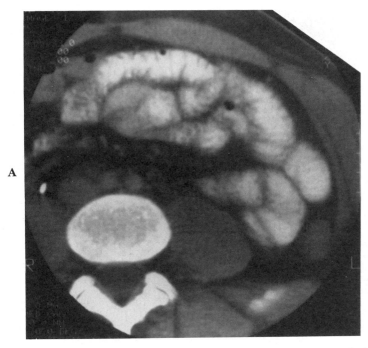

Fig. 5-1. Normal anatomy. **A,** Jejunal loops in the upper abdomen are filled with positive contrast material. Note the feathery mucosal fold pattern and the thin bowel wall.

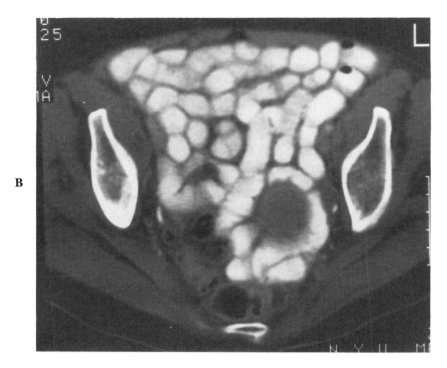

Fig. 5-1, cont'd. B, Ileal loops in the lower abdomen are filled with positive contrast material. The luminal surface is featureless, and the bowel wall itself is barely evident.

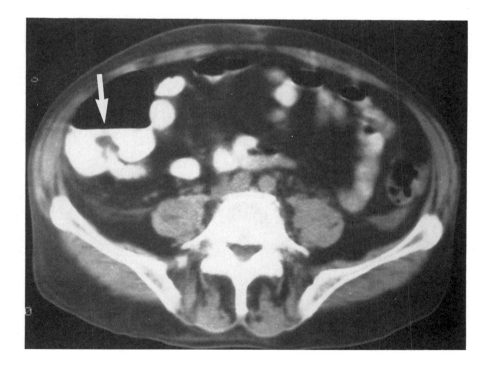

Fig. 5-2. Scan through the lower abdomen demonstrates the terminal ileum entering the cecum *(arrow)*.

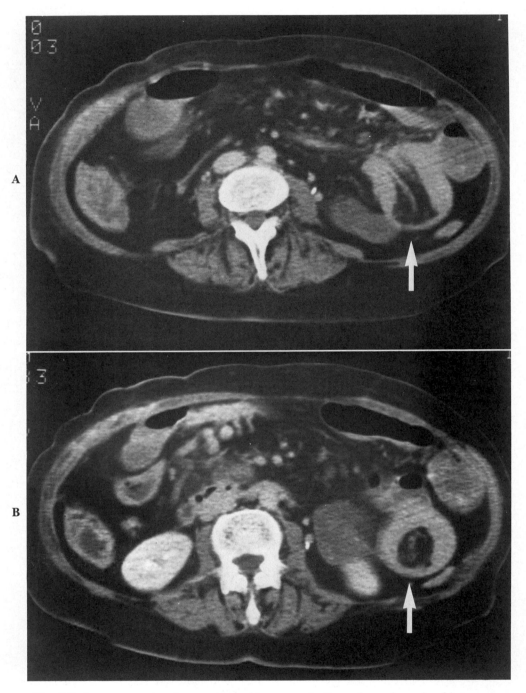

Fig. 5-3. Intussusception in a patient with sprue. **A,** Scan along the axis of intussusception. Mesenteric vessels accompanied by mesenteric fat are seen intussuscepting into a jejunal loop in the left upper quadrant *(arrow)*. **B,** Scan perpendicular to the axis of intussusception. The mesenteric vessels and fat are circumferentially enclosed within the intussuscipiens *(arrow)*. In this patient, there was no mass leading the intussusception.

A knowledge of these basic concepts of mesenteric anatomy explains the characteristic CT appearance of small bowel intussusceptions.[4] Best recognized in either true cross or longitudinal section, the soft-tissue density of the intussuscepting loop is seen centrally, eccentrically surrounded by the fat density of the mesentery and vessels that it carries forward (Figs. 5-3 and 5-4). In turn, the intussusception and its mesentery is enclosed within the intussuscepiens—the inverted wall centrally and the receiving wall peripherally.

A variety of rotational abnormalities may be recognized. In complete nonrotation of the midgut, jejunal loops lie in the right upper quadrant and the colon may be positioned entirely on the left (Fig. 5-4). However, nonrotation of the colon does not necessarily accompany anomalous midgut rotation. Depending on the degree of failure of complete rotation around the mesenteric axis, the ligament of Treitz may be positioned on the right or at midline, but the duodenum is always seen passing dorsal to the mesenteric vessels. A whorled appearance to the mesentery suspending the jejunum (Fig. 5-4, *C*) or to the superior mesenteric artery lying to the left of the superior mesenteric vein (Fig. 5-4, *B*) may be seen in asymptomatic patients with midgut malrotation, but the combination of both signs suggests midgut volvulus.[5]

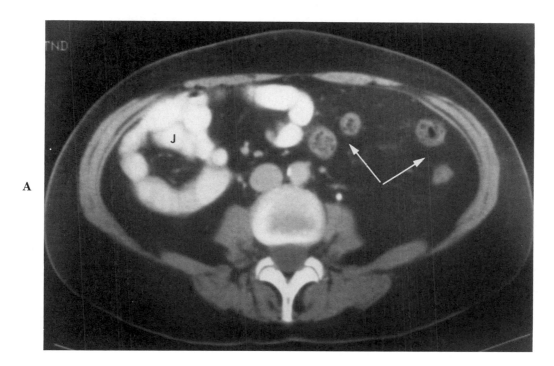

Fig. 5-4. Malrotation. **A,** Scan through the mid-abdomen shows jejunal loops (*J*) positioned on the right side and both ascending and descending colon positioned on the left (*arrows*), indicating complete non-rotation of the midgut.   *Continued.*

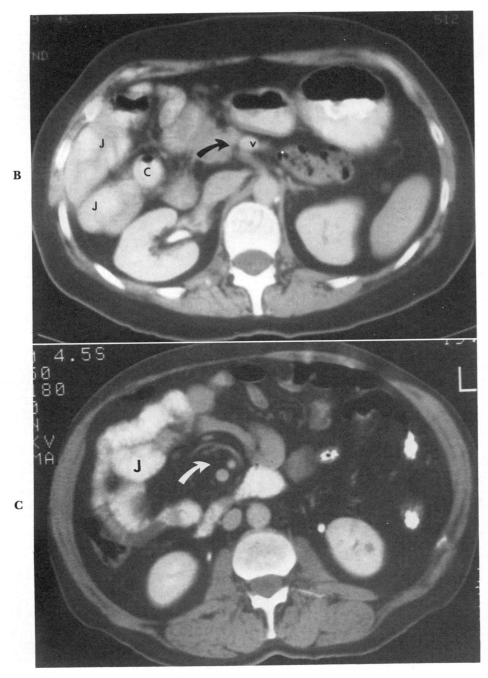

Fig. 5-4, cont'd. B, In another patient, the superior mesenteric artery *(curved arrow)* is seen coursing to the right of the superior mesenteric vein *(V)*, a reversal of their normal relationship. Jejunal loops *(J)* are seen in the right upper quadrant. This patient, who has small bowel malrotation and a normally positioned colon *(C)*, was asymptomatic. **C,** In a third patient, there is a whorled appearance to the mesentery, suspending the jejunum *(J)* in the right upper quadrant *(curved arrow)*. However, the relationship of the superior mesenteric artery to the superior mesenteric vein is normal, there is no volvulus, and the patient was asymptomatic.

PRINCIPLES OF CT DIAGNOSIS

Analysis of the small bowel and mesentery as portrayed by CT requires adherence to an organized framework analogous to that used in analysis of barium studies. First, pathologic findings should be localized to the mucosal surface, bowel wall, or extramural tissues. Whereas barium studies become progressively less efficacious in portraying extraluminal disease in the bowel wall, serosa, mesentery, and peritoneal cavity, CT becomes progressively more useful. Thus mucosal processes remain the province of barium studies, and mural and extramural processes are best analyzed by CT. The advantages and disadvantages of both modalities are complimentary, and often both must be employed for optimal diagnostic potential.

Identification of the segment(s) of bowel involved is important in view of the propensity for different disease processes to involve different portions of the small bowel. Multiplicity of sites of disease or diffuse involvement should be ascertained. Luminal caliber and the status of the stomach and colon are also relevant. Ancillary findings in other abdominal viscera, the status of lymph nodes, and the presence or absence of ascites must also be noted in order to refine the differential diagnosis.

VASCULAR DISEASES

In this section we consider the role of CT in evaluating those processes that affect the mesenteric circulation at the arterial, venous, and capillary levels. In many cases, CT can add specificity to difficult differential diagnostic dilemmas on barium studies by visualizing abnormalities in the mesentery, specifically in the vessels and lymphatics.

Ischemia

Ischemic disease of the small bowel is usually not associated with major vessel occlusions but is rather the result of low flow states from a myriad of causes. This results in edema causing thickening of the bowel wall. Involvement may be diffuse or segmental depending on the site and extent of vascular compromise. Even when segmental, however, relatively long segments of bowel are involved (Fig. 5-5). Generalized ileus or proximal dilation may be associated, and intraluminal fluid content is generally increased.[6] When ischemia is severe, there is blurring of the definition of the bowel wall and ascites (Fig. 5-5, *B*). Although the mucosa may not be displayed, the symmetry and regularity of the bowel wall thickening and the segmental nature of the process usually allow a correct diagnosis.

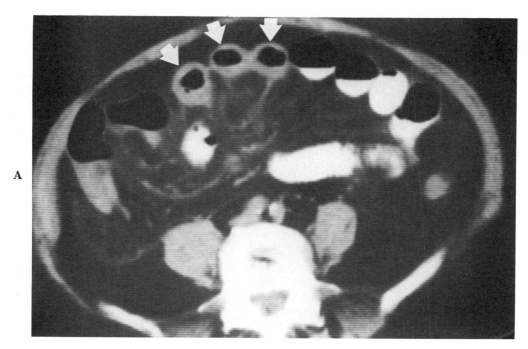

Fig. 5-5. Ischemia. **A,** Several loops of ileum in the right lower quadrant show symmetric circumferential bowel wall thickening *(arrows)*. Accentuation of mesenteric vessels in the region subtending these loops of bowel reflect localized congestion and edema.

Continued.

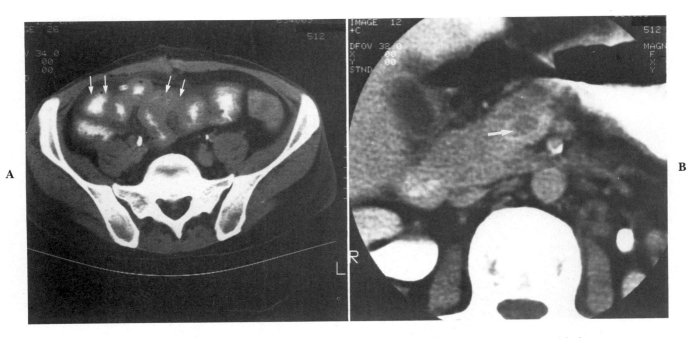

Fig. 5-5, cont'd. B, In another patient, severe ischemic disease is reflected in diffuse bowel wall thickening *(arrows)* and marked accentuation of mesenteric markings. The diffuse, hazy appearance of the mesenteric fat reflects severe edema. This patient, who had a gangrenous bowel, died 48 hours after the CT examination.

Fig. 5-6. Superior mesenteric venous thrombosis. **A,** A CT scan through the mid-abdomen in a febrile patient 10 days following abdominal surgery reveals ascites and diffuse thickening of the intestinal walls of all visualized loops. **B,** A scan through the head of the pancreas reveals thrombosis of the superior mesenteric vein *(arrow).* The cause is presumed to be a hypercoagulable state. The symptoms resolved on anticoagulation, and the bowel resumed a normal appearance on follow-up examinations.

Occlusions of either the arterial or venous superior mesenteric trunks may be differentiated by CT. Intravenous contrast material must be administered. Arterial thrombi are recognized as intraluminal filling defects of different CT density than opacified flowing blood.[3,6] Calcific atherosclerotic plaques related to the aorta and major branch vessels may be seen as well. This finding is not uncommon in the elderly, and it is an isolated abnormality not necessarily associated with bowel ischemia.

Venous thromboses in the superior mesenteric vein, splenic vein, or portal vein appear as low-density intraluminal filling defects, perhaps with a thin, enhanced, surrounding rim representing either enhanced vasa vasorum, inflammatory reaction, or blood flow around the clot (Fig. 5-6). With dynamic scanning techniques and high intravascular contrast levels, collateral vessels may also be recognized. Small intestinal loops subtended by the thrombosed veins show edematous wall thickening, increased fluid content, and blurring of luminal and serosal margins. The mesentery itself also appears "waterlogged."[7]

Pneumatosis intestinalis. Pneumatosis intestinalis is readily recognized on CT as gas collections within the bowel wall, either in linear streaks, bubbles, or cysts. Being extraluminal, the gas is seen peripherally and in dependent as well as nondependent portions of the bowel wall. The use of "lung" window and level settings (wide window, low level) aids in detecting small collections of intraluminal gas[8] (Fig. 5-7). Because there is no overlap of other bowel loops and because CT is so sensitive in identifying gas density, pneumatosis intestinalis is more easily diagnosed on CT than by abdominal radiographs.[8,9] Differentiation of "benign" or "primary" causes from "malignant" or "secondary" causes is also faciliated by CT. A curvilinear rather than cystlike configuration to the intramural gas collections, soft-tissue density thickening of the bowel wall, and enhancement of the wall following intravenous enhancement suggest bowel infarction.[9] In those patients with known ischemic disease, CT is useful in early detection of pneumatosis and the complications of mesenteric or portal venous gas.[10]

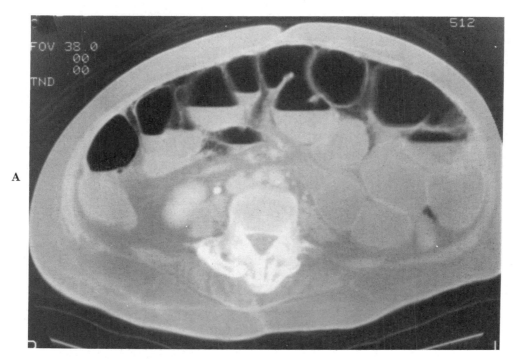

Fig. 5-7. Pneumatosis intestinalis. **A,** A scan through the mid-abdomen demonstrates curvalinear gas collections within the walls of multiple loops of small bowel. This gas is seen in dependent surfaces, appearing to dissect the layers of the wall. "Lung" window and level settings optimally display the finding. *Continued.*

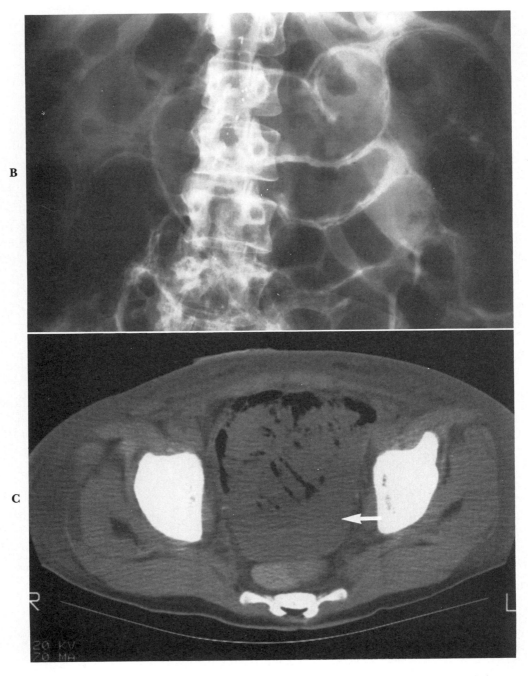

Fig. 5-7, cont'd. B, Supine abdominal film confirms the presence of pneumatosis intestinalis. **C,** Pneumatosis in this patient appears as streaky air collections paralleling the long axis of the bowel and along the valvulae. Fluid is seen in the dependent portion of the peritoneal cavity *(arrow)*. Surgery revealed bowel infarction with leakage of intestinal content into the peritoneal cavity. The cause was an unrelieved, closed loop, obstruction persisting for 2 weeks following appendectomy.

Small vessel disease. Radiation causes a proliferation of fibroblasts in the intestinal submucosa that leads to progressive narrowing of the small vessels, vascular congestion, and ultimately fibrosis of the bowel wall. Doses of 5000 R or greater are necessary to produce these changes. Clinical manifestations may not occur until several months after the completion of the radiation course. CT displays wall thickening that is distributed geographically and that corresponds to the radiation port. The loops have a somewhat straightened appearance. Mucosal folds that appear thickened and crowded and linear streaks of increased density in the mesenteric fat (edema) are also seen (Fig. 5-8).[11]

The vasculitis of systemic lupus erythematosus (SLE) or other collagen vascular diseases similarly involves small vessels. However, resultant bowel ischemia or hemorrhage may be evident. In systemic lupus erythematosus, associated ascites and pleuropericardial effusions may also be seen. CT is used in these patients to assess the extent of bowel involvement and localize other potential sources of acute abdominal pain.

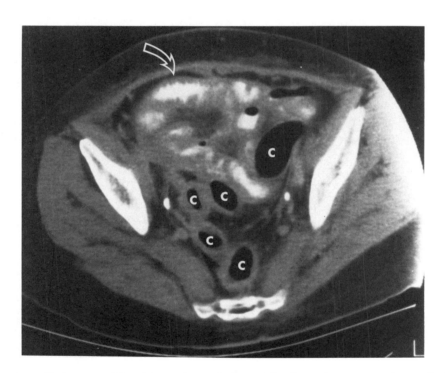

Fig. 5-8. Radiation enteritis. CT scan through the pelvis of a patient 1 year after radiation therapy for colon cancer shows diffuse thickening of the bowel wall of several loops of ileum and rectosigmoid colon *(C)* within the radiation port. Accentuated mucosal fold pattern in the ileum is also apparent *(curved arrow)*.

Intramural hemorrhage. Intramural hemorrhages of the intestine are usually secondary to anticoagulation therapy but may also be seen in bleeding disorders or trauma. Blood is recognized on CT as high-density fluid (60 to 90 H units) reflecting its hemoglobin content. Hemorrhage involving mesenteric loops of small bowel appear as segmental thickening of the bowel wall and mucosal folds.[12] The high-density blood within the bowel wall may not be seen in every case. Extension of hemorrhage into the peritoneal cavity appears as high-density ascites, sometimes with fluid levels representing serum clot layering in a "hematocrit" effect (Fig. 5-9).

Traumatic hemoperitoneum is evident on CT as high-density ascites. Simultaneously, visceral injuries are identified or excluded. For these reasons, in patients with blunt abdominal trauma CT has assumed an important role in diagnostic evaluation. CT has been shown useful in detecting unsuspected jejunal injury that appears as a thickened bowel wall and high-density edema in the local mesentery. Peritoneal lavage is sensitive in detecting intraperitoneal bleeding but, unlike CT, is relatively insensitive in detecting retroperitoneal injuries. In those patients in whom peritoneal lavage would be positive, CT is useful in selecting those patients for whom surgical intervention is necessary from those who can be managed more conservatively. In the absence of significant visceral injury, the mere presence of a small hemoperitoneum in and of itself does not require surgical exploration.[13,13a]

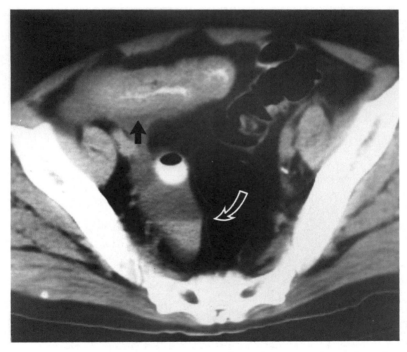

Fig. 5-9. Hemorrhage. Scan through the pelvis of a patient on anticoagulant therapy with acute abdominal pain shows an ileal segment *(arrow)* with a markedly and symmetrically thickened wall and narrowing of the lumen. High-density fluid appears to weep from the segment and layer in the pelvis displaying a serum-clot level *(curved arrow).*

Small bowel edema

Small bowel edema may also be secondary to nonvascular causes such as hypoalbuminemia, cirrhosis, chronic renal disease, or protein loss from the gastrointestinal tract in such conditions as lymphangiectasis, regional enteritis, Ménétrièr's disease, Whipple's disease, or lymphoma. The CT findings include dilation of the bowel lumen, increased intraluminal fluid content, thickening of mucosal folds, and blurring of the definition of both sides of the bowel wall (Fig. 5-10). Mesenteric fat shows diffuse increased soft-tissue density and blurring of the definition of neurovascular bundles (Fig. 5-10) secondary to edema. Ascites usually accompanies these findings.

Diffuse small bowel edema may also be secondary to lymphatic obstruction resulting from metastatic disease to lymph nodes in the root of the mesentery (Fig. 5-11).

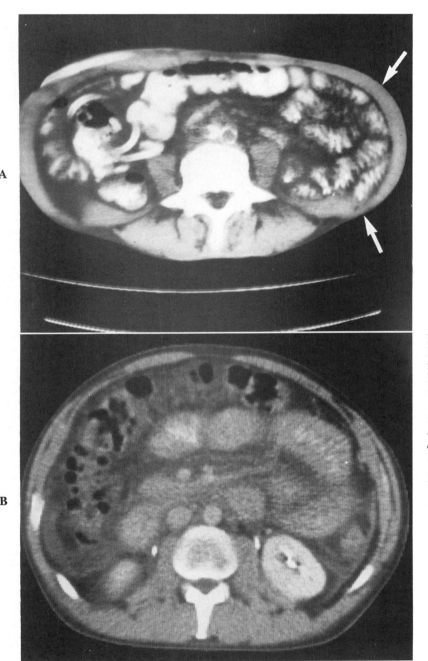

A

B

Fig. 5-10. Small bowel edema resulting from hypoproteinemia. **A,** In this patient with cirrhosis and hypoalbuminemia small bowel loops in the left mid-abdomen show fold and wall thickening indicating edema *(arrows)*. **B,** In another patient with more advanced cirrhosis, small bowel loops are mildly distended. Orally-administered contrast material is diluted by intraluminal fluid, and bowel wall definition is hazy secondary to edema. Mesenteric vascular markings are enlarged and blurred. There is a small amount of ascites in the flanks.

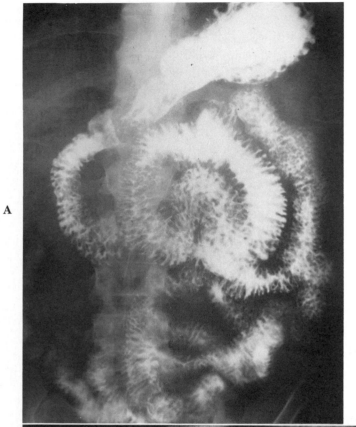

A

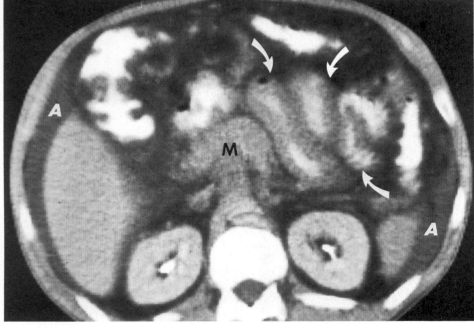

B

Fig. 5-11. Small bowel edema resulting from mesenteric lymphatic obstruction. **A,** Small bowel series shows diffuse symmetric thickening of jejunal folds. **B,** Scan reveals jejunal bowel wall thickening and accentuated mucosal fold pattern reflecting edema *(arrows).* Pathologic soft-tissue mass at the root of the mesentery *(M)* obscures the superior mesenteric artery and superior mesenteric vein, and a small amount of ascites is present *(A).* Percutaneous skinny needle aspiration biopsy of the mass revealed poorly differentiated adenocarcinoma.

INFLAMMATORY DISEASE

In the CT evaluation of inflammatory conditions involving the small bowel, several principles must be kept in mind. First, inflammatory processes confined to the mucosa or to the superficial layers of the bowel wall will probably not be reliably demonstrable by CT. It is only when the full thickness of the bowel wall, serosal surface, or mesentery are involved that CT can be expected to display the process. Bowel wall thickening accompanies transmural inflammation but is a nonspecific finding also seen in ischemic and neoplastic conditions. The fat content of the mesentery provides an excellent barometer of inflammatory processes because the water and cellular content of edema and exudate increase the soft-tissue content of the normally low-density fat. Thus inflammatory reaction takes the form of a cloudy or hazy soft-tissue density or of linear stranding in the fat surrounding an abnormal bowel segment. Bowel loops may appear matted together by serosal adhesions. More severe inflammatory reactions appear as frank fluid-density collections, either loculated in small pockets or as a well-defined abscess. Diffuse peritonitis appears as fluid-density collections interposed between the leaves of the small bowel mesentery; these collections are accompanied by soft-tissue density material associated with the peritoneal surfaces representing inflammatory debris (Fig. 5-12). CT is sensitive to the presence of extraluminal air, either free in the peritoneal cavity or loculated around the involved bowel (see Fig. 5-7). Perforation and fistulization may also be evident as extravasation of orally administered contrast material into the peritoneal cavity (see Fig. 1-1).

In many cases, the specific cause of an intraperitoneal inflammatory process is evident. The presence of a focal, well-defined, soft-tissue density mass amidst an inflammatory reaction suggests underlying neoplasm complicated by infection or perforation. A foreign body, if it is composed of material sufficiently different in CT density than normal abdominal contents, may be visible (Fig. 5-13).[14] Diverticulitis of the small bowel, though unusual, has an appearance analagous to its counterpart in the colon. The proximal small bowel is more commonly affected. The diverticulum itself may be visible as a round structure either filled with orally administered contrast material, gas, or inflammatory debris. The adjacent fat shows characteristic inflammatory changes ranging from increased hazy and linear soft-tissue density to frank abscess collection (Fig. 5-14).

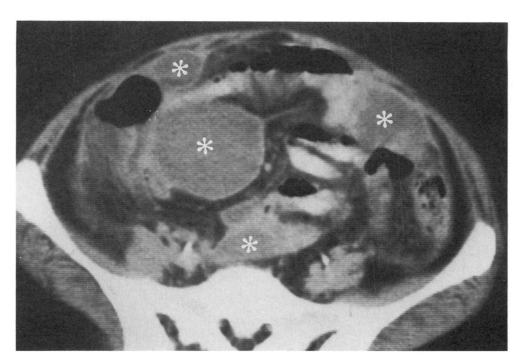

Fig. 5-12. Interloop abscesses. Scan through the lower abdomen shows multiple, loculated pockets of fluid displacing bowel loops (*). The mesentery shows inflammatory-type changes. CT localizes and characterizes the extent and nature of the inflammatory process.

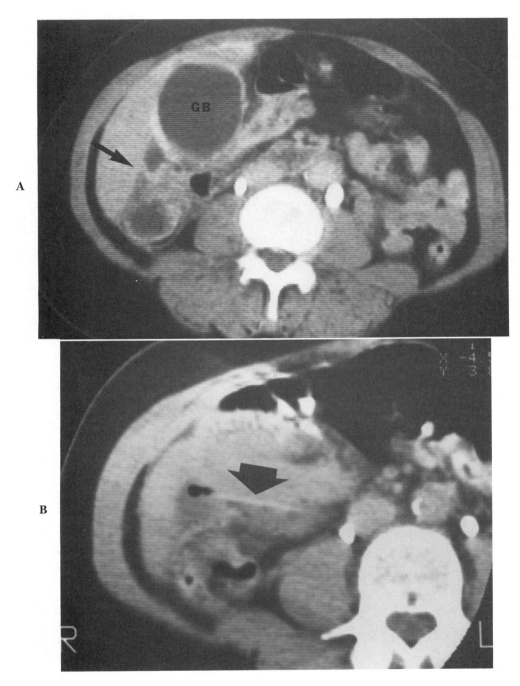

Fig. 5-13. Foreign body perforation. **A,** CT scan through the upper abdomen shows a
severe inflammatory process in the subhepatic region; matted bowel loops, small pockets
of fluid, and obscuration of mesenteric fat are seen *(arrow)*. The gallbladder is distended
(GB). **B,** Magnified scan obtained at a level just caudal to **A** shows a thin linear density
amidst the inflammatory reaction that proved at surgery to be a toothpick perforating the
jejunum *(arrow)*. A small amount of extraluminal gas is noted in an abscess cavity immediately to the right of the foreign body.

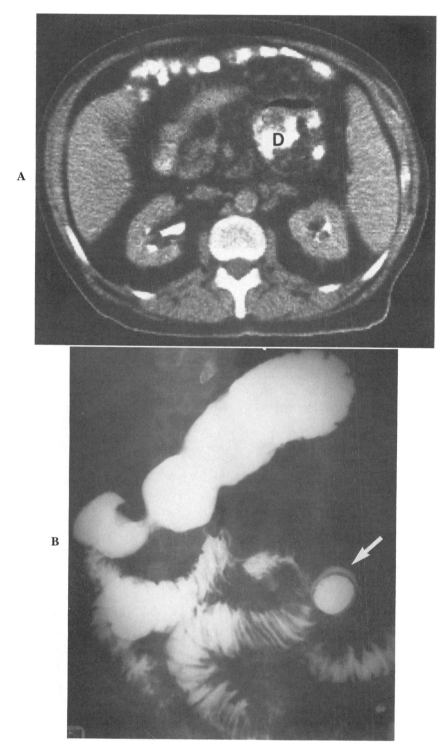

Fig. 5-14. Jejunal diverticulitis. **A,** A large diverticulum arising from the proximal jejunum is partially filled with orally-administered contrast material *(D)*. There are inflammatory changes in the surrounding mesentery, appearing as ill-defined areas of increased attenuation. **B,** Small bowel series outlines the diverticulum and shows inflammatory tethering of adjacent small bowel loops *(arrow)*.

Acute pancreatitis can effect the small bowel in a number of ways. In addition to its local effects on the adjacent duodenum, more severe pancreatic inflammation may also directly extend along the root of the mesentery to involve proximal loops of jejunum. Intestinal wall thickening and luminal narrowing are characteristic features that accompany the phlegmon extending from the gland (Fig. 5-15).[15]

The CT findings in sprue, as one would expect from experience with conventional barium studies, include dilation of the bowel, particularly the small bowel, increased fluid content, and perhaps mucosal fold thickening. The proximal small bowel tends to appear most involved (Fig. 15-16). Intussusception without a leading mass may be evident (Fig. 5-3). CT demonstration of mild to moderate lymphadenopathy in the mesentery or retroperitoneum is not a rare finding and does not necessarily imply associated lymphoma or carcinoma. Indeed lymphadenopathy, like the clinical malabsorption picture and the findings on barium study, may regress following institution of a gluten-free diet.[13] Nevertheless, the CT demonstration of adenopathy at initial appearance of sprue or as a new finding accompanying clinical deterioration warrants a high index of suspicion for superimposed malignancy.[16]

Adenopathy is a more characteristic feature in Whipple's disease or intestinal lipodystrophy. Being laden with fat and fatty acids, the involved nodes appear low in denity on CT.[17,18] Intestinal folds are thickened, and there may be increased secretions but the bowel is usually not dilated. Extra-intestinal findings evident on abdominal CT may also include ascites, splenomegaly, pleuropericarditis, and sacroilitis.

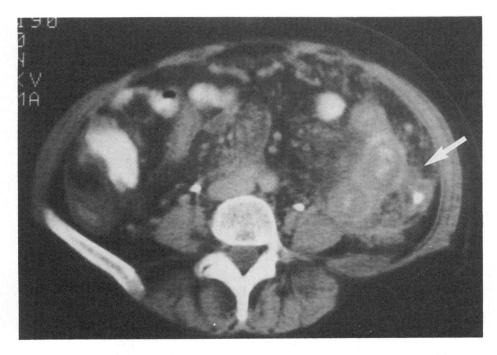

Fig. 5-15. Effect of acute pancreatitis on the small bowel. In this patient with severe, necrotizing pancreatitis, phlegmon extended caudally into the mesentery where hazy and linear soft-tissue density changes are apparent. Jejunal loops and the descending colon show marked edematous wall thickening secondary to inflammatory reaction *(arrow)*. Note the "double halo" appearance.

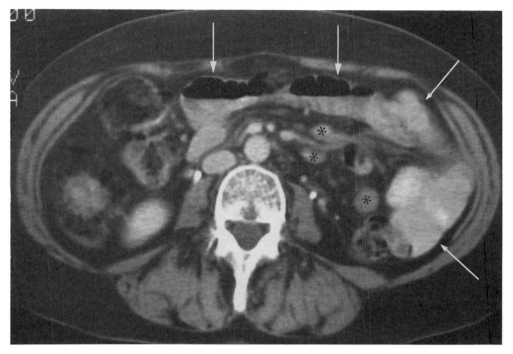

Fig. 5-16. Sprue. Scan through the mid-abdomen shows dilation of jejunal loops *(arrows).* Notice the thin wall and widely spaced valvulae conniventes. The caliber of the loop may be confused with the transverse colon; compare with stool-filled colon seen immediately adjacent. Mildly enlarged lymph nodes in the mesentery (*). Clinical evaluation and jejunal biopsy confirmed the presence of sprue.

INFECTIOUS DISEASE

More patients with infectious diseases of the small bowel are being studied with CT because of an increased incidence of these organisms in an increasingly larger immunocompromised patient population. CT demonstrates several features of diagnostic importance. Relevant observations include mucosal fold thickness, luminal diameter, volume of secretions, and distribution of abnormalities within the bowel. Ancillary findings that pertain to the differential diagnosis, such as adenopathy or ascites, are also imaged.

Tuberculosis within the abdomen almost always includes adenopathy, particularly in a mesenteric or peripancreatic distribution.[19] Splenomegaly, and less often hepatomegaly, are often associated. When present, ascites is often of high density and complicated by peritoneal nodularity, thickening, or enhancement. In patients with AIDS, tuberculosis, especially secondary to *Mycobacterium avium-intracellulare,* is common. Vincent[20] and Nyberg[21] have described the pseudo-Whipple complex in AIDS patients with *Mycobacterium avium-intracellulare.* Thus one may expect to find thickened intestinal folds associated with mesenteric adenopathy on CT scans in these patients (Fig. 5-17).

Cryptosporidia and *Isospora belli* (Fig. 5-18) are enteric protozoans that occur in patients with this unique immune defect.[22] These patients have refractory diarrhea that leads to severe fluid and electrolyte disturbances. CT plays a role in evaluating the overall status of the abdomen in these patients. Changes in the jejunal fold pattern should be looked for and appropriate cultures obtained.

Disseminated histoplasmosis, another granulomatous infection, may also include mesenteric adenitis (Fig. 5-19). The infections mentioned above have been considered diagnostic of AIDS.

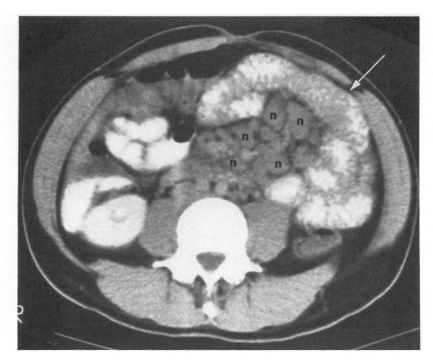

Fig. 5-17. Pseudo-Whipple's disease in AIDS. Scan through the mid-abdomen shows wall and fold thickening of small bowel loops *(arrow)* and marked mesenteric adenopathy *(n)*. This patient with AIDS suffered systemic infection with *Mycobacterium avium-intracellulare.*

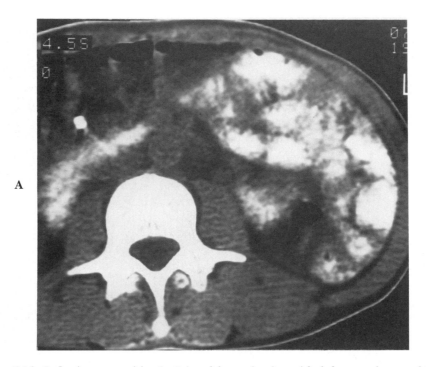

Fig. 5-18. Infectious enteritis. **A,** Jejunal loops in the mid-abdomen show a thickened disorganized fold pattern and poor mixing of orally administered contrast material with intraluminal fluid.

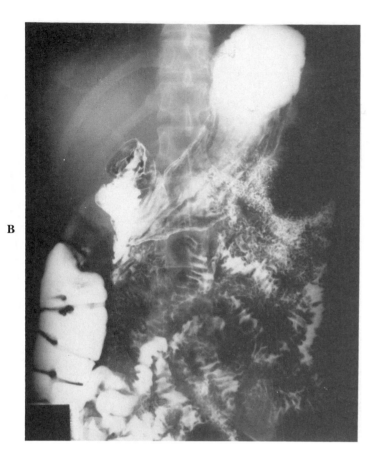

B

Fig. 5-18, cont'd. B, Small bowel series shows a thickened and irregular fold pattern in the small bowel with increased secretions and rapid transit. The etiologic agent in this AIDS patient was *Isospora belli*.

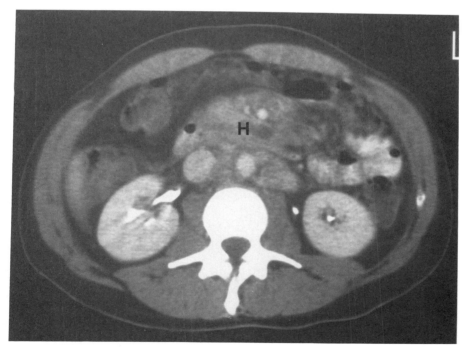

Fig. 5-19. Abdominal histoplasmosis in AIDS. In the mid-abdomen, mesenteric adenopathy surrounds the superior mesenteric artery and superior mesenteric vein *(H)*. Mild inflammatory changes involve the entire mesentery. Needle aspirate revealed *Histoplasma capsulatum* on fungal stains.

REGIONAL ENTERITIS (CROHN'S DISEASE)

The transmural involvement characteristic of regional enteritis and its proclivity for extraluminal complication such as fistula or abscess make CT an important diagnostic modality complimentary to barium studies in the evaluation of these patients. As in conventional barium studies, several different manifestations, of regional enteritis may be recognized on CT.

Nonstenotic involvement has a nonspecific appearance with thickening and blunting of folds sometimes with evidence of increased secretions (Fig. 5-20). The bowel wall itself may also appear slightly thickened.

Stenotic forms display several characteristic CT appearances. The most common site of involvement is the distal ileum. The frequency of disease in the proximal small bowel tends to decrease in relation to increasing distance from the ileocecal valve. However, jejunal and even duodenal involvement may occur with or without involvement of the distal small bowel. When disease is limited to the ileocecal region, CT demonstrates matting together of the terminal ileum and adjacent colon, narrowing or obliteration of the lumen, and thickening and poor definition of the respective bowel walls with inflammatory changes in the surrounding fat (Fig. 5-21). (See also Figs. 8-14 to 8-17.)

Another appearance characteristic of Crohn's enteritis is sharply delimited "skip" areas intervening between normal and diseased segments (Fig. 5-22). Actual ulcerations and cobblestone appearance are not routinely visualized on CT, but hyperplastic pseudopolyps may sometimes be recognized, especially if "lung" window and level settings are used. The lumen may be so narrow as to appear obliterated, the CT equivalent of the "string" sign[23] (Fig. 5-22, B). Dilation may be noted proximal to areas of disease. The inflamed mucosa and bowel wall may show significant enhancement following intravenous contrast material administration,[24] and the intensity of this enhancement correlates with the clinical activity of disease.[25]

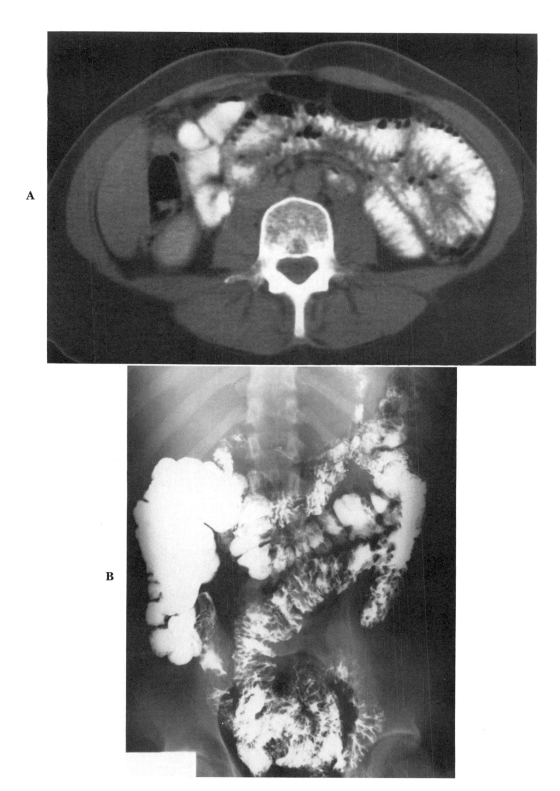

Fig. 5-20. Non-stenotic regional enteritis. **A,** Mid-abdominal scan shows mildly dilated jejunal loops with a prominent mucosal fold pattern. **B,** Overhead radiograph from concurrent small bowel series confirms mild dilation of the jejunum with accentuated fold pattern. Patient had recrudescence of regional enteritis following previous ileal resection.

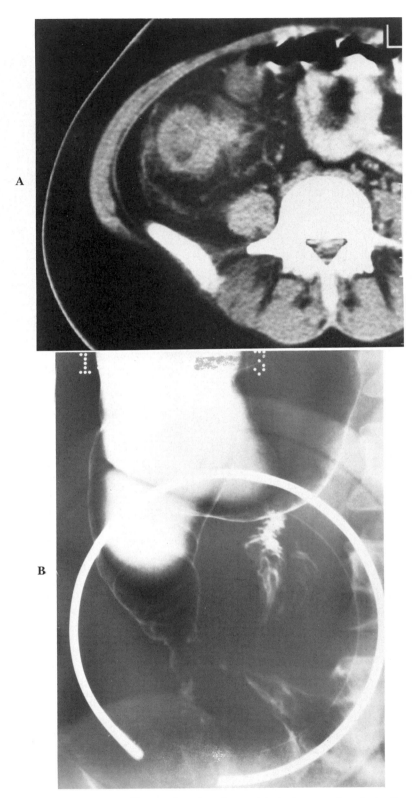

Fig. 5-21. Stenotic form of ileocecal regional enteritis (subacute phase). **A,** Magnified scan of the right lower quadrant shows matting together of the terminal ileum and cecum, thickening and poor definition of their walls and the underlying lumen, and inflammatory changes in the surrounding fat. **B,** Spot radiograph confirms typical findings of Crohn's disease with narrowed and shortened cecum and stenotic and ulcerated terminal ileum paralleled by short fistulous tracts.

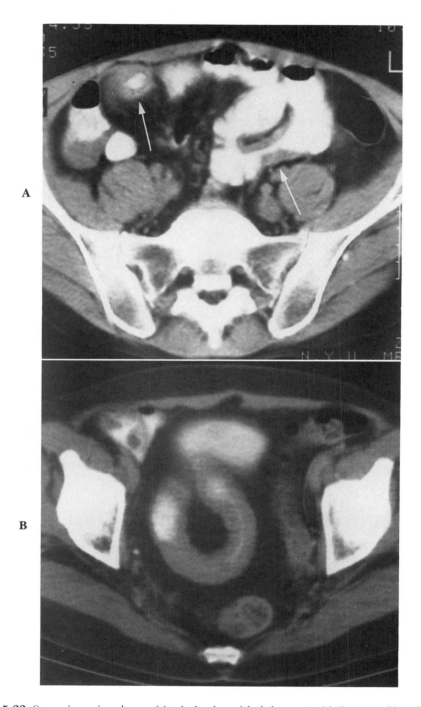

Fig. 5-22. Stenotic regional enteritis. **A,** In the mid-abdomen, "skip" areas of involvement are seen narrowing the lumen and thickening the bowel wall of discontinuous segments *(arrows).* **B,** In the pelvis, the ileal lumen is narrowed in a "string" configuration and the surrounding bowel wall is thickened.

A "double halo" configuration of involved bowel loops has been described[26] (Fig. 5-23). (See also Figs. 8-7 to 8-9.) The intestinal lumen and its contents are surrounded by an inner ring of low attenuation, near water density, representing inflamed and edematous mucosa. Surrounding this ring is an outer ring of higher-attenuation and soft-tissue density that purportedly represents thickened and fibrotic muscularis and serosa. Originally described as a specific finding in Crohn's disease, this appearance has been seen in radiation enteritis, ischemia, mesenteric venous thrombosis, and acute pancreatitis (see Figs. 5-15 and 5-42, A). In our experience, this finding is present in less than 50% of patients with Crohn's disease. In the colon, the "double halo" may be seen in radiation colitis, ulcerative colitis, and pseudomembranous colitis.

Extraluminal manifestations of regional enteritis are particularly amenable to CT analysis.[27] CT is especially useful to further analyze the separa-tion of bowel loops seen on barium studies. In mild cases this separation may be seen secondary merely to thickening of the bowel walls of adjacent involved loops (Fig. 5-24). With more advanced involvement, the mesenteric fat surrounding the involved bowel loops may appear hypertrophied and mass-like,[26,27] the so-called "creeping fat" that surgeons and pathologists have classically described (Fig. 5-23). Mesenteric adenopathy is often visable (Fig. 5-23). Fat density may be near normal, but in more advanced cases, especially with superimposed acute inflammation, the fat takes on increased soft-tissue, hazy density with linear streaks and bands running throughout. The fibro-fatty proliferation may effect the retroperitoneum leading to ureteral encasement and obstruction.[28] Frank abscess formation adjacent to involved bowel segments can also be identified by CT (Fig. 5-25). Abscesses appear as loculated fluid collections; occasionally air fluid levels or gas bubbles may be seen within them.

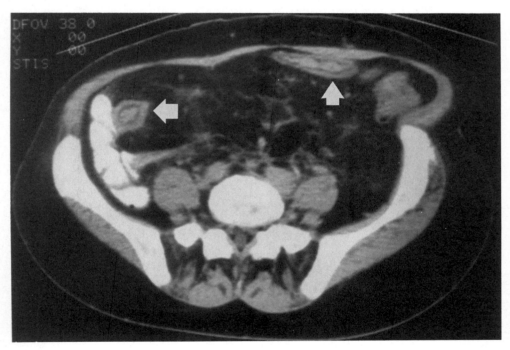

Fig. 5-23. Halo sign in Crohn's disease. In the lower abdomen, loops of bowel in cross and longitudinal section demonstrate a low-density "halo" surrounding the lumen that is in turn surrounded by a rim of thickened hyperemic bowel wall *(arrows)*. Note also the proliferation of mesenteric fat.

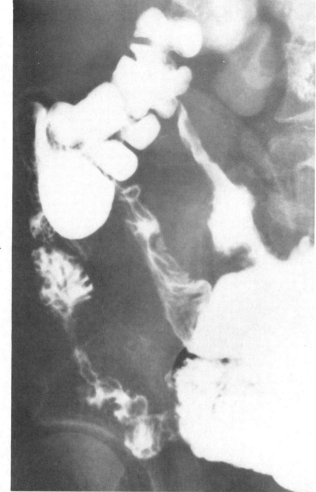

A

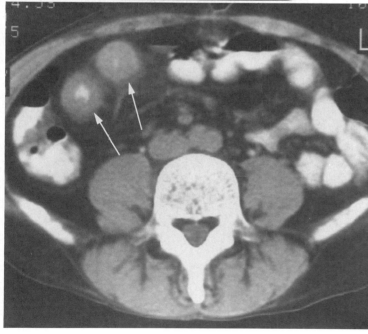

B

Fig. 5-24. Separation of bowel loops in Crohn's disease. **A,** Ileal loops in the right lower quadrant show luminal abnormalities characteristic of Crohn's disease and separation of the bowel loops by mass effect. **B,** Scan through this region shows the mass effect to be secondary to the marked transmural bowel wall thickening of the involved loops *(arrows)*, rather than to abscess.

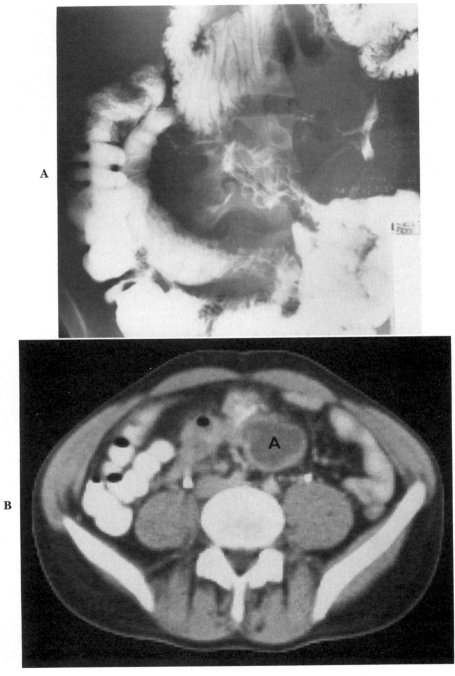

Fig. 5-25. Interloop abscess in Crohn's disease. **A,** Spot radiograph of the right lower quadrant in a patient with regional enteritis. Radiograph shows marked luminal narrowing and separation of bowel loops. **B,** Scan through this region reveals an interloop abscess *(A)*. Fluid collection is the cause of the mass effect seen in **A.**

Although perforation is rarely seen, fistulae are an integral part of the disease process (Fig. 5-21). The high spatial and contrast resolution of CT allows minute amounts of extraluminal gas to be identified, affording important correlative information to gastrointestinal studies in outlining the full extent of fistulae.[24,29,30] In areas of severe involvement, matting together of diseased loops and extramural inflammatory mass may make identification of fistulae difficult; precise mapping of the tracts is better delineated by barium studies. However, extraluminal fistulous tracts to other organs, such as the bladder, vagina or perineum or skin, are particularly well demonstrated. The presence of a fistulous tract may be inferred from visualizing extraluminal gas or contrast surrounded by a stellate-appearing, ill-defined region of increased density in the adjacent fat. Extra-alimentary abscesses in the liver, body wall musculature (Fig. 5-26), or subcutaneous tissues are also well demonstrated by CT. The unique postoperative complications of Crohn's disease such as stomal recurrence, peristomal abscess (Fig. 5-27), and blind loop syndrome (Fig. 5-28) may be detected on CT; these are difficult to diagnose solely on barium studies. An additional role for CT exists in those patients with extremely painful perianal and perineal disease in whom enema examination or endoscopy cannot be performed.[27]

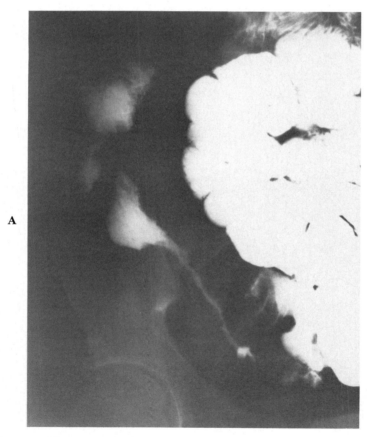

Fig. 5-26. Extra-alimentary abscess in Crohn's disease. **A,** Overhead radiograph from small bowel series shows terminal ileitis and right lower quadrant mass effect.

Continued.

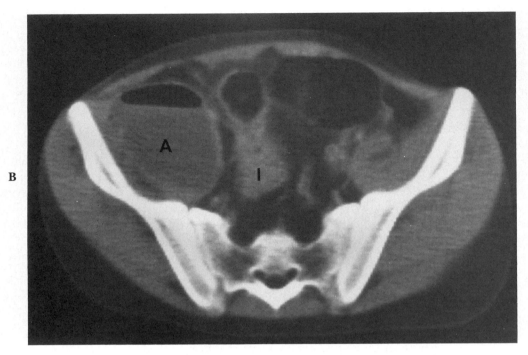

Fig. 5-26, cont'd. B, Scan through the lower abdomen shows a large abscess in the right psoas muscle containing a gas/fluid level *(A)*. Note the adjacent abnormal ileal loop *(I)*.

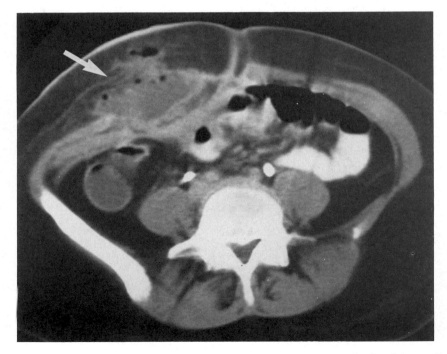

Fig. 5-27. Peristomal abscess in recurrent Crohn's disease. Scan obtained immediately cephalad to an ileostomy stoma demonstrates bubbles of gas and liquid pus in an abscess in the subcutaneous tissues and body wall *(arrow)*.

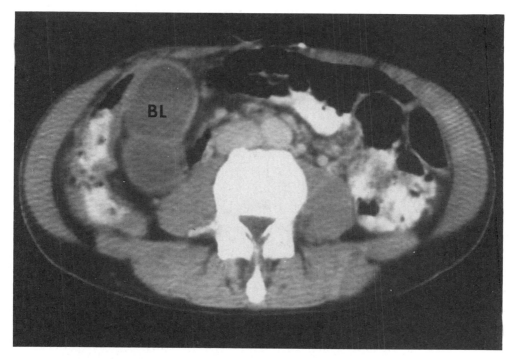

Fig. 5-28. Postoperative blind loop. In this patient with Crohn's disease and multiple previous small bowel resections, CT demonstrates a well-defined, peanut-shaped, fluid-filled structure in the right lower quadrant *(BL)*, which proved at surgery to be a blind loop with stasis and secondary infection.

NEOPLASIA

Small intestinal neoplasms, although much less common than gastric or colonic lesions, are not rare. Lymphoma, adenocarcinoma, carcinoid, leiomyomatous tumors, and metastatic foci are the neoplasms most frequently encountered in the small intestine. In a single examination, CT can demonstrate the tumor itself and evaluate possible sites of spread involving lymph nodes, other abdominal viscera, omentum and peritoneal surfaces, bones, lungs, and mediastinum. Associated mechanical bowel obstruction may also be evident. In preoperative patients with obvious widespread neoplasia or in postoperative patients with suspected recurrent disease, CT has evolved as an important tool to guide percutaneous biopsy of appropriate sites and thereby avoid unnecessary exploratory surgery.

Lymphoma

CT of the abdomen has become a widely used modality in initial and follow-up evaluation of lymphoma, primarily because of its ability to demonstrate lymphadenopathy and solid organ in-volvement. However, gastrointestinal involvement is the initial presentation of non-Hodgkin's lymphoma in 5% to 20% of cases,[31,32] and secondary gastrointestinal involvement is common, found at autopsy in up to 50% of cases. Gastrointestinal lymphoma is multicentric in 10% to 50% of cases.[31] The small bowel closely follows the stomach as the most common focus of disease, and histology is most often histiocytic, diffuse form.[33] Although half of the patients with gastrointestinal disease will have only vague nonspecific abdominal complaints,[34] the presence of gastrointestinal involvement changes the clinical stage and therefore can have important therapeutic implications.

The distribution of lymphoma in the small bowel roughly approximates the distribution of lymphoid tissue, being most common in the ileocecal area and progressively less common proximally. CT staging of gastrointestinal lymphoma is based on the presence of tumor confined to the bowel wall (Stage I), limited to local nodes (Stage II), accompanied by wide-spread nodal disease (Stage III), or disseminated to bone marrow, liver, or other organs (Stage IV). With these distinctions in

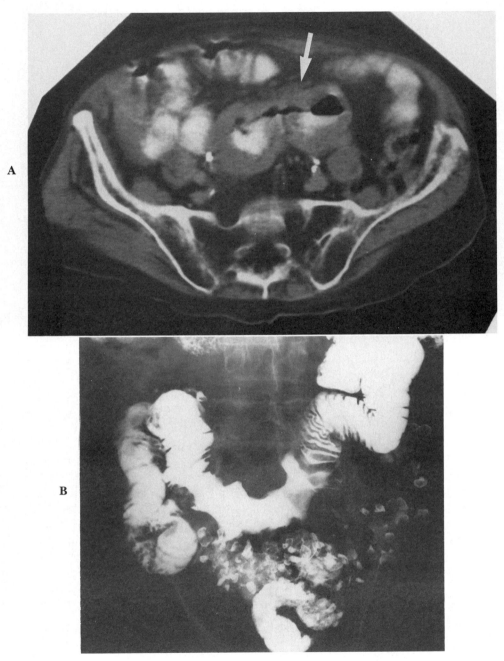

Fig. 5-29. Lymphoma. **A,** A well-defined segment of small bowel in the lower abdomen shows wall thickening and a dilated ulcerated lumen *(arrow)*. **B,** Small bowel series shows the presence of an ulcerated lesion in the ileum without proximal obstruction. Surgery confirmed localized lymphoma.

mind, the role of CT in staging of gastrointestinal lymphoma becomes clear. By demonstrating the full thickness of bowel wall involvement and by evaluating the site(s) of disease in abdominal nodes and solid viscera, accurate staging is accomplished in a single examination.

Although it is usually a manifestation of systemic disease and accompanied by mesenteric and retroperitoneal lymphadenopathy,[34,35] lymphoma limited to the bowel wall may appear as intraluminal polypoid masses, multiple nodules, or segments of mural infiltration. CT recognition of these forms depends on adequate delineation of the bowel lumen with contrast so that wall thickening can be appreciated. In the mural infiltration form, the bowel wall is thickened either in a nodular or concentric manner (Fig. 5-29). Endoexoenteric forms of small bowel lymphoma may appear as large masses with only a small intramural component (Fig. 5-30). Bowel wall lesions tend to be relatively homogeneous in tissue density. Intravenous contrast material enhances the lesions only moderately and usually less so than leiomyomatous or epithelial tumors. Although low-density areas of necrosis may be seen (Fig. 5-31), the presence of fluid-density material related to the tumor mass raises the possibility of bowel perforation and superimposed abscess. Irregular air collections reflect ulceration.[36]

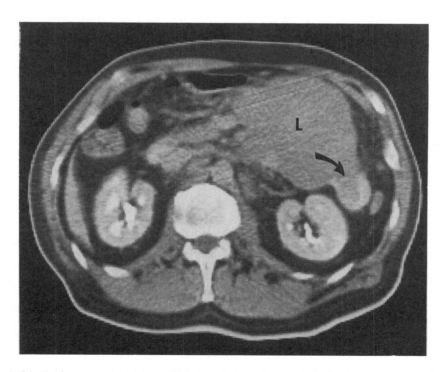

Fig. 5-30. Endoexocentric form of histiocytic lymphoma. A bulky homogeneous density mass in the left upper quadrant has a small intramural component arising from the jejunum *(curved arrow)* and a larger mesenteric component extending to the superior mesenteric artery and superior mesenteric vein *(L)*.

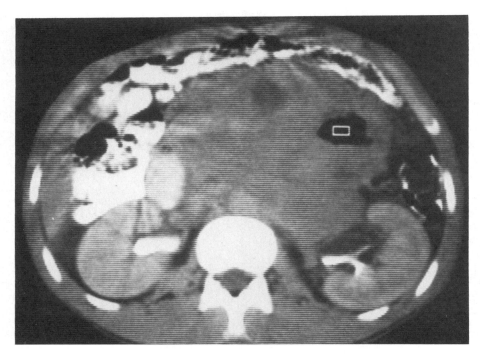

Fig. 5-31. Lymphoma. A conglomerate mantle of mesenteric and retroperitoneal adenopathy surrounds a proximal jejunal loop *(cursor)*. The finding of a dilated, air-filled cavity not only suggests ulceration but also allows prediction of direct intestinal involvement rather than simply extrinsic displacement.

Mechanical obstruction associated with small bowel lymphoma is more likely secondary to intussusception of polypoid masses or nodules (Fig. 5-32) than to the relatively unusual, annular, constricting forms of lymphoma growth. In contrast, aneurysmal dilation of the lumen characteristic of lymphoma may be recognized as a central or eccentric collection of gas or contrast within an ulcerated mass.[36] Thinning of the bowel wall secondary to tumor growth, necrosis, and tissue sloughing has also been reported. Associated perforation, abscess formation, and fistula may also be demonstrable with CT, providing important correlative information to conventional barium studies.[33]

The mesentery may be involved by lymphoma in several characteristic patterns. Small bowel involvement is usually accompanied by mesenteric and/or retroperitoneal adenopathy, and this ancillary finding assists in the differential diagnosis of segmental small bowel lesions. Discrete mesenteric lymph node masses may displace but not involve loops of small bowel. These masses surround mesenteric vessels but leave intact a thin rim of preserved perivascular fat in a "sandwich" configuration (Fig. 5-33). This feature is of diagnostic importance since mesenteric masses of other causes rarely adopt such a configuration.[37] Mesenteric lymphoma may also appear as an ill-defined confluent mass engulfing and encasing multiple loops of adjacent bowel (Fig. 5-34) or as a conglomerate mantle of retroperitoneal/mesenteric mass (Fig. 5-31). When lymphomatous mesenteric masses do not respect the boundary of perivascular fat, bolus enhancement of mesenteric vessels may be necessary to localize the tumor within the mesentery (Fig. 5-35).

Calcification in mesenteric masses is rare and is usually seen only after treatment by radiation or chemotherapy (Fig. 5-36). We have also encountered calcification in masses of Burkitt's lymphoma in two patients with AIDS (Fig. 5-37).

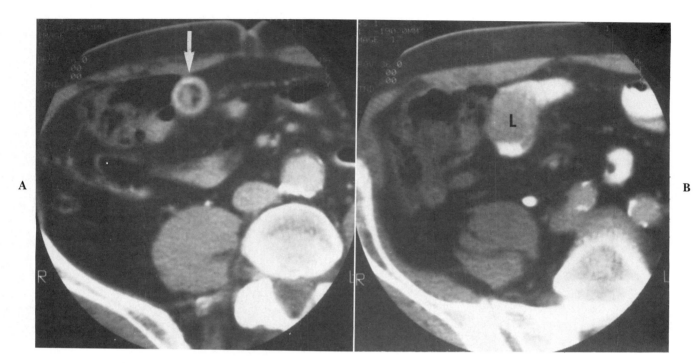

Fig. 5-32. Lymphoma with enteroenteric intussusception. **A,** Magnified scan of the right lower quadrant shows in cross-section mesenteric vessels and fat intussuscepting into an ileal loop *(arrow)*. **B,** Slightly caudad, the lymphomatous mass leading the intussusception is identified *(L)*.

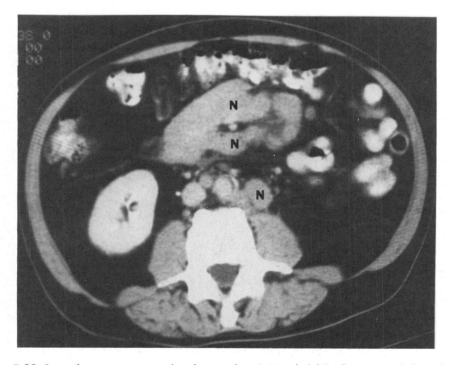

Fig. 5-33. Lymphoma—mesenteric adenopathy. A "sandwich" of mesenteric lymphoma *(N)* surrounds the mesenteric fat and vessels. Retroperitoneal adenopathy is also present.

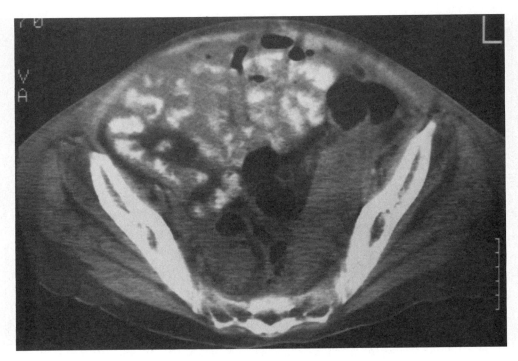

Fig. 5-34. Lymphoma—mesenteric infiltration. A scan through the lower abdomen shows a confluent mesenteric mass engulfing and infiltrating adjacent ileal loops.

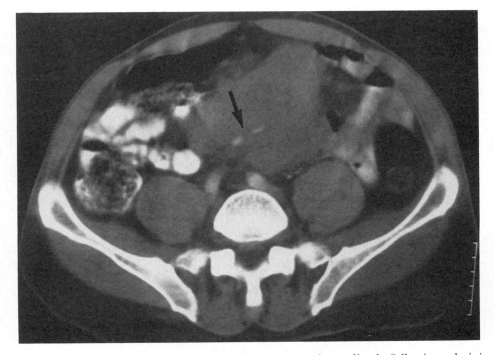

Fig. 5-35. Lymphoma—mesenteric mass. Dynamic scan immediately following administration of a bolus of intravenous contrast material reveals a homogeneous, soft-tissue density mass encasing mesenteric vessels (*arrow*).

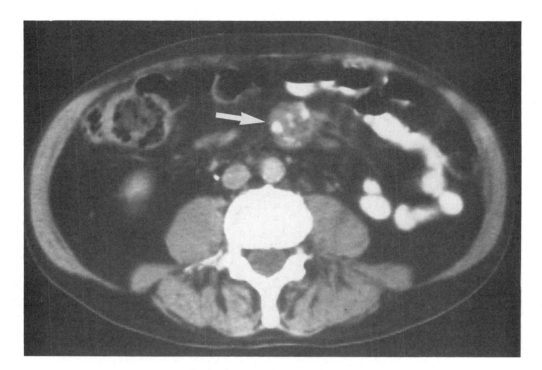

Fig. 5-36. Calcified mesenteric lymphoma following chemotherapy. A scan through the mid-abdomen reveals a shrunken, focally calcified, mesenteric mass—a remnant of treated lymphoma *(arrow)*. Follow-up scans are necessary to assess further shrinkage or growth of any residual viable tumor.

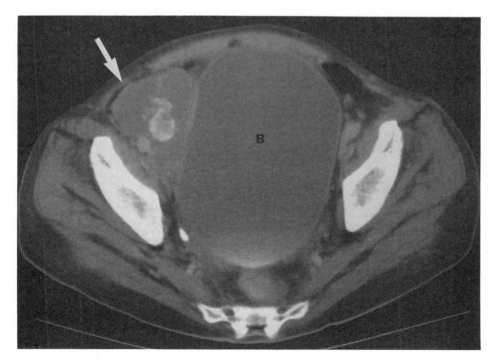

Fig. 5-37. Burkitt's lymphoma—AIDS. CT scan through the right lower quadrant reveals a well-marginated, side-wall mass with central calcification *(arrow)* adjacent to the urinary bladder *(B)*. Needle biopsy revealed a Burkitt's lymphoma. Calcification has been seen in two of three patients with Burkitt's lymphoma complicating AIDS studied to date.

Leiomyoma and leiomyosarcoma

Leiomyomatous tumors of the gastrointestinal tract arise in the muscular or submucosal layers of the bowel wall. Since growth tends to be exophytic rather than intraluminal, small lesions may go undetected on endoscopy or barium studies and can grow to a large size before the diagnosis is apparent.

On CT small lesions appear as round, well circumscribed masses of homogeneous density associated with the bowel wall. When larger, the tumors can be seen compressing and displacing adjacent loops of bowel or the stomach. Ulcerations may be extensive and deep and fill with gas or orally-administered contrast material (Fig. 5-38). The soft-tissue component of the tumor usually shows marked enhancement with intravenous contrast material. CT can demonstrate the frequently occurring, central tumor necrosis as a low-density central area, especially when intravenous contrast material has been administered.[38] Calcification in primary and metastatic foci has been reported but is rare. Lymph node metastases in the mesentery, omentum, or retroperitoneum are seen only in a minority of cases. Metastatic disease tends to involve the liver, and secondary hepatic deposits are often cystic or of low density with solid tumor nodules associated.[39] Other sites of hematogenous dissemination include the lung, spleen, bones, and soft tissues.

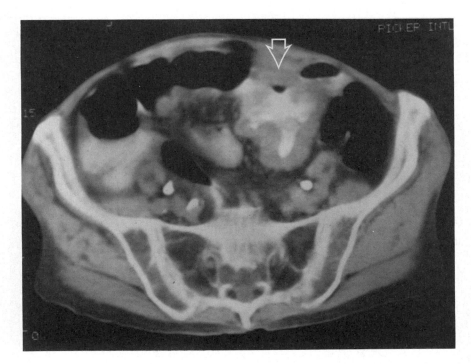

Fig. 5-38. Leiomyosarcoma. A bulky exophytic mass is seen growing from the proximal jejunum. The irregular appearance of the oral contrast material reflects deep ulceration (*arrow*).

Although most leiomyosarcomas tend to be encapsulated, huge infiltrating lesions may rarely occur. They are similar in appearance to lymphoma, but a bolus injection of contrast material can usually differentiate highly vascular leiomyosarcoma from less vascular lymphoma.

It is not always possible to distinguish benign from malignant leiomyomatous tumors radiologically or pathologically. CT criteria that suggest malignancy include large size (greater than 6 cm), necrotic or heterogeneous tissue density, and ulceration or fistula formation.[40] Multiple satellite masses throughout the abdomen indicate peritoneal seeding (Fig. 5-39). This is the most common mode of dissemination of small bowel leiomyosarcoma.

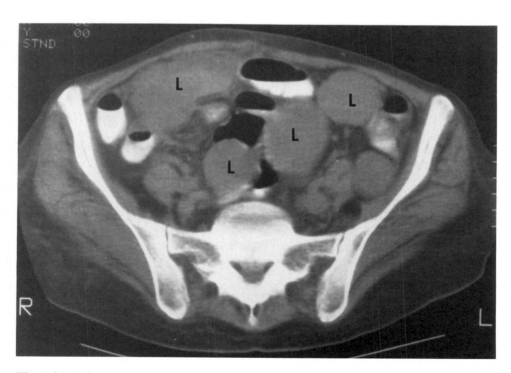

Fig. 5-39. Leiomyosarcoma. Multiple, homogeneous, soft-tissue density masses *(L)* represent intraperitoneal metastases of previously resected ileal leiomyosarcoma. This mode of spread is the most common pattern of metastases of small intestinal leiomyosarcoma.

Carcinoid tumors

Carcinoid tumors are the most common primary neoplasms of the small intestine but many are discovered only as incidental findings at surgery or necroscopy.[41] Most come to attention because of abdominal pain, obstructive symptoms, or the relatively rare carcinoid syndrome associated with liver metastases.

Radiologic features of carcinoid tumors are diverse, reflecting the variety of growth patterns and associated tissue responses. Since the Kulchitsky cells, from which carcinoid tumors arise, lie deep in the bowel mucosa, the primary lesion may not present as a mucosal mass. Therefore barium studies are often nondiagnostic. Angiography, although it may suggest the diagnosis, is invasive and is limited in demonstrating the full extent of disease. CT portrays the bowel, mesentery, lymph nodes, and liver in a single examination and is therefore extremely useful in detecting and staging carcinoid tumors as well as in following them postoperatively or during chemotherapy.

Primary carcinoid lesions are usually not apparent on CT but may be seen as soft-tissue masses associated with the bowel wall (Fig. 5-40). More common and characteristic findings are related to the desmoplastic response in the mesentery incited by the primary tumor. In these cases the primary neoplasm may not be seen but displacement or kinking of adjacent bowel loops or a stellate radiating pattern of mesenteric neurovascular bundles reflects its presence[42-45] (Fig. 5-41). Walls of adjacent bowel loops may be segmentally thickened secondary to the chronic ischemia as a result of encasement of mesenteric vessels by the desmoplastic reaction incited by the tumor (Fig. 5-42). Differential diagnosis includes retractile mesenteritis and desmoplastic carcinoma or lymphoma.[42] With carcinoids, mesenteric masses reflect direct extension or metastases to local lymph nodes, occasionally as the only evident site of disease.[43] Dystrophic calcification related to tumor necrosis in involved nodes as well as in liver metastases has been described[43,45] but is rare. Ascites secondary to peritoneal seeding is a late finding associated with advanced disease. Liver metastases are common at the time of CT diagnosis but are not always associated with the carcinoid syndrome. In our experience, metastatic liver disease is associated with marked hepatomegaly. Usually hypodense and easily detectable on precontrast scans, liver metastases may become isodense with hepatic parenchyma on slow infusion contrast scans. Therefore, while contrast scans improve diagnostic efficacy in analyzing the primary disease and mesenteric and retroperitoneal involvement, some centers have stressed the importance of non-contrast scans for patients in whom knowledge of the number and size of metastases are critical for therapy.[44]

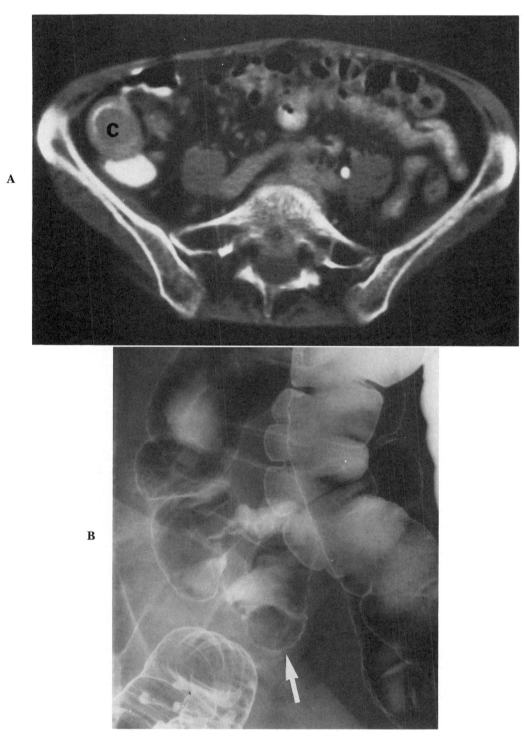

Fig. 5-40. Carcinoid. **A,** A scan through the lower abdomen identifies a homogeneous, well-defined, soft-tissue density mass *(C)* in a distal ileal loop. There is no small bowel obstruction. **B,** Spot radiograph from barium enema examination outlines the egg-shaped mass *(arrow)* in the terminal ileum, proven at surgery to represent intramural carcinoid.

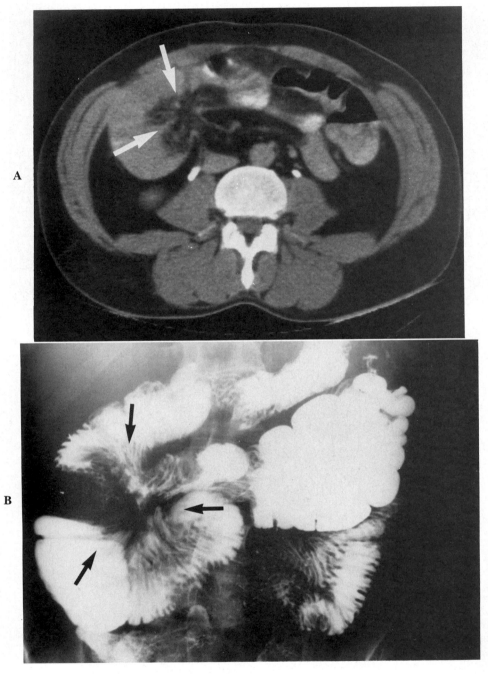

Fig. 5-41. Carcinoid—mesenteric changes. **A,** CT scan through the mid-abdomen shows dilated loops of ileum suspended from the mesentery with neurovascular markings accentuated in a stellate configuration *(arrows).* A terminal ileal carcinoid had been resected 2 months previously. **B,** Small bowel series shows angulated, kinked loops, partial obstruction, and separation of the involved bowel loops *(arrows).*

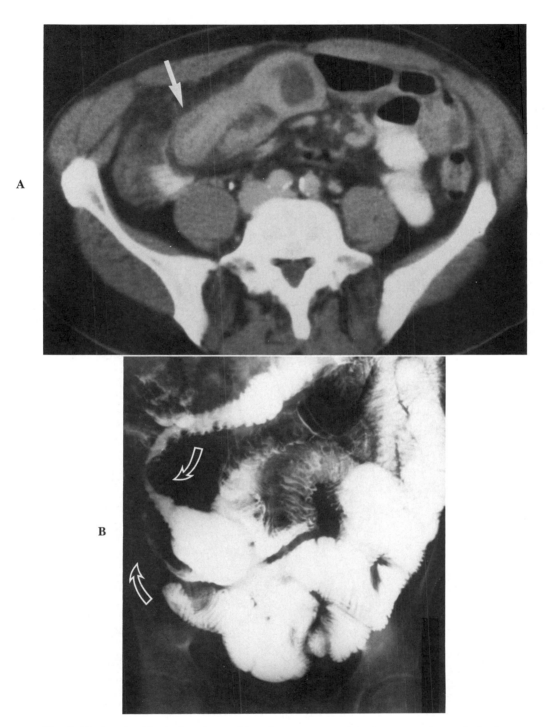

Fig. 5-42. Carcinoid—ischemia resulting from mesenteritis. **A,** A scan through the lower abdomen 1 year following resection of an ileal carcinoid shows dilated ileal lumen abruptly terminating in a segment with marked wall thickening, obliteration of the lumen, and desmoplastic changes in the adjacent mesentery *(arrow)*. Note the "double halo" appearance. **B,** Small bowel series demonstrates ischemic changes in the distal ileum and high-grade obstruction *(curved arrows)*. Several other loops suspended by the involved mesentery show angulation and narrowing. No tumor was found at surgery.

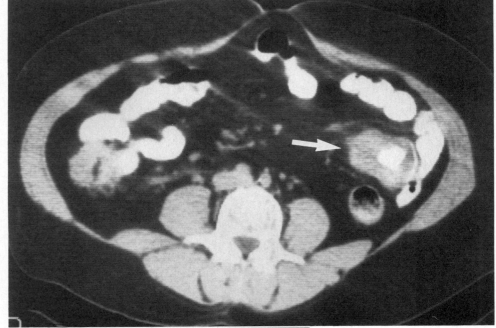

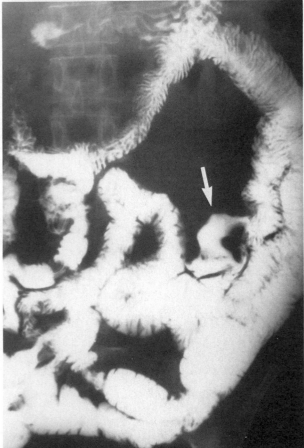

Fig. 5-43. Primary small bowel adenocarcinoma. **A,** Scan through the mid-abdomen shows a slightly heterogeneous density mass asymmetrically surrounding the lumen of a jejunal loop *(arrow).* **B,** Small bowel series shows an annular constricting lesion in the jejunum with mucosal destruction *(arrow).*

Primary adenocarcinoma

Primary adenocarcinoma arises in the small bowel much less frequently than in the stomach or colon, but its growth patterns are similar. The neoplasms may arise in villous tumors or grow de novo as polypoid masses or annular stenotic lesions. As yet, no series of these lesions studied by CT has been published. In our experience, with contrast outlining and distending the bowel lumen, the lesions can be identified as focal masses thickening the bowel wall and compromising the lumen either concentrically or asymmetrically (Fig. 5-43). The lesions may be heterogeneous in tissue density and show moderate enhancement following intravenous contrast administration. Occasionally, primary adenocarcinoma may appear as a large well-defined mass without bowel obstruction. Liver, peritoneal surfaces, and ovaries may be secondarily involved. The proximal bowel may be dilated secondary to obstruction. Associated bulky adenopathy is less commonly seen than in lymphoma but lymph node metastases may be found in 60% of cases at surgery.[47]

Metastatic disease

Metastatic involvement to the small bowel can be secondary to intraperitoneal seeding, hematogenously disseminated tumor emboli, or direct extension from an adjacent mass.[48] The CT appearance will reflect these pathologic mechanisms as well as growth characteristics allowing for differential diagnosis.

Intraperitoneal seeding is most often secondary to primary tumors of the ovary, breast, or gastrointestinal tract. Metastatic deposits appear as soft-tissue density nodules or sheets of tissue thickening bowel walls and mesenteric leaves, and are most readily evident in the greater omentum beneath the anterior body wall (Fig. 5-44). Compared to conventional barium upper gastrointestinal and small bowel examinations, CT is far superior in detecting mesenteric or omental neoplastic disease.[49]

Ascites either free or loculated usually accompanies peritoneal seeding. Ascitic volume is quite variable, from small collections seen only in the dependent portions of the peritoneal cavity to voluminous tense ascites. Dynamic flow of ascitic fluid tends to be toward recesses of the lower small bowel mesentery in the right lower quadrant.[50] Implants growing here appear as soft-tissue masses separating ileal loops. Luminal contours may be narrowed and irregular (Fig. 5-45, A and B), and in those primaries that stimulate a strong desmoplastic response, fixation and angulation of loops with resultant obstruction may also be seen. Alternatively, tumor deposits can grow to a large size, displacing adjacent loops of bowel without causing obstruction.

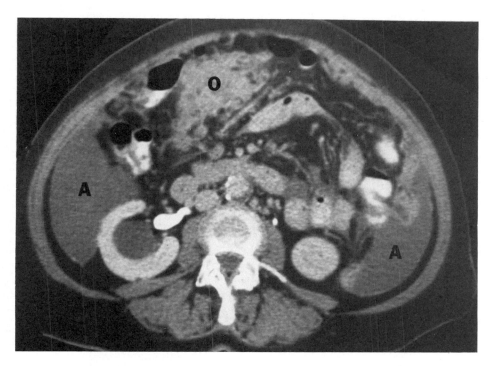

Fig. 5-44. Peritoneal metastases. Omental mass *(O)*, reticulonodular changes permeating the mesenteric surfaces, and ascites *(A)* reflect metastatic breast carcinoma. Right hydronephrosis is present as well.

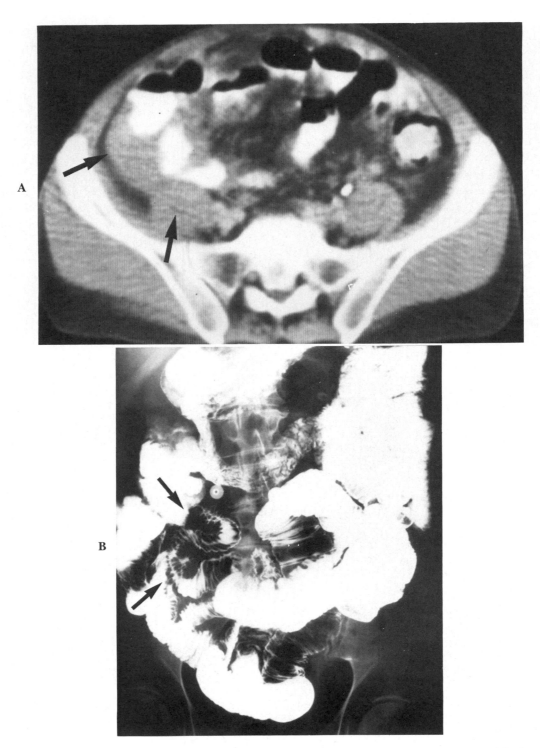

Fig. 5-45. Metastases and peritoneal seeding. **A,** A confluent mass surrounds several ileal loops in the right lower quadrant *(arrows).* **B,** Small bowel series demonstrates extrinsic spiculation of the mucosal contours of terminal ileal loops secondary to peritoneal seeding from gastric cancer *(arrows).*

Pseudomyxoma peritonei is a form of peritoneal carcinomatosis secondary to a primary mucin-producing cystadenocarcinoma of the appendix or ovary whose cystic components or metastatic foci have ruptured freely into the peritoneal cavity. The resultant seeding and growth of gelatinous tumor masses have a characteristic CT appearance. Ascites is diffuse and tends to be voluminous. Peritoneal implants along the liver margin result in a characteristic scalloped contour.[51] Septations can often be discerned coursing through the ascites, and well-defined cystic masses may also be evident. Soft-tissue density thickening of the peritoneal and omental surfaces reflects the more solid non-mucin components of the tumor. The primary appendicular mucocele or ovarian mass may also be evident (Figs. 5-46 and 6-78).

Hematogenous dissemination of tumor to the small bowel is most commonly associated with melanoma, carcinoma of the breast or lung, or Kaposi's sarcoma. Deposition is usually in the submucosa and multiple sites are often involved (Fig. 5-47). As on barium studies, when a metastatic deposit grows to circumferentially involve the bowel wall, its appearance mimics primary malignancy (Fig. 5-48). Melanoma deposits may be enormous and extensively ulcerated (Fig. 5-49). Breast tumor deposits may appear as linitis plastica in the small bowel as well as in the stomach, with symmetric wall thickening and apparent rigidity and luminal narrowing. Presumably because of the dense cellular content of the metastatic infiltrate, intravenous contrast material may markedly enhance the involved bowel wall.

Direct invasion from contiguous extra-alimentary primary tumors may also involve the small bowel (Fig. 5-50). Primary malignancies of the ovary, uterus, or prostate may grow directly into adjacent small bowel loops in the pelvis, usually the ileum. Pancreatic, colonic, or renal carcinoma may extend directly to involve the adjacent retroperitoneal duodenum or transverse mesocolon, or traverse mesenteric reflections into adjacent small bowel loops.

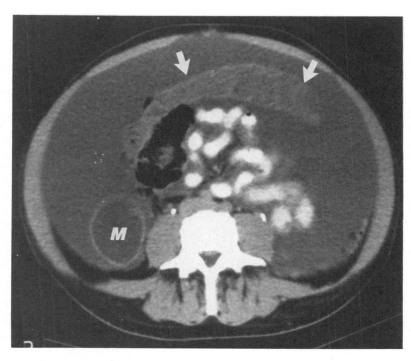

Fig. 5-46. Pseudomyxoma peritonei—ruptured appendicular mucocele. CT scan of the mid-abdomen demonstrates massive ascites, solid implants along the greater omentum *(arrows)*, and a cystic mucocele of the appendix *(M)*. Notice the expanded almost bubbly appearance of the omentum (compare to Fig. 5-44).

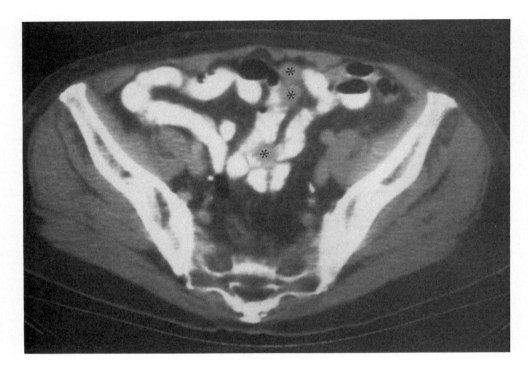

Fig. 5-47. Metastases and hematogeneous seeding. A scan through the pelvis shows multiple, soft-tissue density nodular masses (*) inpinging on the lumen of the ileum, which is well outlined by positive contrast material. Primary neoplasm was oat cell carcinoma of the lung.

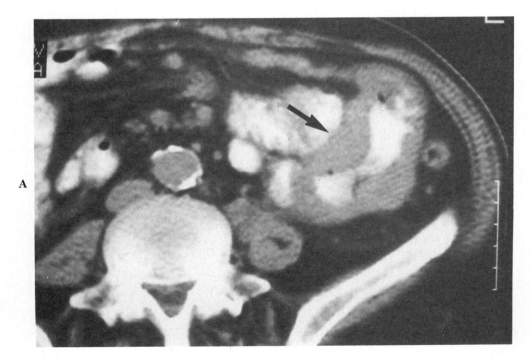

Fig. 5-48. Metastatic hypernephroma. **A,** Magnified scan of the left upper quadrant shows marked, symmetric wall thickening of a jejunal segment and effacement of the normal mucosal pattern *(arrow)*. (Compare to Fig. 5-43.)

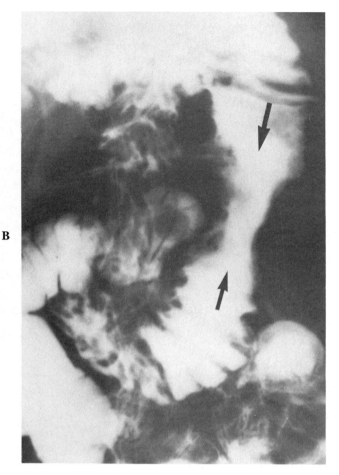

B

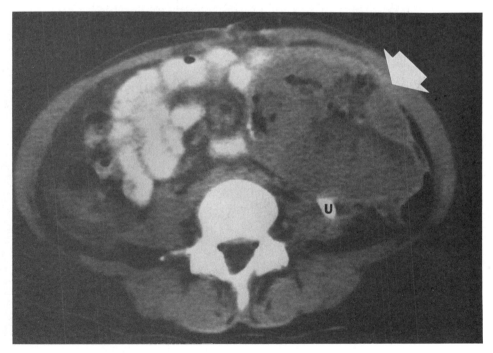

Fig. 5-48, cont'd. B, Spot radiograph from small bowel series confirms the presence of an ulcerating annular lesion with moderate constriction of the lumen *(arrows)*. Surgery revealed metastatic hypernephroma; nephrectomy had been performed 4 years previously.

Fig. 5-49. Metastatic melanoma. A scan through the mid-abdomen demonstrates an enormous heterogeneous density mass with bubbles of gas within *(arrow)*. Left ureter *(U)* is obstructed. Ascites is present in the right paracolic gutter. Invasive melanoma of the skin had been resected 5 years previously.

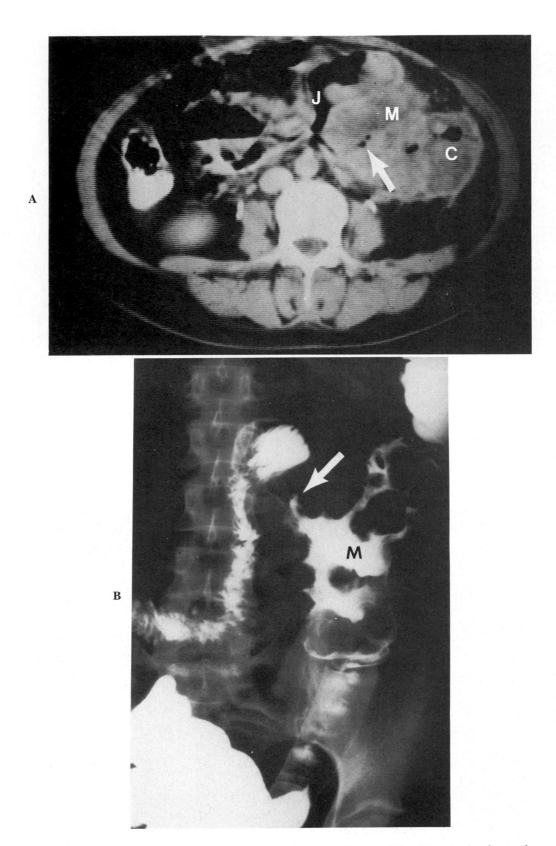

Fig. 5-50. Direct invasion by adjacent malignancy. **A,** A mass (M) arising in the descending colon (C) extends to displace and distort a jejunal segment (J). Bubbles of extraluminal gas lie within the mass *(arrow).* **B,** Water-soluble contrast enema outlines an adenocarcinoma of the colon *(M)* with perforation and fistulization to the jejunal loop *(arrow).*

MISCELLANEOUS MESENTERIC MASSES

Mesenteric cysts appear as round, well-circumscribed, homogeneous density masses, perhaps with a thick wall displacing but not invading adjacent structures.[52] CT density may be near that of water, but more commonly density is in the soft-tissue range because of the protein content of the cyst fluid. Fluid levels related to fatty and water density components may be present (Fig. 5-51). Being avascular, there is no change in density following intravenous contrast media administration.

Hematomas in the mesentery may appear as either well-defined collections or as pockets of fluid interspersed between the leaves of the mesentery (Fig. 5-52). CT density is variable, depending on the degree of clot formation and on the age of the hematoma. Especially when acute, a high-density component reflecting hemoglobin content can usually be identified.[53,54]

Solid primary mesenteric tumors are usually of mesenchymal origin. Fibromatous neoplasms are the most common, but lipomas, smooth muscle tumors, fibrous histiocytomas (Fig. 5-53), neural tumors, and hemangiomas may be encountered as well.

In the case of lipomatous tumors, a specific diagnosis can often be made by CT because of the characteristic low-density content of fatty elements.[55] Non-tumoral lipmatosis usually involves the pelvis or retroperitoneum but may also extend peripherally into the lower extremity.[56,57] Simple lipomas arising in the bowel wall or mesentery are quite uncommon, appearing as well-defined, homogeneous density, noninvasive, and usually solitary masses, although CT demonstration of diffuse intestinal lipomatosis has been reported.[58] Inflammatory conditions in the abdominal fat, such as, lipodystrophy or panniculitis, have also been demonstrated on CT.[59] Liposarcomas can present a confusing appearance, ranging from predominantly fat, water, and soft-tissue density elements to entirely soft-tissue density aggressive masses.[55] Especially in view of the often indolent nature of even malignant fatty tumors, CT is extremely useful in pre-operative planning and post-surgical follow-up of these lipomatous lesions.

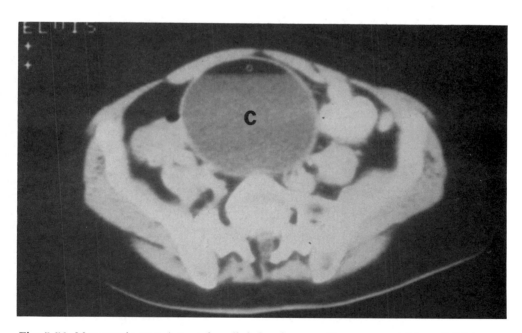

Fig. 5-51. Mesenteric cyst. A round, well-defined mass with an appreciable wall thickness is displacing but not involving small bowel loops in the lower abdomen. Fluid levels of fatty density *(O)* and water density material *(C)* are present.

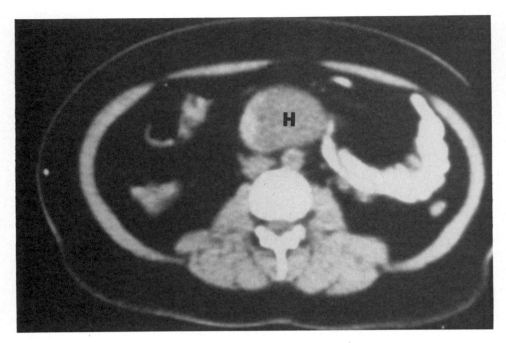

Fig. 5-52. Mesenteric hematoma. A round, well-defined mass is present in the mid-abdomen but does not affect bowel loops *(H)*. There are soft-tissue density and high-density components representing fresh hematoma in this anticoagulated patient.

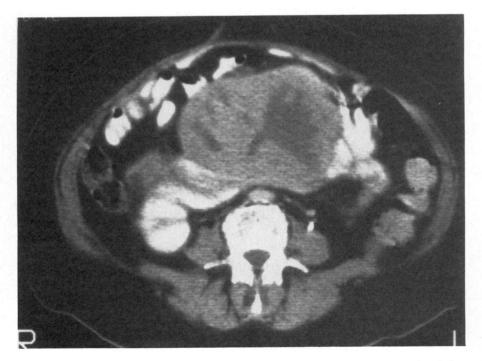

Fig. 5-53. Fibrous histiocytoma—mesentery. A large, well-defined mass in the abdomen displaces multiple small bowel loops. Low-density areas within represent necrosis.

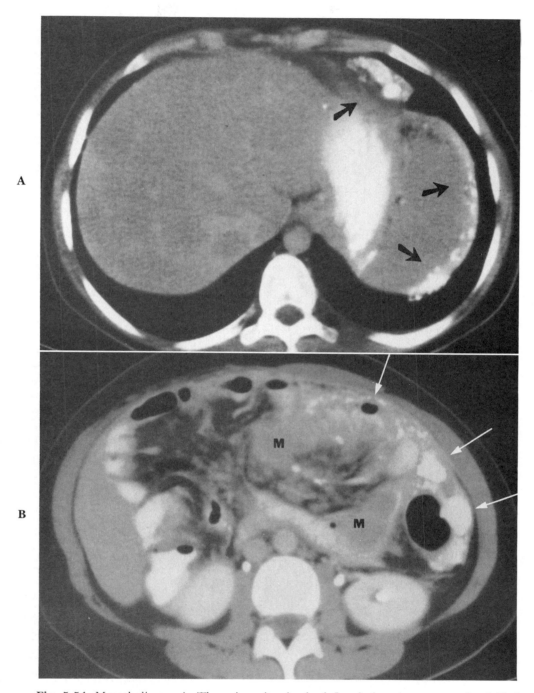

Fig. 5-54. Mesothelioma. **A,** There is ascites in the left subphrenic space, and calcified nodules and sheets of tissue thicken the peritoneal surfaces *(arrows)*. **B,** In the mid-abdomen, a calcified mass in the left pericolic gutter beneath the anterior body wall displaces and distorts adjacent loops of bowel *(arrows)*. Mesenteric adenopathy, partially calcified, is also present *(M)*. The patient is a 23-year-old female who has carried this diagnosis for 10 years.

Peritoneal mesothelioma has two distinct CT appearances. Aggressive malignant mesothelioma displays a nodular, irregular thickening of the peritoneal surfaces, localized masses, or infiltrating sheets of tissue.[60] There may be small foci of calcification. Most patients have ascites that is close to water in density. Mesenteric involvement is also common and may result in a stellate configuration of the neurovascular bundles, or in soft-tissue it may result in pleated thickening of the mesenteric leaves. Growth into the omentum may also occur.

More benign forms of mesothelioma appear less infiltrative, with multiple, discrete, extensively calcified masses and loculated pockets of ascites (Fig. 5-54). Patients with this form of disease may have a long indolent course.

Peritoneal desmoid tumors may be recognized in patients with Gardner syndrome (Fig. 5-55, *A* and *B*) and rarely, in the general population as well. Particularly in the Gardner's syndrome patient with abdominal complaints following colectomy, CT is the modality of choice in identifying these lesions and in differentiating them from other processes such as abscess or adhesions.[61,62] Another feature of Gardner's syndrome are diffuse fibromatous changes in the mesentery (Fig. 5-55, *C*).

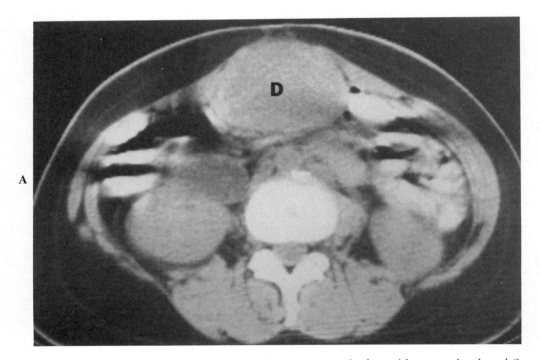

Fig. 5-55. Gardner's syndrome. **A,** This large, mesenteric desmoid tumor developed 2 years following colectomy *(D)*.

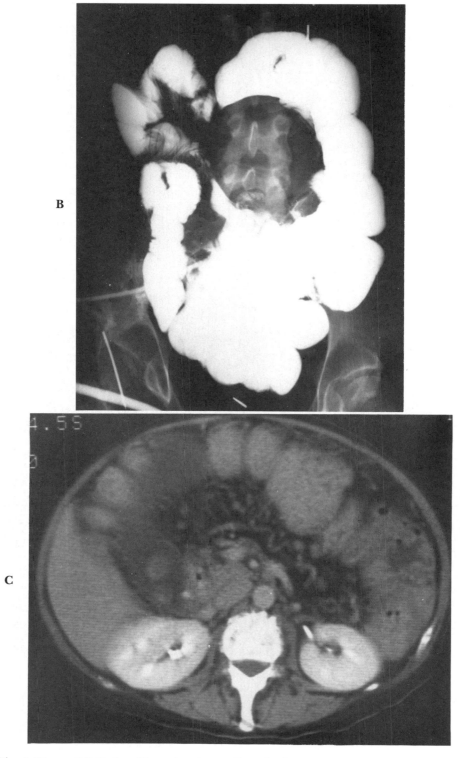

Fig. 5-55, cont'd. B, Small bowel series outlines the large mesenteric mass that displaces small bowel loops. **C,** In another patient with Gardner's syndrome, fibromatosis in the mesentery is evidenced by diffuse reticulonodular changes.

SMALL BOWEL OBSTRUCTION

CT can be extremely useful in confirming the presence of small bowel obstruction and often in revealing its cause. As in analysis of plain abdominal radiographs, small bowel obstruction is confirmed by identifying a normal caliber colon and normal caliber small bowel distal to the point of obstruction. Ileus or pseudo-obstruction can usually be reliably distinguished from true mechanical obstruction.

Inflammatory, vascular, and neoplastic (Fig. 5-56) abdominal processes relating to the small bowel may be recognized on CT in association with small bowel obstruction. However, the most common cause of small bowel obstruction is post-operative adhesions, and unfortunately, these cannot be readily visualized. Balthazar[63] has re-ported a case of closed loop obstruction in which CT showed evidence of fluid-filled, distended, small bowel loops, abrupt transition with collapsed distal intestinal loops, and a grossly distended fluid-filled U shaped loop as diagnostic of closed loop obstruction. In this case, the plain radiographs were normal. In contrast, volvulus secondary either to adhesions, malrotation, internal hernia, or other causes has a characteristic CT appearance (Fig. 5-57). Dilated loops, usually with thickened hyperemic walls secondary to ischemia, are seen twisted around the axis of their mesenteric vascular supply. Transudative or hemorrhagic ascites may be present as well (Fig. 5-58). A paraduodenal internal hernia has been demonstrated by CT as a sac-like mass of dilated small bowel loops in the retroperitoneum.[64]

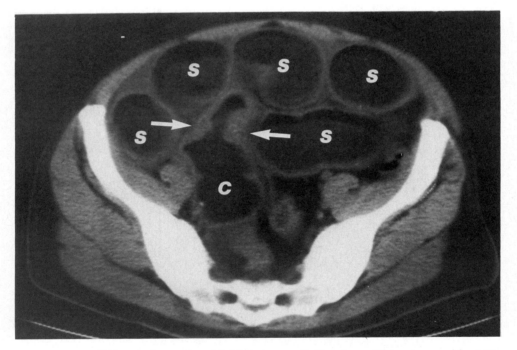

Fig. 5-56. Small bowel obstruction. Multiple loops of dilated small bowel are evident *(S)*. The thickened caliber of the wall and associated stasis are indicative of a high-grade, mechanical obstruction with approaching vascular compromise. An annular constricting adenocarcinoma *(arrows)* of the colon *(C)* is identified as the cause of the bowel obstruction. (Courtesy Dr. R. Surapeneni, M.D., Brooklyn Veterans Administration Hospital, Brooklyn, New York.)

Body wall hernias are a common cause of mechanical small bowel obstrucuon, and CT is useful in revealing the precise site and type of hernia and its contents. Ventral body wall hernias are most commonly seen postoperatively. The more unusual ventral body wall hernias of the spigelian type have also been demonstrated by CT.[65] The defect in the body wall occurs at a weak point along the lateral border of the rectus muscle, approximately midway between the umbilicus and symphysis pubis at the fold of Douglas (Fig. 5-59). Inguinal hernias can usually be distinguished from femoral hernias by locating the hernia sac as either anterior to the inguinal ligament in the former (Fig. 5-60) or posterior to the inguinal ligament alongside the femoral vessels in the latter.

More unusual body wall hernias may present more of a clinical problem. CT examination has reportedly demonstrated a femoral hernia with the hernia sac containing small bowel and omentum extending upward over the inguinal ligament and tracking along the superior epigastric vessels to appear as a lower abdominal mass.[66] CT has also been useful in demonstrating the unusual obturator hernia containing small bowel projecting between the pectineus and external obturator muscles[67,68] (Fig. 5-61).

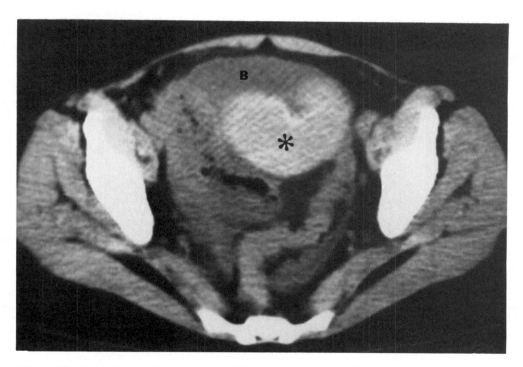

Fig. 5-57. Closed loop obstruction. A dilated sausage-shaped bowel loop contains high-density hemorrhagic fluid (*). A closed loop obstruction has resulted from adhesions (*B*, bladder). (Courtesy Dr. S. Gross, Muhlenberg, New Jersey.)

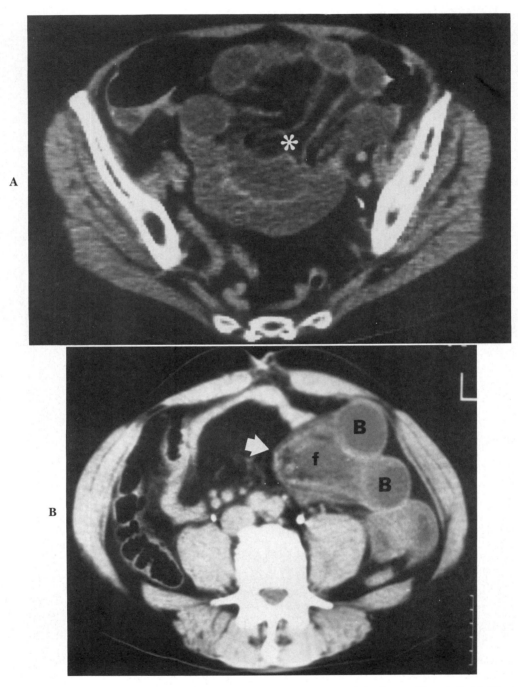

Fig. 5-58. Small bowel volvulus. **A,** A scan through the pelvis shows dilated, fluid-filled loops of ileum with mesenteric vascular bundles radiating to a single point around which volvulus has occurred (*). At surgery the small adhesive band responsible was identified and lysed. **B,** In another patient, dilated jejunal loops *(B)* are seen twisted about their mesenteric vascular supply *(arrow)*. Ascites *(f)* is present between the mesenteric leaves.

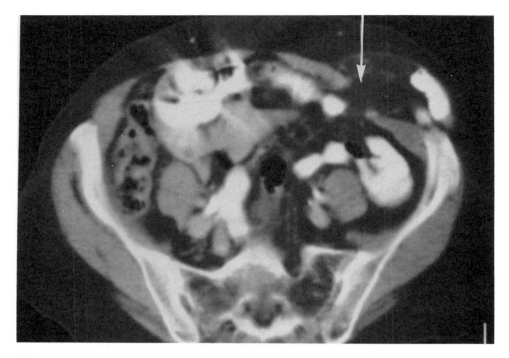

Fig. 5-59. Spigelian hernia. Small bowel loop and mesenteric fat are seen herniating through a defect in the ventral body wall at the lateral margin of the rectus muscle, the spiegelian line *(arrow).*

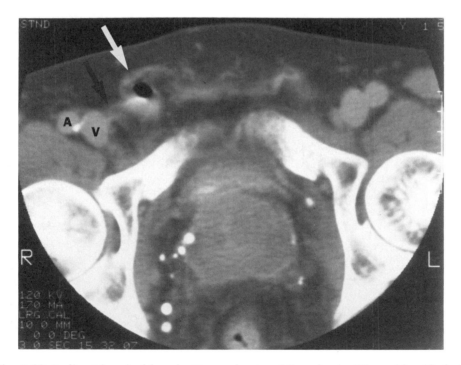

Fig. 5-60. Indirect inguinal hernia. Femoral artery *(A)* and vein *(V)* are identified. Anteromedially, a loop of small bowel containing gas and contrast material is present in a hernia sac in the inguinal canal *(white arrow).* The inguinal ligament is faintly discerned *(black arrow).*

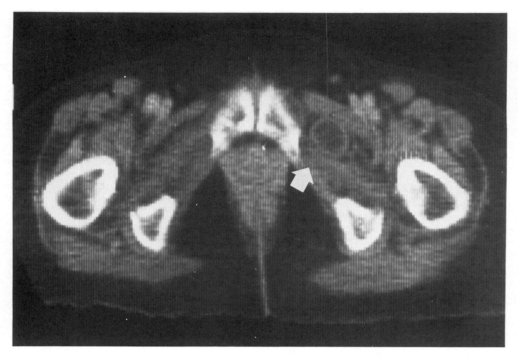

Fig. 5-61. Obturator hernia. In this patient with small bowel obstruction, a scan at the level of the obturator foramen shows a fluid density mass between the peripheral pectinus muscle and the central obturator externus muscle. This represents the hernia sac *(arrow).*

REFERENCES

1. Megibow, A.J., Zerhouni, E.A., Hulnick, D.H., et al.: Air contrast techniques in gastrointestinal computed tomography, AJR **145:**418, 1985.
2. Shapiro, J., and Rubin, J.: CT appearance of the inferior mesenteric vein, J. Comput. Assist. Tomogr. **8:**877-880, 1984.
3. Silverman, P.M., Kelvin, F.M., Korobkin, M., et al.: Computed tomography of the normal mesentery, AJR **143:**953-957, 1984.
4. Curcio, C.M., Feinstein, R.S., Humphrey, R.L., et al.: Computed tomography of entero-enteric intussusception, J. Comput. Assist. Tomogr. **6:**969-974, 1982.
5. Fisher, J.K.: Computed tomographic diagnosis of volvulus in intestinal malrotation, Radiology **140:**145-146, 1981.
6. Federle, M.P., Chun, G., Jeffrey, R.B., et al.: Computed tomographic findings in bowel infarction, AJR **142:**91-95, 1984.
7. Nichols, D.M.: Computed tomography in acute mesenteric vein thrombosis, J. Comput. Assist. Tomogr. **8:**171-172, 1984.
8. Connor, R., Jones, B., Fishman, E.K., et al.: Pneumatosis intestinalis: role of computed tomography in diagnosis and management, J. Comput. Assist. Tomogr. **8:**269-275, 1984.

9. Kelvin, F.M., Korobkin, M., Rouch, R.F., et al.: Computed tomography of pneumatosis intestinalis, J. Comput. Assist. Tomogr. **8:**276-280, 1984.
10. Fisher, J.K.: Computed tomography of colonic pneumatosis intestinalis with mesenteric and portal venous air, J. Comput. Assist. Tomogr. **8:**573-574, 1984.
11. Fischman, E.K., Zinreich, E.S., Jones, B., et al.: Computed tomographic diagnosis of radiation ileitis, Gastrointest. Radiol. **9:**149-152, 1984.
12. Plojoux, O., Hauser, H., and Wettstein, P.. Computed tomography of intramural hematoma of the small intestine, Radiology **144:**559-561, 1982.
13. Federle, M.P.: Computed tomography of blunt abdominal trauma, Radiol. Clin. North Am. **21:**461-475, 1983.
13a. Wing, V.W., Federle, M.P., Morris, J.A., et al.: The clinical impact of CT for blunt abdominal trauma, AJR **145:**1191-1195, 1985.
14. Strauss, J., Balthazar, E.J., and Naidich, D.P.: Jejunal perforation by a toothpick: CT demonstration, J. Comput. Assist. Tomogr. **9:**812-814, 1985.
15. Jeffrey, R.B., Federle, M.P., and Laing, F.C.: Computed tomography of mesenteric involvement in fulminant pancreatitis, Radiology **147:**185-188, 1983.

16. Jones, B., Bayless, T.M., Fishman, E.K., et al.: Lymphadenopathy in celiac disease: compted tomographic observations, AJR **142**:1127-1132, 1984.

17. Li, D.K.B., and Rennie, C.S.: Abdominal computed tomography in Whipple's disease, J. Comput. Assist. Tomogr. **5**:249-252, 1981.

18. Rijke, A.M., Falke, T.H.M., and deVries, R.R.P.: Computed tomography in Whipple disease, J. Comput. Assist. Tomogr. **7**:1101-1102, 1983.

19. Hulnick, D.H., Megibow, A.J., Naidich, D.P., et al.: Abdominal tuberculosis evaluated by computed tomography, Radiology **157**:199-205, 1985.

20. Vincent, M.E., and Robbins, A.H.: Mycobacterium avium intracellulare complex enteritis; Pseudo-Whipple's disease in AIDS, AJR **144**:921-922, 1985.

21. Nyberg D.A., Federle, M.P., Jeffrey, R.B., et al.: Abdominal CT findings of disseminated *Mycobacterium Avium-Intracellulare* in AIDS, AJR **145**:297-299, 1985.

22. Berk, R.N., Wall, S.D., McCardle, C.B., et al.: Cryptosporidiosis of the stomach and small intestine in patients with AIDS, AJR **143**:549-554, 1984.

23. Schnur, M.J., and Weiner, S.N.: The "string sign" on computerized tomography, Gastrointest. Radiol. **7**:43-46, 1982.

24. Berliner, L., Redmond, P., Purow, E., et al.: Computed tomography in Crohn's disease, Am. J. Gastroenterol. **77**: 548-553, 1982.

25. Engelholm, L., and DeToeuf, J.: Personal communication, August 1985.

26. Frager, D.H., Goldman, M., and Beneventano, T.C.: Computed tomography in Crohn's disease, J. Comput. Assist. Tomogr. **7**:819-824, 1983.

27. Goldberg, H.I., Gore, R.M., Margulis, A.R., et al.: Computed tomography in the evaluation of Crohn's disease, AJR **140**:277-282, 1983.

28. Megibow, A.J., Bosniak, M.A., Ambos, M.A., et al.: Crohn's disease causing hydronephrosis, J. Comput. Assist. Tomogr. **5**:509-511, 1981.

29. Gore, R.M., and Goldberg, H.I.: Computed tomographic evaluation of the gastrointestinal tract in diseases other than primary adenocarcinoma, Radiol. Clin. North. Am. **20**:781-796, 1982.

30. Goldman, S.M., Fishman, E.K., Gatewood, O.M.B., et al.: CT in the diagnosis of enterovesical fistulae, AJR **144**: 1229-1233, 1985.

31. Brady, L.W.: Malignant lymphoma of the gastrointestinal tract, Radiology **137**:291-298, 1980.

32. Zornoza, J., and Dodd, G.D.: Lymphoma of the gastrointestinal tract, Semin. Roentgenol. **15**:272-287, 1980.

33. Lewin, K.J., Ranchod, M., and Dorfman, R.F.: Lymphomas of the gastrointestinal tract: a study of 117 cases presenting with gastrointestinal disease, Cancer **42**:693-707, 1978.

34. Megibow, A.J., Balthazar, E.J., Naidich, D.P., et al.: Computed tomography of gastrointestinal lymphoma, AJR **141**: 541-547, 1983.

35. Burgener, F.A., and Hamlin, D.J.: Histiocytic lymphoma of the abdomen: radiographic spectrum. AJR **137**:337-342, 1981.

36. Pagani, J.J., and Bernardino, M.E.: CT-radiographic correlation of ulcerating small bowel lymphomas, AJR **136**:998-1000, 1981.

37. Mueller, P.R., Ferrucci, J.T., Harbin, W.P., et al.: Appearance of lymphomatous involvement of the mesentery by ultrasonography and body computed tomography: the "sandwich" sign, Radiology **134**:467-473, 1980.

38. Clark, R.A., and Alexander, E.S.: Computed tomography of gastrointestinal leiomyosarcoma, Gastrointest. Radiol. **7**: 127-129, 1982.

39. McLeod, A.J., Zornoza, J., and Shirkhoda, A.: Leiomyosarcoma: computed tomographic findings, Radiology **152**: 133-136, 1984.

40. Megibow, A.J., Balthazar, E.J., Hulnick, D.H., et al.: CT evaluation of gastrointestinal leiomyomas and leiomyosarcomas, AJR **144**:727-731, 1985.

41. Bancks, N.H., Goldstein, H.M., and Dodd, G.D.: The roentgenologic spectrum of small intestinal carcinoid tumors, AJR **123**:274-280, 1975.

42. Siegel, R.S., Kuhns, L.R., Borlaza, G.S., et al.: Computed tomography and angiography in ileal carcinoid tumor and retractile mesenteritis, Radiology **134**:437-440, 1980.

43. Picus, D., Glazer, H.S., Levitt, R.G., et al.: Computed tomography of abdominal carcinoid tumors, AJR **143**:581-584, 1984.

44. McCarthy, S.M., Stark, D.D., Moss, A.A., et al.: Computed tomography of malignant carcinoid disease, J. Comput. Assist. Tomogr. **8**:846-850, 1984.

45. Cockey, B.M., Fishman, E.K., Jones, B., et al.: Computed tomography of abdominal carcinoid tumor, J. Comput. Assist. Tomogr. **9**:38-42, 1985.

46. Balthazar, E.J.: Carcinoid tumors of the alimentary tract, Gastrointest. Radiol. **3**:47-56, 1978.

47. Ochsner, S., and Kleckner, M.S.: Primary malignant neoplasms of the duodenum and small bowel, JAMA **163**:413-417, 1957.

48. Meyers, M.A.: Intraperitoneal spread of malignancies. In Meyers, M.A.: Dynamic radiology of the abdomen, New York, 1977, Springer-Verlag New York Inc.

49. Levitt, R.G., Sagel, S.S., and Stanley, R.J.: Detection of neoplastic involvement of the mesentery and omentum by computed tomography, AJR **131**:835-838, 1978.

50. Meyers, M.A.: Metastatic seeding along the small bowel mesentery, AJR **123**:67-73, 1975.

51. Seshul, M.B., and Covlam, C.M.: Pseudomyxoma peritonei: computed tomography and sonography, AJR **136**: 803-806, 1981.

52. Bernardino, M.E., Jing, B.S., and Wallace, S.: Computed tomography diagnosis of mesenteric masses, AJR **132**:33-36, 1979.

53. Whitley, N.O., Bohlman, M.E., and Baker, L.P.: CT patterns of mesenteric disease, J. Comput. Assist. Tomogr. **6**:490-496, 1982.

54. Raghavendra, B.N., Grieco, A.J., Balthazar, E.J., et al.: Diagnostic utility of sonography and computed tomography in spontaneous mesenteric hematoma, Am. J. Gastroenterol. **77**:570-573, 1982.

55. Waligore, M.P., Stephens, D.H., Soule, E.H., et al.: Lipomatous tumors of the abdominal cavity: CT appearance and pathologic correlation, AJR **137**:539-545, 1981.

56. Gerson, E.S, Gerzof, S.G., and Robbins, A.H.: CT confirmation of pelvic lipomatosis: two cases, AJR **129**:388-340, 1977.

57. Lewis, V.L., Shaffer, H.A., Williamson, B.R.J.: Pseudotumoral lipomatosis of the abdomen, J. Comput. Assist. Tomogr. **6**:79-82, 1982.

58. Ormson, M.J., Stephens, D.H., and Carlson, H.C.: CT recognition of intestinal lipomatosis, AJR **144**:313-314, 1985.

59. Katz, M.E., Heiken, J.P., Glazer, H.S., et al.: Intraabdominal panniculitis: clinical radiographic, and CT features. AJR **145**:293-296, 1985.

60. Whitley, N.O., Brenner, D.E., Antman, K.H., et al.: CT of peritoneal mesothelioma: analysis of eight cases, AJR **138:** 531-535, 1982.

61. Baron, R.L., and Lee, J.K.T.: Mesenteric desmoid tumors, Radiology **140:**777-779, 1981.

62. Magid, D., Fishman, E.K., Jones, B., et al.: Desmoid tumors in Gardner syndrome: use of computed tomography, AJR **142:**1141-1145, 1984.

63. Balthazar, E.J., Bauman, J.S., Megibow, A.J.: CT diagnosis of closed loop obstruction, J. Comput. Assist. Tomogr. **9:** 953-955, 1985.

64. Harbin, W.P.: Computed tomographic diagnosis of internal hernia, Radiology **143:**736, 1982.

65. Balthazar, E.J., Subramanyam, B.R., and Megibow, A.J.: Spigelian hernia: CT and ultrasonography diagnosis, Gastrointest. Radiol. **9:**81-85, 1984.

66. Lewin, J.R.: Femoral hernia with upward extension into abdominal wall: CT diagnosis, AJR **136:**206-207, 1981.

67. Meziane, M.A., Fishman, E.K., and Siegelman, S.S.: Computed tomographic diagnosis of obturator foramen hernia, Gastrointest. Radiol. **8:**375-377, 1983.

68. Megibow, A.J., and Wagner, A.G.: Case report: obturator hernia, J. Comput. Assist. Tomogr. **7:**350-352, 1983.

Chapter Six

COLON

Emil J. Balthazar

Although CT is a valuable radiographic method of identifying and evaluating colonic lesions, it should not be regarded as competitive but as complimentary to colonoscopy and barium enema examination. Conventional examinations of the colon should be performed in all cases in which the presence, extent, origin, or nature of the pathologic process is questionable at the time of the CT examination. CT examination of the colon accomplishes three main functions: (1) CT can diagnose or suggest the presence of intrinsic colonic pathology hither-to unsuspected clinically; (2) CT evaluates the nature and the extent of a known colonic lesion and attempts to stage colonic malignancies; and (3) CT determines the presence, location, and severity of complications associated with colonic lesions (i.e., perforation, abscess, peritonitis). The ability of CT to precisely define colonic wall thickness as well as to visualize pericolic fat and mesenteric and fascial planes represents a novel addition to the radiographic imaging modalities. CT is of invaluable help to the clinician in planning the appropriate medical or surgical therapy.

TECHNIQUE

The sensitivity and to some degree specificity of CT depends on the quality and type of examination performed. Multiple factors play crucial roles in achieving an adequate examination, such as the CT equipment used, the scanning time, the competence of the radiologist monitoring the examination, and the patient's ability to cooperate in avoiding respiratory or body motion. In addition, the quality of the examination improves greatly when the colonic lumen is well visualized. To achieve this goal the colon should be prepared to eliminate fecal material, and the colonic lumen should be filled and distended with a contrast agent. Colonic preparation is performed by using one of the many commercially available products employed for barium enema examinations. We use a 24 hour, clear fluid diet and an oral cathartic bowel preparation.* Patients who are not previously prepared can be adequately cleansed with 2000 ml of a water cleansing enema containing 20 ml of liquid bisacodyl.

Visualization of the colonic lumen is achieved in some institutions by rectally administering a positive contrast material that consists of dilute barium or dilute, water-soluble contrast.[1,2] Oral administration of 20 to 50 ml of diatrizoate meglumine the night before the examination has been suggested and tried in our institution with limited success. Lack of colonic distention and an uneven and unreliable visualization of the distal colonic segments are the main shortcomings of this technique. We consider air insufflation the simplest and most reliable way to distend the colon and evaluate intraluminal or intramural pathology.[3,4] The density difference between the air-filled lumen, colonic wall, and pericolic fat allows for a reliable assessment of the colonic wall thickness as well as the detection of smaller intraluminal colonic lesions. Before the examination is started, the rectum is cannulated using a simple, small (20 French), red rubber catheter with a bulb attached for insufflation. Other commercially available rectal air tips can be used. Air is slowly insufflated into the colon until the patient feels the urge to defecate. Glucagon (0.5 mg) can be administered to help retention, reduce discomfort, and facilitate patient cooperation. All patients receive 500 ml of oral contrast material approximately 45 minutes before scanning time to opacify distal ileal loops.† Unless

*Fleet Kit No. 1 manufactured by C.B. Fleet Co. Inc.
†E-Z CAT manufactured by E-Z-M Company, Westbury, New York.

there is a history of allergy or renal insufficiency, intravenous contrast material is administered as a rapid bolus/rapid infusion just before and during scanning. A scout film is obtained, and the entire abdomen is scanned generally using 10 mm sections at 15 mm intervals. If colonic pathology is detected or has been realized previously, selected 10 × 10 mm, or for subtle lesions 5 × 5 mm, sections are repeated. At this time, depending on the location, morphology, and extent of pathologic process, the colon can be examined in the lateral decubitus or prone position. For instance, to achieve adequate air distention of the rectum, the prone position is preferred. If the colon is not sufficiently distended, additional air can be slowly insufflated at any time. (For further details see Chapter One.)

Imaging is performed using standard windows of 300 to 500 H units. When colonic pathology is suspected, a careful survey of the region of interest, employing wide window widths (1000 to 2000 H units) and window levels (−200 to −500 H units) can better delineate intraluminal pathology and visualize small lesions.

CT examination of the colon can be performed using different techniques, depending on the local circumstances, the time available for scanning, and the habits and preferences of the radiologist.[1] Unless a definite effort to clean, distend, and visualize the colonic lumen is made, reliable, high-quality examinations should not be expected. We perform these examinations mainly on patients with known colonic lesions, high clinical suspicion of colonic or pericolic pathology, and known or suspected pelvic pathology.[4] In our experience, air insufflation of the colon is relatively well accepted by patients, the procedure is reliable and safe, there is no significant time lost, and there is no danger of leakage of positive contrast material on the table. This examination provides the best means to image the true thickness of the bowel wall and to identify small intraluminal lesions. Air insufflation should not be performed in patients with an acute abdomen when a colonic perforation or impending perforation is suspected.

NORMAL COLON

During the abdominal CT examination, the colon is easily identified, particularly when the lumen is filled with contrast material or air. Depending on the position and orientation of different colonic segments, the CT images show ring-like structures in the vertical segments (ascending and descending colon and rectum) and tubular structures oriented transversely or anteroposteriorly in the transverse colon and sigmoid colon respectively (Fig. 6-1). When the colon is at least partially distended, the normal colonic haustrations can be identified (Fig. 6-1). The cecum is more anteriorly located, and because of its mobility it may be visualized either in the right lower quadrant or more medially in the abdomen. Recognition of the cecum is facilitated by the visualization of the contrast-filled terminal ileum or occasionally by visualization of the ileocecal valve (Fig. 6-2). Fatty infiltration and lipomas of the ileocecal valve can be diagnosed by visualizing low-density tissue (Fig. 6-2). During routine examinations, the normal appendix is seen infrequently. Depending on its orientation, the appendix appears as a small, ring-like, or tubular structure sometimes containing air (Fig. 6-3). The presence of air in the appendix without any associated abnormalities is not indicative of appendicitis and should be considered a normal finding (Fig. 6-3). Fecal material appears as intraluminal, mottled, soft-tissue and air density that can usually be differentiated from the homogeneous appearance of a colonic tumor (Figs. 6-3 and 6-4). The dependent location of fecal material helps in this differentiation. Impacted, long-standing fecalomas may occasionally calcify or be impregnated by barium. They exhibit a high-density peripheral ring and a characteristic mottled central core.[5] The pericolic fat, connective tissue, and mesenteric attachments appear as homogeneous structures having a fat density and a few thin enhancing vascular channels. The normal transverse mesocolon and greater omentum are usually not well visualized. However, on good quality scans one can identify the mesosigmoid and when present a mesocecum.

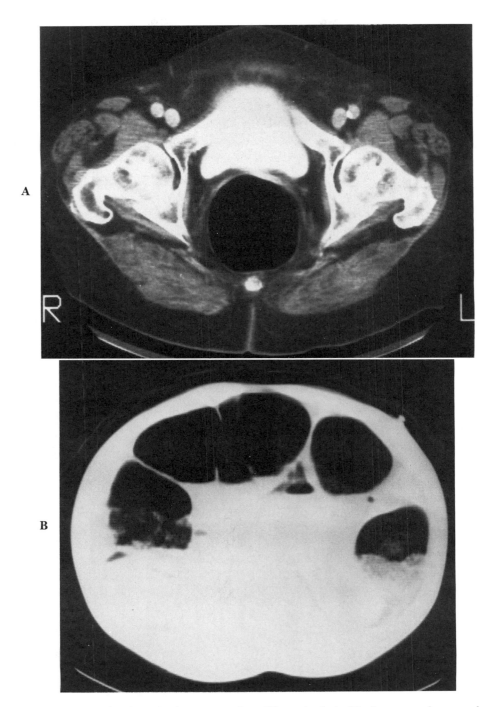

Fig. 6-1. Normal colon. **A,** A cross section (10 mm) of air-filled rectum shows a sharp inner and outer contour and a normal wall thickness. The image was obtained with a window width of 500 H units and a window level of +8 H units. **B,** Air-filled transverse colon with residual fecal material. This image was obtained with lung window settings (window width 1200 H units and window level −532 H units) to enhance visualization of intraluminal lesions. Haustrations are seen partially traversing the colonic lumen.

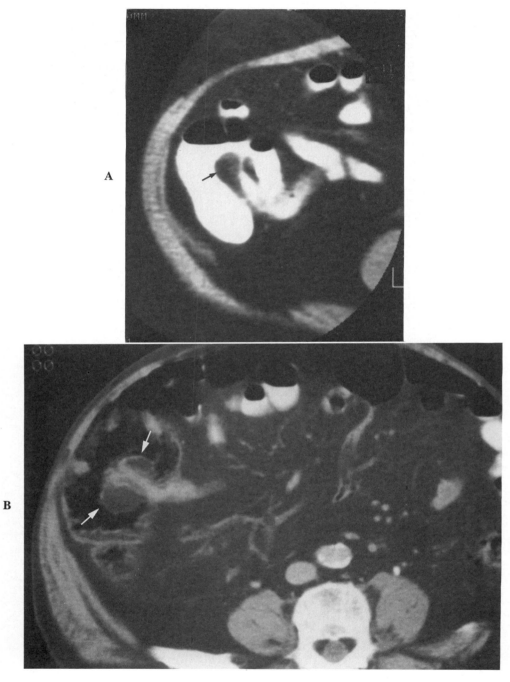

Fig. 6-2. Normal ileocecal valve. **A,** A magnified view showing the terminal ileum entering the cecum and surrounded by fatty infiltration of the ileocecal valve *(arrow)*. Note the clean and homogeneously lucent pericecal fat. **B,** The terminal ileum and fatty infiltration of the ileocecal valve are demonstrated *(arrows)* on an air-filled cecum.

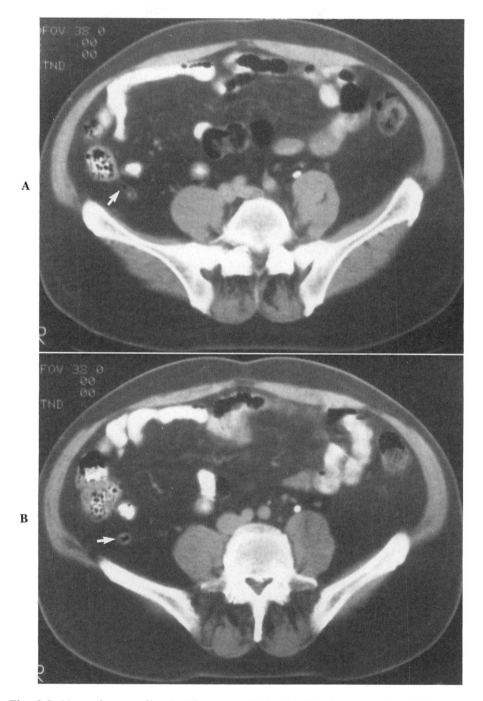

Fig. 6-3. Normal appendix. **A,** The appendix is visualized as a small tubular structure arising from the tip of a collapsed barium- and fecal-filled cecum *(arrow).* **B,** Cross section through a normal air-filled appendix *(arrow)* showing a thin-walled, small structure containing air. Note the normal periappendicular fat with a fine linear branching pattern, representing mesenteric vessels.

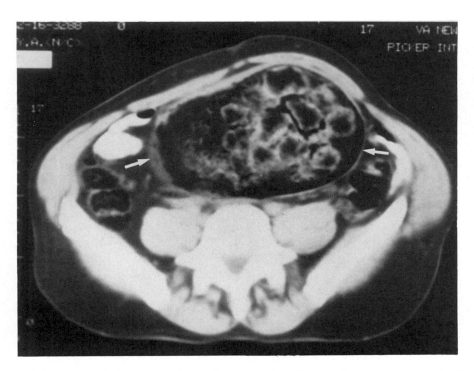

Fig. 6-4. Impacted fecaloma of the sigmoid colon. The patient was admitted with a palpable abdominal mass. A distended sigmoid colon filled with mottled soft-tissue and air densities is seen elevating the anterior abdominal wall *(arrows)*. (Courtesy Dr. R. Gordon, Veterans Administration Hospital, New York, New York.)

The rectum is about 12 to 15 cm in length, with the upper part having the same diameter as the sigmoid. The lower part below the peritoneal reflection widens to form the rectal ampulla and ends in an abruptly narrow anal canal.[6,7] Peritoneum covers the anterior surface of the upper rectum and reflects anteriorly over the posterior wall of the bladder in males or of the vagina in females to form the rectovesical pouch or Douglas' pouch. The level of the peritoneal reflection is not fixed; it is raised when the rectum or the bladder are distended. The floor of Douglas' pouch is usually situated about 2.5 cm above the prostate or about 7.5 cm above the anal orifice.[6] Peritoneum and pelvic floor muscles divide the lower pelvis into three compartments (Fig. 6-5): (1) the peritoneal cavity above the peritoneal reflection; (2) the subperitoneal space between the peritoneum and levator ani muscles; and (3) the ischiorectal fossa inferior and lateral to the levator ani.[6,7] The lower two thirds of the rectum is enveloped by extraperitoneal connective and adipose tissue. Within the subperitoneal space, a fascial plane called the perirectal fascia encloses the perirectal fatty tissue and separates it from the more periph-

erally located pararectal connective tissue (Fig. 6-5). The degree of development of the perirectal fascia varies in different individuals and in its normal appearance it is only rarely visualized on CT examinations[7] (Fig. 6-6). Its visualization depends on its thickness and on the density differences between this fascial plane and the two subperitoneal compartments adjacent to it. The perirectal space (capsula adiposa rectalis) contains the superior hemorrhoidal vessels and, because of the abundant amount of fatty tissue, has an homogeneous, low-density appearance on CT. A somewhat increased inhomogeneous density is normally present within the pararectal space, which contains the middle hemorrhoidal vessels and a larger proportion of fibroblasts and collageneous fibers. Alteration of the normal anatomical relationships of these structures helps in early CT recognition of inflammatory or neoplastic involvement of perirectal and pararectal spaces (Fig. 6-6). For a more detailed description of the normal CT anatomy of the lower pelvis and perineum the reader can consult recently published papers by Grabbe et al.[7] and Tismado et al.[8]

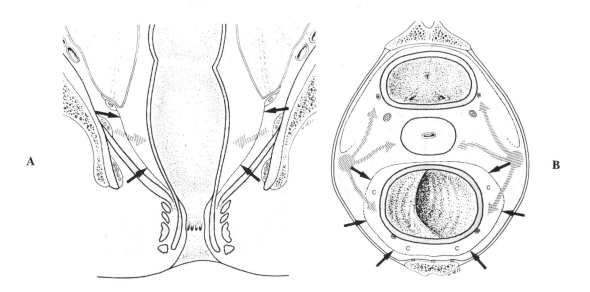

Fig. 6-5. Diagram of the rectum and perirectal compartments. **A,** Coronal and **B,** transverse sections. Capsula adiposa rectalis *(C)* enclosed by the perirectal fascia *(arrows).* Note the position of the peritoneal reflection and of the levator ani muscles dividing the lower pelvis into three compartments. (From Grabbe, E., et al.: The perirectal fascia: morphology and use in staging of rectal carcinoma, Radiology **149:**241-246, 1983.)

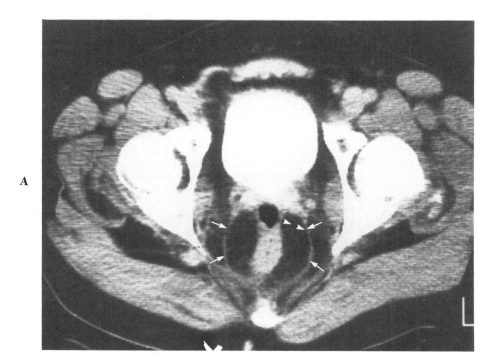

Fig. 6-6. The perirectal fascia divides the perirectal connective tissue into perirectal and pararectal compartments. **A,** Normal appearance with a well-developed perirectal fascia *(arrows).* Note the homogeneously lucent perirectal space (capsula adiposa rectalis).

Continued.

B

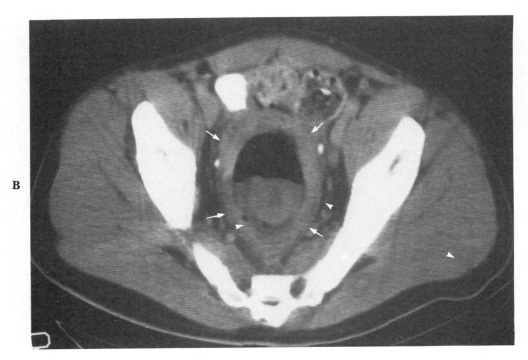

Fig. 6-6, cont'd. B, Foreign body perforation of the rectum, leading to severe perirectal inflammation that obliterates the perirectal space *(arrows)*. The finding is not specific; it can be seen with tumor infiltration (see Fig. 6-82, *C*).

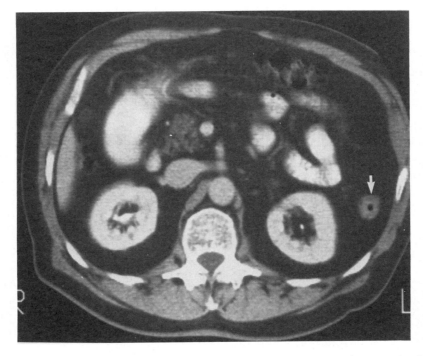

Fig. 6-7. Normal collapsed descending colon showing an apparent increase in the wall thickness *(arrow)*. The inner and outer contours are sharp and the pericolic fat homogeneously lucent.

When the colonic lumen is filled with air, an accurate measurement of the true thickness of the wall of the colon can be made (see Fig. 6-1). The presence, extent, and configuration of a thick bowel wall are the most important CT criteria in the evaluation of colonic pathology.[9,10] Measurements of colonic wall at different levels in normal individuals have shown thicknesses between 0.9 and 2.6 mm with a standard deviation of 0.4 mm.[9] There are no significant variations in the wall thickness of different colonic segments, including the rectum. A slight increase in the wall thickness of collapsed colonic segments is often seen (Fig. 6-7). It is safe to assume that when the colon is distended, its wall thickness does not exceed 3 mm, while on a collapsed colon it is not greater than 5 mm.[9,10] In addition, the wall of the colon is homogeneously dense and has a perfectly symmetrical configuration with a sharp inner and outer contour (Figs. 6-1 and 6-7).

INFLAMMATORY DISEASE OF THE COLON

CT findings in inflammatory diseases of the colon are dependent on the quality of the examination and on the severity of the inflammatory process. Established parameters, such as the site and length of involvement, universal versus segmental disease, and rectal or associated small bowel involvement, should be carefully evaluated. In addition, the thickness of the bowel wall, the existence and degree of associated pericolic abnormalities, and distant complications, such as abscesses, should be looked for. Barium enema remains the procedure of choice in visualizing mucosal disease, superficial ulcers, and small filling defects, while CT has proved far superior in diagnosing pericolic and mesenteric abnormalities.

Based on their CT appearance, the syndrome of acute colitis can be divided and described as two separate entities.

Mild to moderate colitis

In patients with superficial mucosal disease, CT findings are either totally absent or minimal and unimpressive. Among the eight patients with ulcerative colitis reported by Gore et al.[11] six (75%) demonstrated slight symmetrical thickening of the colonic wall within a range of 3 to 9 mm with a mean of 7.8 mm. The wall of the colon is sometimes inhomogeneously attenuated, and a "target" configuration on cross section may be seen in the rectum.[11] This sign refers to the inner layer having a lucent appearance compared with the higher density of the peripheral circumferential layer. Superficial edematous and inflammatory changes probably explain this finding. In the more severe cases, an ill-defined hazy, or dirty appearance of the perirectal fat may be seen (Fig. 6-8). In our experience the majority of cases of ulcerative colitis have shown minimal CT findings. Slight thickening of the wall, never exceeding 1 cm, is present mainly at levels where the colonic lumen is narrowed and the inflammatory process more severe (Fig. 6-9). The wall of the colon is generally homogeneous in density and the subtle, mucosal changes and superficial ulcerations expected are not seen on CT.

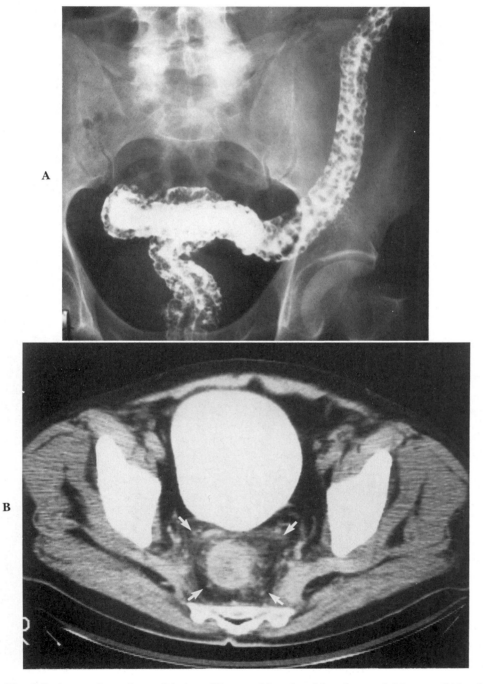

Fig. 6-8. Acute ulcerative colitis in a 57-year-old male with a 6-month history of bloody diarrhea. **A,** Barium enema shows a diffusely ulcerated mucosa of the rectum and distal colon. **B,** Pericolic inflammation appearing as ill-defined, streaky and hazy densities involving the perirectal fat *(arrows)*. The rectal lumen is not seen, and the rectal wall thickness can not be reliably evaluated.

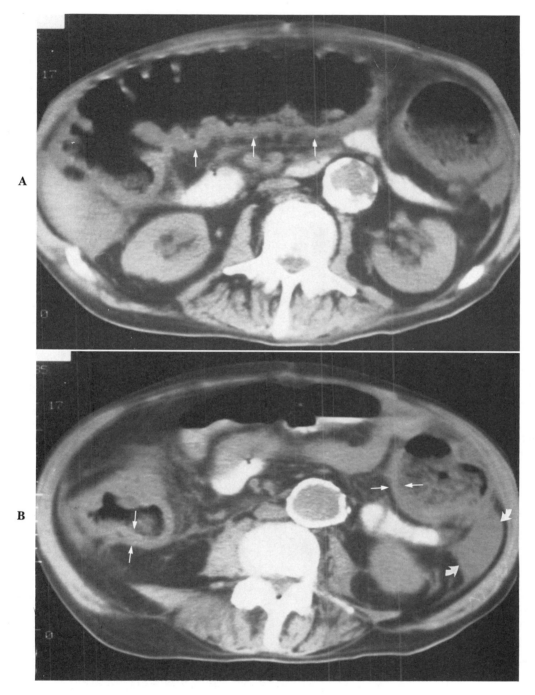

Fig. 6-10. Pseudomembranous colitis with diffuse colonic involvement in a 69-year-old male on antibiotic therapy. **A,** An irregular lumen, ulcerated mucosal surface, and circumferential wall thickening of the transverse colon and splenic flexure *(arrows)*, is demonstrated. **B,** Homogeneous circumferential thickening of the right and left colon and pericolic inflammatory changes are seen *(arrows)*. In addition, there is fluid in the peritoneal cavity *(curved arrows)*.

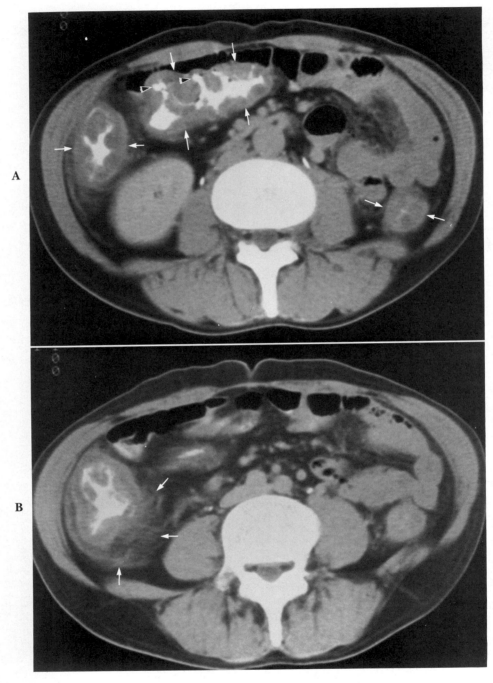

Fig. 6-11. Hemorrhagic cytomegalovirus colitis in young homosexual male with AIDS. **A** and **B,** Circumferential thickening of the wall of the colon *(arrows)* and deep intramural ulcerations filled with barium are visualized *(arrowheads)*. The density of the wall is not homogeneous, and inflammatory infiltration of the pericolic fat is present *(arrows in* **B***)*.

Ischemic colitis. Slight segmental thickening of the wall of the colon, particularly on the left side, is the expected CT finding (Fig. 6-12). The degree of wall thickening is variable. It may be symmetrical or it may appear as slightly lobulated and associated with an irregular narrowed colonic lumen similar to thumbprinting described on barium enema examination.[17] At this stage of evolution the ischemic process mimics other forms of segmental or diffuse inflammatory colitis.

When bowel infarction develops, CT examination may show in addition curvilinear collections of intramural gas, portal and mesenteric venous air, and blood clots in the superior mesenteric artery or vein (see Fig. 6-80). These findings were present in several cases of bowel infarction recently reported.[18] Although intrahepatic portal venous gas is not in itself pathognomonic of bowel infarction, its association with intramural bowel pathology is virtually diagnostic. It should be noted that intramural gas, cystlike or curvilinear in appearance, may be seen in the benign forms of pneumatosis intestinalis without infarction. CT is more sensitive than conventional radiographs in detecting intravascular or intramural air.[18] The diagnosis of ischemic bowel should be made only in symptomatic patients and in the proper clinical context. Intestinal infarction carries a mortality of 80% to 92%,[19,20] mainly because of delays in the clinical diagnosis. A close survey for signs of bowel ischemia or infarction during CT examination can lead to an earlier diagnosis and proper surgical treatment.

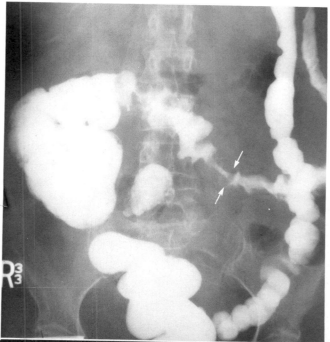

A

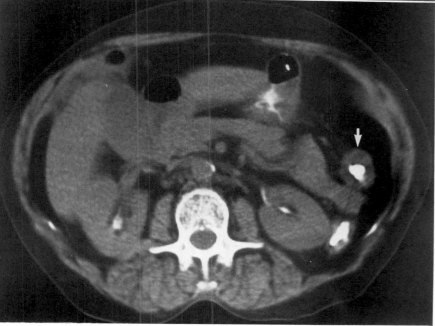

B

Fig. 6-12. Ischemic colitis in a 74-year-old female. **A,** Barium enema shows segmental involvement of the transverse colon and splenic flexure (*arrows*). **B,** CT shows circumferential thickening, particularly of the anterior limb of splenic flexure (*arrow*).

Radiation colitis. CT findings indicative of radiation injury are seen mainly in the pelvis following external and/or internal radiation treatment for malignancies. We have observed CT abnormalities in patients in whom the radiation dose exceeded 4000 rads. The expected findings are related to the amount of radiation, the size of the treatment field, and the time of the examination in the natural evolution of radiation injury. In the acute phase, during and immediately following radiation, the obliterative arteritis resulting in tissue ischemia produces an acute proctitis. CT at this time shows a narrowed, partially distensible rectum with slight wall thickening and a submucosal circumferential lucency similar to the "target sign" described in ulcerative colitis[11] (Fig. 6-13). In the chronic phase with the development of intramural fibrosis, the rectal wall becomes thicker and homogeneous in density, the lumen is narrowed, and associated perirectal abnormalities are present (Fig. 6-14). Proliferation of the perirectal fat with widening of the presacral space greater than 1 cm has been described.[21] There is thickening of the perirectal fascia, and an increased amount of fibrotic tissue is seen, particularly in the pararectal space, creating a "halo effect."[21] The process is symmetrical and similar findings may be seen involving ileal loops and small bowel mesentery.[22] The visualization of a well-defined, soft-tissue mass either in the wall of the rectum or in the perirectal space is incompatible with the diagnosis of radiation injury alone and should be considered suggestive of residual or recurrent pelvic malignancy.

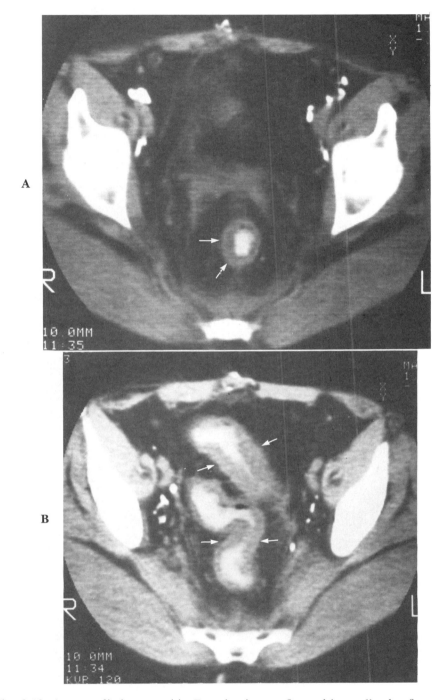

Fig. 6-13. Acute radiation proctitis. Examination performed immediately after completion of radiation for cervical carcinoma. **A,** Slight thickening of the rectal wall with the "target sign" configuration *(arrows).* **B,** Luminal narrowing, thickening of the rectosigmoid *(arrows),* and haziness of the perirectal fat are demonstrated. Findings are similar to acute colitis. There is residual contrast material in the pelvic nodes from a lymphangiogram.

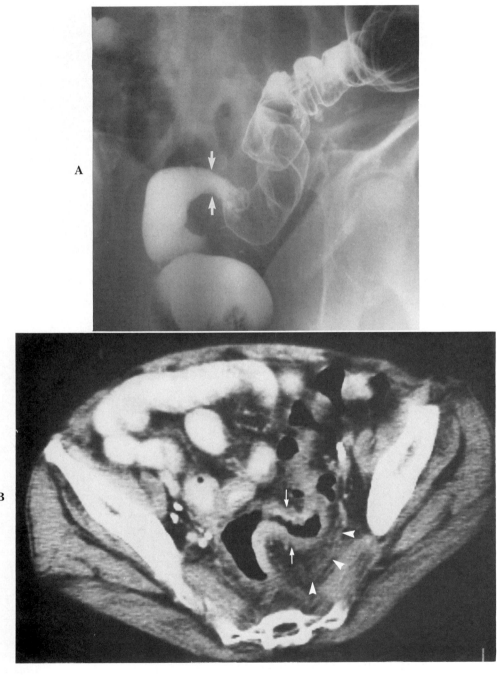

Fig. 6-14. Chronic radiation injury of the sigmoid colon 1 year after external and internal radiation for cervical carcinoma. **A,** Barium enema reveals smooth narrowing of a segment of the sigmoid colon *(arrows)*. **B,** CT shows circumferential and homogeneous wall thickening *(arrows)* and luminal narrowing. Fibrotic changes give a dirty appearance to the pericolic fat *(arrowheads)*.

Granulomatous (Crohn's) colitis

The chronic, granulomatous, inflammatory process in Crohn's disease is characterized by transmural inflammation as well as by associated pericolic and mesenteric abnormalities. Although barium studies and endoscopic examinations are the primary means to evaluate mucosal disease, CT by virtue of its superior contrast resolution has the potential to evaluate bowel wall, mesentery, and adjacent organs. CT is not recommended as a primary diagnostic modality in Crohn's disease. It is, however, extremely useful in assessing the extramucosal and mesenteric manifestations of the disease as well as its common complications. Patients with unexplained clinical complaints (fever, leukocytosis, etc.) and those with suggestive mesenteric changes on barium studies (separation of loops, mass effect) benefit most by the CT examination. The following CT findings are indicative or very suggestive of Crohn's disease[23-28]:

Bowel wall disease. Segmental or skip areas of symmetrical wall thickening measuring 1 to 2 cm from the luminal to serosal surface when assessed transaxially or longitudinally are seen (Figs. 6-15 and 6-16). This finding was present in 23 of 28 cases (82%) reported by Goldberg et al.[23] The bowel wall has generally a homogeneous density[23]; it can occasionally exhibit an inner circumferential lucency enveloped by a denser peripheral zone given the appearance of a "double halo" on cross section[24] (Fig. 6-17). In our experience this finding is seldom seen, is visualized only at certain levels within the diseased bowel, and it is not pathognomonic. It is probably produced by the inflammatory reaction, by edema, and by the deposition of fat in the submucosa. Contrast enhancement of the wall of the diseased colon occurs particularly after a bolus injection. This finding is seen in other forms of inflammatory or ischemic colitis. Luminal narrowing and variable degrees of proximal dilation may be present. Superficial ulcers, cobblestoning, and small pseudopolyps are usually not detected by CT. Deeper transmural ulcerations and larger pseudopolyps may be seen (Fig. 6-18).

Text continued p. 302.

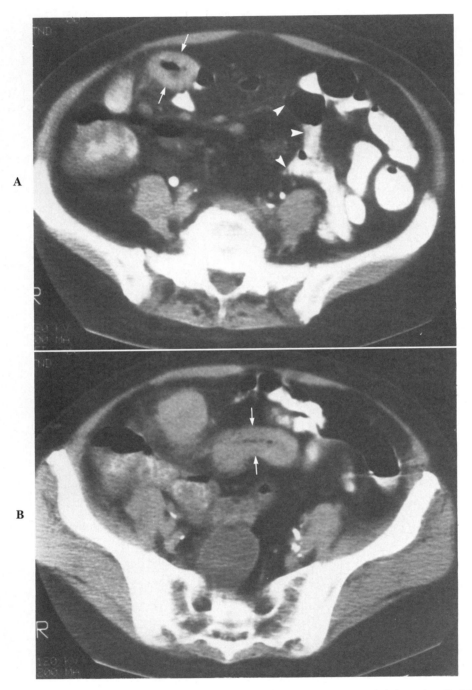

Fig. 6-15. Crohn's disease. Skip areas of symmetrical, circumferential, bowel wall thickening is seen in cross section (**A**) and longitudinal section (**B**) *(arrows)*. Note the proliferation of mesenteric fat with increased density compressing small bowel loops *(arrowheads)*. (Courtesy Dr. E. Gallagher, Lawnwood Medical Center, Ft. Pierce, Florida.)

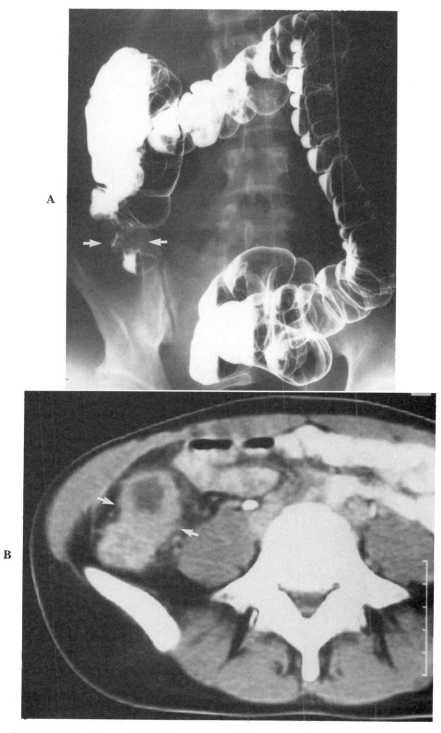

Fig. 6-16. Crohn's disease. **A,** Barium enema shows narrowing and spasticity of the cecum *(arrows).* **B,** Circumferential thickening of the wall of the cecum and pericecal inflammatory reaction (strands and dirty fat) are demonstrated *(arrows).*

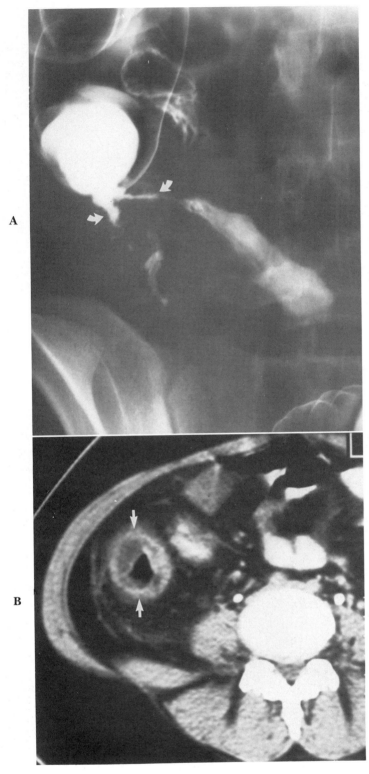

Fig. 6-17. Crohn's disease with a "double halo" sign. **A,** Barium enema demonstrates inflammation with deformity and shrinkage of the cecum and the "string sign" in the terminal ileum *(curved arrows).* **B,** On CT the bowel wall is inhomogeneously thickened with an inner lucency enveloped by a denser peripheral zone *(arrows).* Haziness and small strands are present in the mesentery adjacent to the involved bowel.

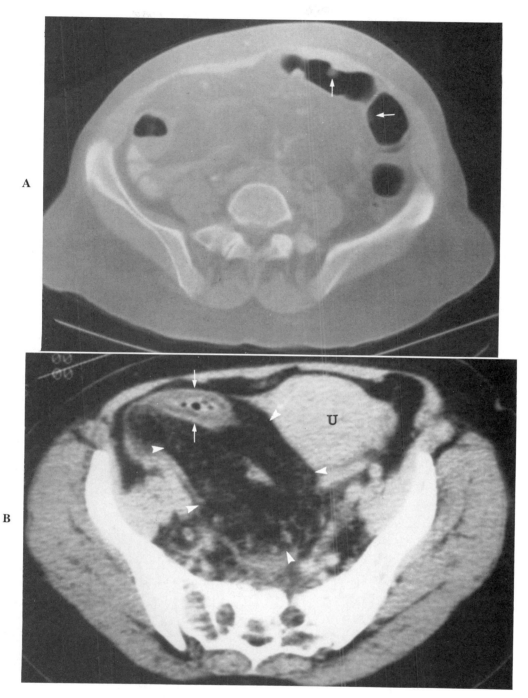

Fig. 6-18. A 58-year-old female with proven granulomatous colitis. **A,** Pseudopolyps are seen in the transverse colon *(arrows)*. The image was obtained with a window width of 2000 H units and a window level of 47 H units. **B,** The sigmoid colon has a thick wall and demonstrates the "double halo" sign *(arrows)*. There is massive proliferation of pelvic fat that acts as a mass, displacing the uterus *(U)* anteriorly and to the left. Increased density with multiple linear strands in the fat represents the "creeping mesenteric fat" sign *(arrowheads)*.

Continued.

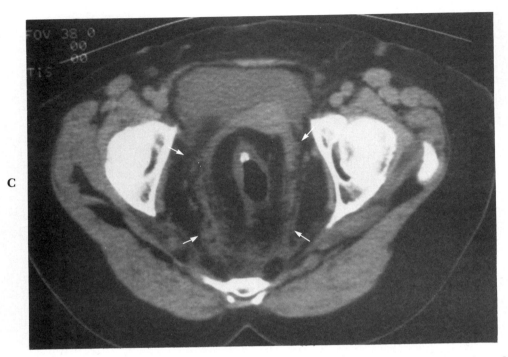

Fig. 6-18, cont'd. C, There is circumferential thickening of the rectal wall, thickening of the perirectal fascia, and an increase in linear and hazy densities in the perirectal and pararectal space *(arrows).* This appearance is similar to some cases of radiation proctitis.

Mesenteric disease. Associated mesenteric abnormalities are commonly seen in Crohn's disease. Fibrofatty proliferation of the mesenteric fat is seen in about 40% of cases.[23] It appears as an enlarged, poorly defined fatty mass with a slightly higher attenuation compared with the homogeneous lower attenuation of the normal mesenteric fat (−100 to −150 H units). When excessive deposition of fat occurs, intestinal loops, the urinary bladder, and even solid organs such as the uterus may be displaced by the mass effect (Fig. 6-18).

Inflammatory involvement of the mesentery, which is sometimes referred to as the "creeping fat sign," appears as streakiness with a dirty or hazy appearance of the mesenteric fat (Fig. 6-18). It has been suggested that the association of "creeping mesenteric fat" with the double halo sign should be considered diagnostic of Crohn's disease.[24] However, this association is rarely seen, and the diagnosis of creeping fat is difficult to establish since it may resemble other mesenteric inflammatory reactions. Mesenteric reactive lymphadenopathy is actually present in the majority of patients with Crohn's disease. It was visualized on CT in 18% of cases in Goldberg's series.[23]

Complications. Abscess, sinus tracts, fistulae, and small bowel obstruction are among the more common and clinically significant complications of Crohn's disease. Mesenteric and/or retroperitoneal abscesses are seen in septic individuals and are characterized by a poorly encapsulated fluid collection (Fig. 6-19). It has a variable density (10 to 30 H units), and it may contain air or contrast material. Although the air may be produced by gas-forming bacteria, the demonstration of positive contrast material in an abscess cavity indicates a fistulous tract or a localized sealed-off perforation. Fistulae and sinus tracts can be identified sometimes in spite of barium studies that appear normal. Enterocolic, enterocutaneous, and perineal fistulae and sinus tracts can be visualized (Fig. 6-20). Detection of bubbles of air in the urinary bladder or vagina adjacent to a disease sigmoid or ileal loop is diagnostic of a fistulous tract. Other expected complications such as fatty infiltration of liver, gallstones, renal stones, small bowel obstruction, carcinoma of the colon, and ureteral obstruction with secondary hydronephrosis can be diagnosed.[27]

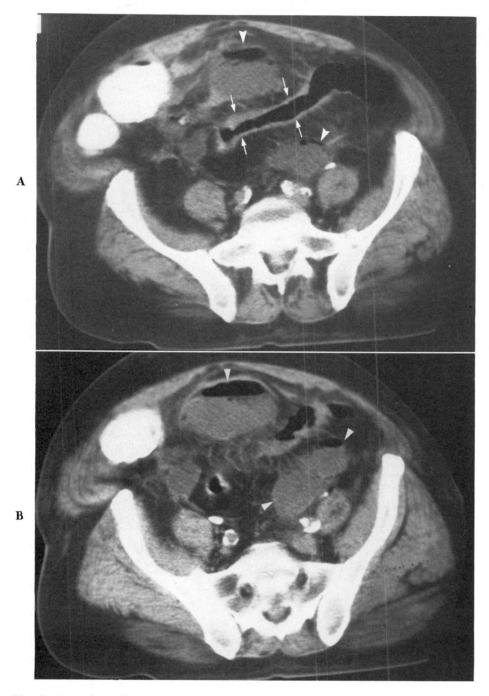

Fig. 6-19. Crohn's disease with mesenteric abscess. **A** and **B,** Granulomatous disease of the sigmoid colon showing a narrowed lumen and a thick, homogeneously dense bowel wall *(arrows).* Poorly encapsulated fluid collections with air-fluid levels representing abscesses are visualized *(arrowheads).* Barium enema showed Crohn's disease of the sigmoid colon but no abscesses.

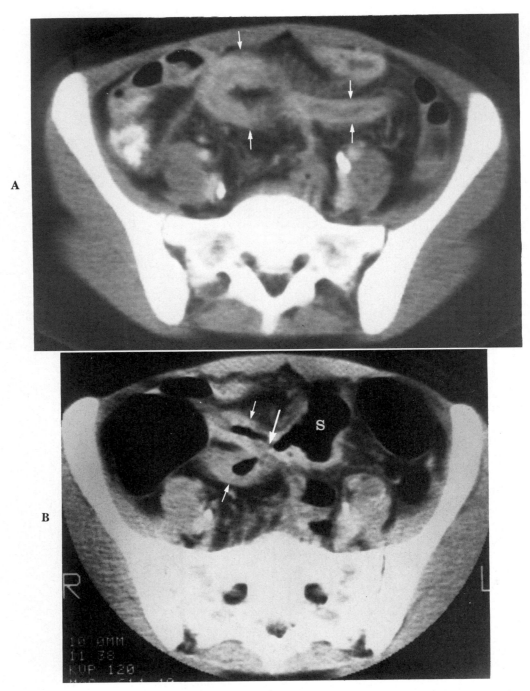

Fig. 6-20. Crohn's disease of the terminal ileum with ileocolic fistula. **A,** Homogeneous thickening of the wall of a segment of the distal small bowel *(arrows).* The mesentery is increased in density and contains linear strands. **B,** A thickened small bowel loop *(arrows)* adjacent to the air-filled sigmoid colon *(S)* with loss of intervening fat plane is seen. Ileosigmoid fistula *(long arrow)* was documented on barium enema examination.

The differential CT diagnosis includes other forms of segmental, inflammatory, or ischemic colitis, colonic tuberculosis (Fig. 6-21), diverticulitis, appendicitis, and rarely infiltrating carcinoma with sealed-off perforation. The association of an abnormally thickened bowel wall detected at different levels in the ileum and colon with adjacent mesenteric abnormalities is very suggestive of Crohn's disease. When the diagnosis is not already known, it should be confirmed by barium studies.

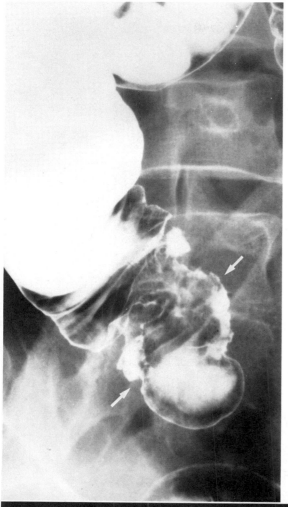

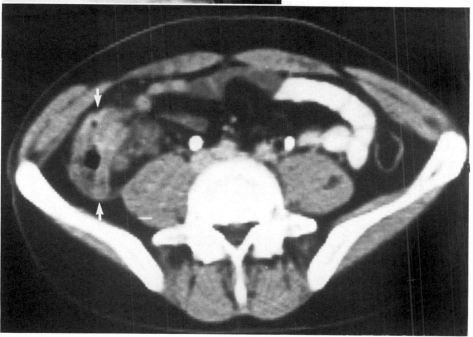

Fig. 6-21. Cecal tuberculosis in a 42-year-old male. **A,** Thickened nodular mucosal folds, superficial ulcers, and an irregular contour is seen in the cecum *(arrows).* **B,** CT demonstrates symmetrical and inhomogeneous thickening of the cecal wall *(arrows).* Findings are similar to granulomatous colitis.

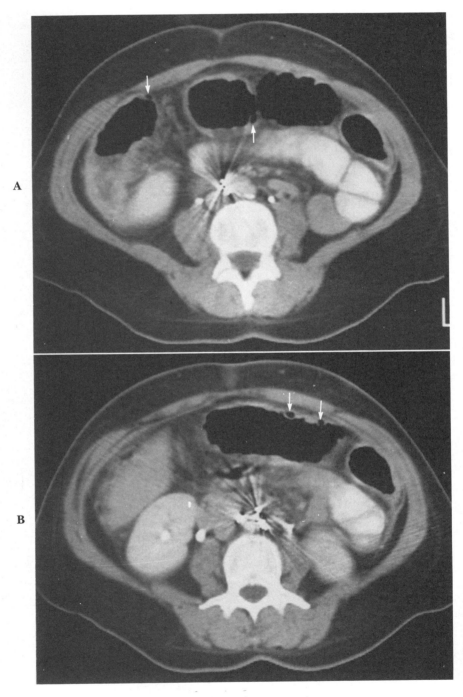

Fig. 6-22. For legend see opposite page.

TOXIC DILATION OF THE COLON

This is an acute, life-threatening complication of acute colitis. It is characterized by transmural inflammation, paralysis and/or destruction of the muscular and neural elements, and impending colonic perforation. It may occur in specific bacterial infections or in amoebic, ischemic, or granulomatous (Crohn's) colitis, but it is most commonly associated with ulcerative colitis. Plain film radiographs remain the fastest and most convenient method to secure the diagnosis. CT examination shows a distended colon filled with a large amount of fluid and air, an irregular, nodular contour, and a distorted haustral pattern.[29] The colonic wall is thin or minimally thickened and small collections of intramural air may be seen (Fig. 6-22). Pericolic air may occur in walled-off perforations. Associated abdominal abscess or free air in the peritoneal cavity indicates perforation or peritonitis.

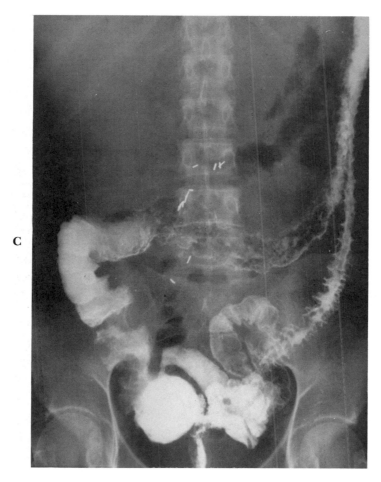

Fig. 6-22. Toxic dilation of the colon in a 41-year-old woman with Crohn's disease. **A** and **B,** Dilated, air-filled, transverse colon has a scalloped contour. Small, soft-tissue indentations and intramural air are identified *(arrows)*. **C,** A barium enema performed later demonstrates diffuse colitis. (Courtesy Dr. B. Siskind, Yale University Hospital, New Haven, Connecticut.)

DIVERTICULITIS

The extramural location of the inflammatory process in diverticulitis explains the inherent diagnostic limitations of contrast enema examination and the great potential advantages provided by CT. The significance and role of CT in the initial diagnosis, evaluation, and management of patients with diverticulitis is being evaluated.[30-32] In addition to the known conventional radiographic findings of diverticula, colonic obstruction, sinus tracts, fistulas, and communicating abscesses, CT evaluates the colonic wall, mesenteric fat, and peritoneal cavity. In our experience CT proved particularly helpful in the detection of the complications of severe diverticulitis; in the diagnosis of mild forms that may not be recognized by conventional means; and in ruling out diverticulitis clinically suspected in symptomatic individuals. It is a noninvasive means of evaluation that may be used initially in septic patients with signs of peritoneal irritation in whom contrast enemas are contraindicated.

The incidence of various CT findings in a series of 43 patients with proven diverticulitis is shown in Table 6-1.[30] Diverticula are visualized in most cases of diverticulitis (Fig. 6-23). Their presence, as well as a distorted luminal contour and muscular hypertrophy, are findings characteristic of uncomplicated diverticulosis (Fig. 6-23) and are not clinically significant. In diverticulitis, thickening of the bowel wall is seen in the majority of patients (Figs. 6-23 and 6-24). It ranges from 4 to 12 mm. It is circumferential, focal, and usually symmetrical. In chronic cases a pericolic soft-tissue mass representing the extension of a walled-off, organized, inflammatory process is sometimes present (Fig. 6-25). Localized, ill-defined, hazy densities associated with linear strands located in the adjacent pericolic fat are the most common and considered the most reliable signs of diverticulitis (Figs. 6-23 and 6-26). In the mild forms these inflammatory changes are minimal, while in severe forms of diverticulitis they may be diffuse and accompanied by extraluminal pockets of fluid scattered throughout the pelvis (Fig. 6-27). Abscesses appear as loculated fluid collections that sometimes contain air. They are usually located adjacent to a colonic segment (Fig. 6-28) but may be distant in the retroperitoneal space, psoas muscle, or liver. Fluid and/or air in the peritoneal cavity indicates diffuse peritonitis if no other diagnostic tests or known pathologic processes can explain these findings (Fig. 6-27). Intramural sinus tracts and fistula to urinary bladder, vagina, or small bowel can be identified by demonstrating linear fluid collections or pockets of air in the adjacent hollow organs. The bladder may show focal wall thickening adjacent to the inflamed sigmoid colon or in proximity of an abscess.[32] Other associated complications, such as colonic obstruction and ureteral obstruction with hydronephrosis, can be recognized.

Text continued p. 316.

Table 6-1. CT findings in 43 cases of diverticulitis

Finding	Number of patients	Percentage
Inflammation of pericolic fat	42	98%
Diverticula	36	84%
Thickened bowel wall	30	70%
Intramural sinus tracts	4	9%
Abscess	20	47%
Peritonitis	7	16%
Fistula	6	14%
Colonic obstruction	5	12%
Ureteral obstruction	3	7%

From Hulnick, M.A., et al.: Computed tomography in the evaluation of diverticulitis, Radiology **152:**491-495, 1984.

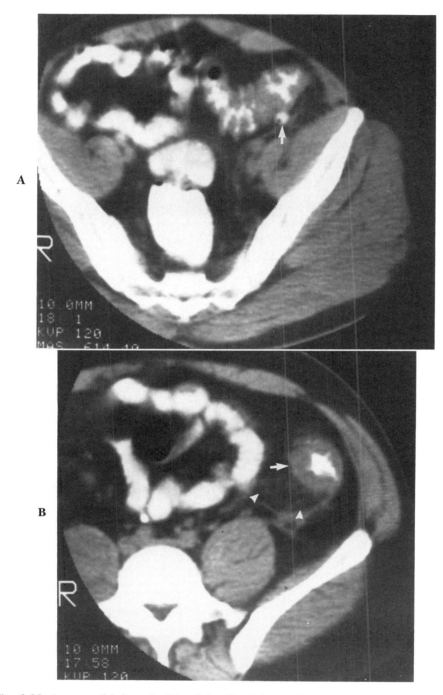

Fig. 6-23. Acute, mild diverticulitis of the distal descending colon. **A,** The sigmoid colon shows a distorted lumen, muscle hypertrophy, and an isolated diverticulum *(arrow)*. **B,** There is circumferential thickening more marked on the medial aspect in the descending colon *(arrow)*. Fine, localized, hazy densities and linear strands are located in the adjacent pericolic fat *(arrowheads)*.

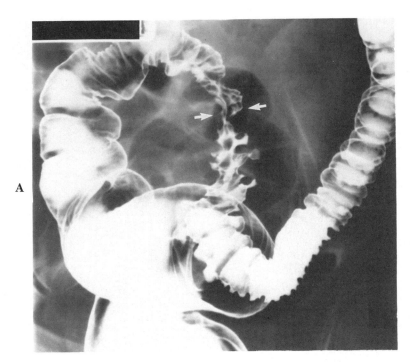

Fig. 6-24. Diverticulitis of the sigmoid colon in a 46-year-old man. **A,** Barium enema shows the sigmoid colon with a normal ascending (right) limb and narrowing, distortion, and diverticula of the descending (left) limb *(arrows)*. **B,** High CT section shows the adjacent two limbs. Note wall thickening of the left limb *(arrows)* compared to the right. **C,** A lower CT cut shows significant luminal narrowing and wall thickening of the affected segment *(arrows)* compared with the normal left segment *(arrowheads)*.

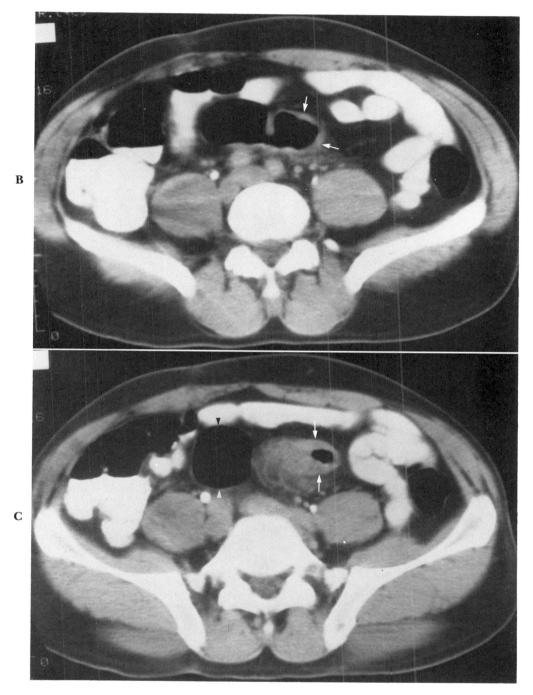

Fig. 6-24. For legend see opposite page.

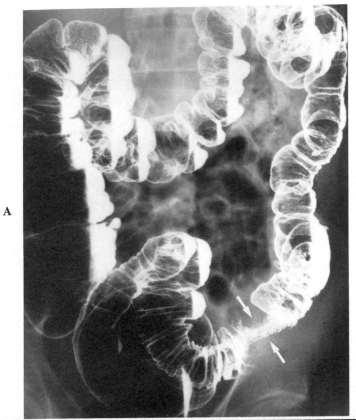

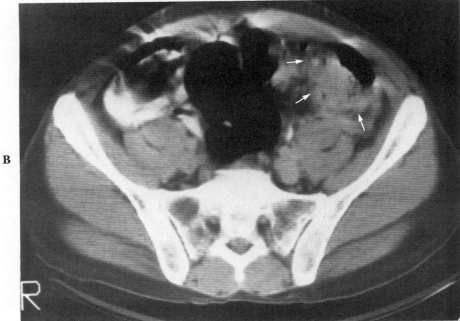

Fig. 6-25. The patient is a 52-year-old man who had a previous episode of acute diverticulitis. Barium enema and CT performed 5 months later. **A,** A narrowed segment of the sigmoid colon with preservation of mucosal folds *(arrows)* is seen. **B,** An eccentric, ill-defined pericolic, soft-tissue mass is visualized *(arrows)*. The pathological specimen showed intramural and pericolic, organized, inflammatory mass secondary to diverticulitis. The CT appearance alone mimics colonic carcinoma.

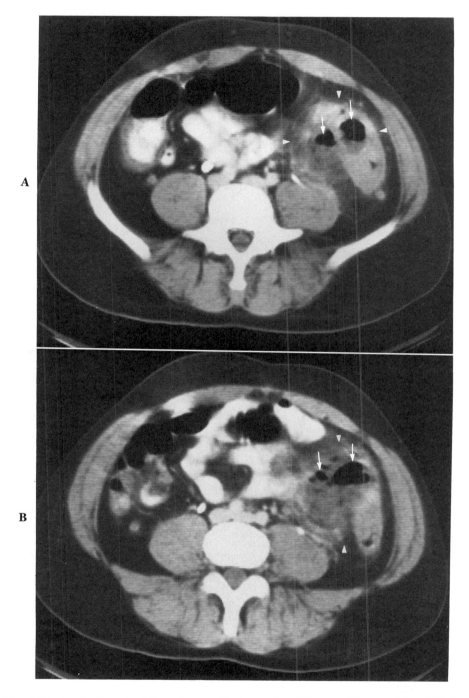

Fig. 6-26. Acute diverticulitis and pericolic abscess in a 30-year-old man with a 102 degree fever, increased white blood count, and peritoneal signs. Barium enema was contraindicated. **A** and **B,** The descending colon reveals severe pericolic inflammation (haziness and dirty fat) *(arrowheads)* and several pockets of air with air-fluid levels *(arrows)*. At surgery a pericolic abscess secondary to a perforated diverticulum was drained.

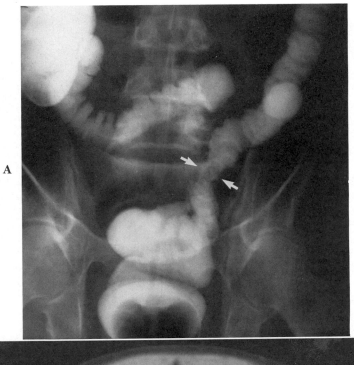

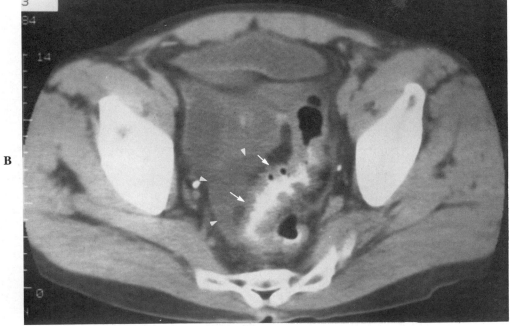

Fig. 6-27. Diverticulitis with pelvic peritonitis. **A,** Hypaque enema reveals slight narrowing of the sigmoid colon *(arrows)*. **B,** CT shows a thick-walled sigmoid, few diverticula, and an irregular lumen *(arrows)*. Pericolic inflammatory changes and fluid collection are seen in the pelvis *(arrowheads)*. Surgery revealed acute diverticulitis with perforation and peritonitis.

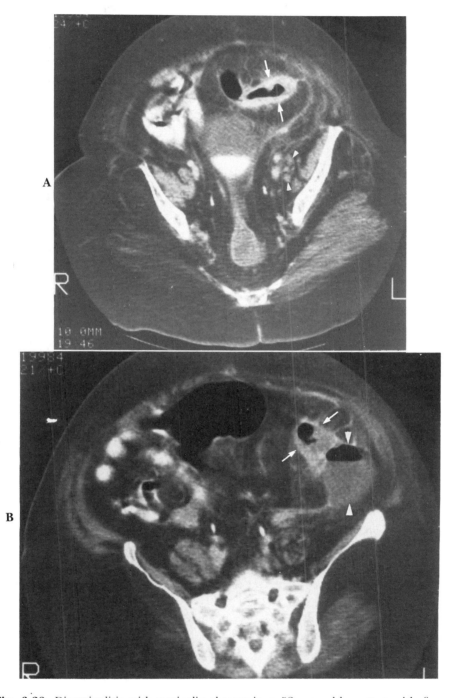

Fig. 6-28. Diverticulitis with pericolic abscess in a 52-year-old woman with fever and severe, left lower quadrant tenderness. A contrast enema was not performed. **A,** Circumferential wall thickening of the sigmoid colon *(arrows)* with pericolic mesenteric inflammation and inflammatory nodes is visualized *(arrowheads)*. **B,** The proximal sigmoid shows thickening of the wall *(arrows)*, and the adjacent abscess appears as a loculated, air-fluid collection *(arrowheads)*. The abscess was surgically drained.

CT OF APPENDICITIS

The role of CT in the diagnosis and evaluation of patients with appendicitis is currently being investigated.[33-35] Although its specificity and sensitivity are not yet established, it appears that CT is particularly useful in diagnosing severe forms of appendicitis associated with phlegmons, periappendicular abscess, and fistulizations. Similar to other more conventional radiographic methods, it is performed mainly in patients with atypical complaints but without localizing signs, fever, or leukocytosis.[33] CT should be considered a valuable adjunct to conventional barium studies in the evaluation of appendicular pathology. It may demonstrate focal inflammation in some patients despite normal barium enema; it shows pathology directly rather than inferentially; it provides a more exact evaluation of the extent and location of intra-abdominal disease. Inflammation confined only to the appendix may not be detected by CT and a negative study does not exclude appendicitis.

The expected CT findings in acute appendicitis are as follows:

1. Circumferential symmetrical thickening of the wall of the appendix (Figs. 6-29 and 6-30). This is a valuable and specific sign. However, the appendix is seldom visualized during CT examination.

2. Linear and streaky densities involving the pericecal, mesenteric, or pelvic fat. An associated pericecal soft-tissue mass indicative of an appendicular phlegmon may be seen. The mass has no distinct capsule and it is accompanied by blurring and thickening of the surrounding fascial planes (Fig. 6-31).

3. Appendicolith in the right lower quadrant appearing either as a homogeneous or ring-like calcified density (Fig. 6-32). When associated with other CT findings this is an extremely valuable and specific sign of appendicitis. Appendicoliths have been reported on plain films in 7% to 12% of adults and in 50% of children with appendicitis.[34] They were identified in 4 of 5 cases in one series[33] and were seen on CT in 9 of 36 consecutive cases (25%) in our institution.

4. Pericecal, mesenteric, or pelvic abscess appears as a poorly encapsulated single or multiloculated fluid collection (Fig. 6-33). The collection is extraluminal, it may displace adjacent structures, and it may contain bubbles, of air or extravasated contrast material. Its location remote from the right lower quadrant in the left pelvis (Figs. 6-33 and 6-34), upper abdomen, subhepatic space, or posterior to the ascending colon (Fig. 6-35) makes its origin sometimes difficult to identify.

It should be remembered that because of the mobility of the right colon and cecum as well as the variations in the size and position of the appendix, abscesses of appendicular origin often have an unexpected intraperitoneal or retroperitoneal location.

Chronic appendicular phlegmon may induce mesenteric lymphadenopathy and thickening of the wall of the cecum and distal ileum similar to Crohn's disease (Fig. 6-36). Appendicocolic, appendicovesicle, or appendicotubo-ovarian fistulas are rarely seen.[36] The differential diagnosis includes cecal or sigmoid diverticulitis, foreign body perforation, and tubo-ovarian abscess (Fig. 6-37).

Text continued p. 326.

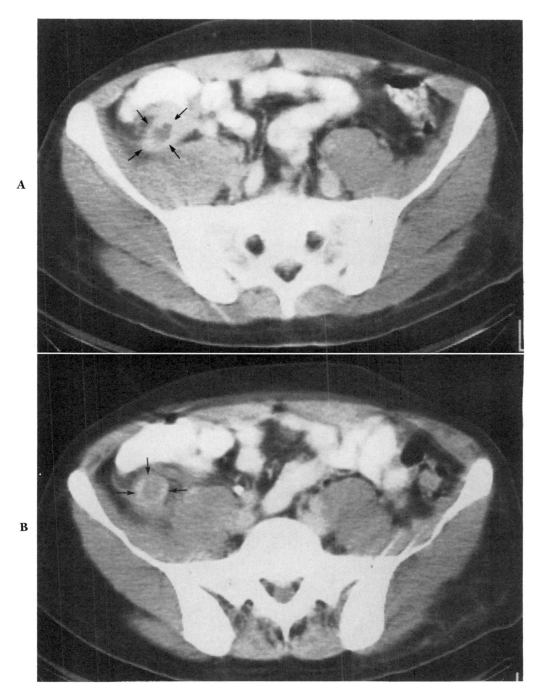

Fig. 6-29. Acute hemorrhagic appendicitis. **A** and **B,** The enlarged and thickened appendix *(arrows)* and periappendicular inflammation is seen. Surgery revealed a thick-walled, inflamed, and hemorrhagic appendix measuring 8.5 × 1.3 cm. There was no periappendicular abscess.

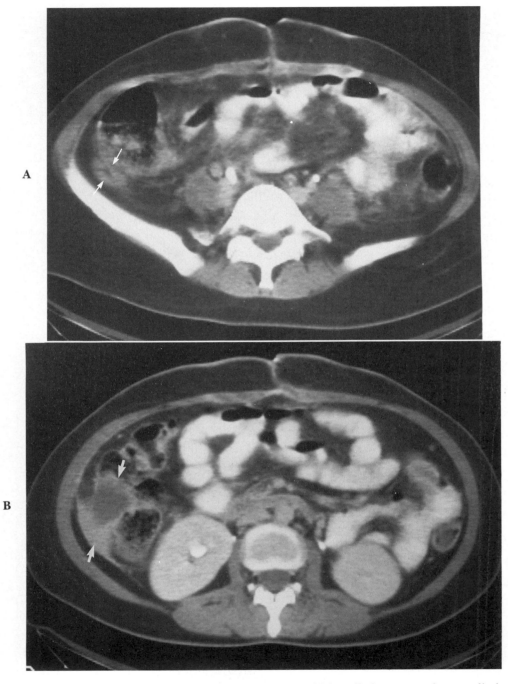

Fig. 6-30. Retrocecal appendicitis and abscess. **A,** A thick-walled, retrocecal appendix is visualized *(arrows)*. **B,** A collection of partially encapsulated fluid is seen lateral to the proximal ascending colon *(arrows)*. Surgery revealed a perforated retrocecal appendix and abscess.

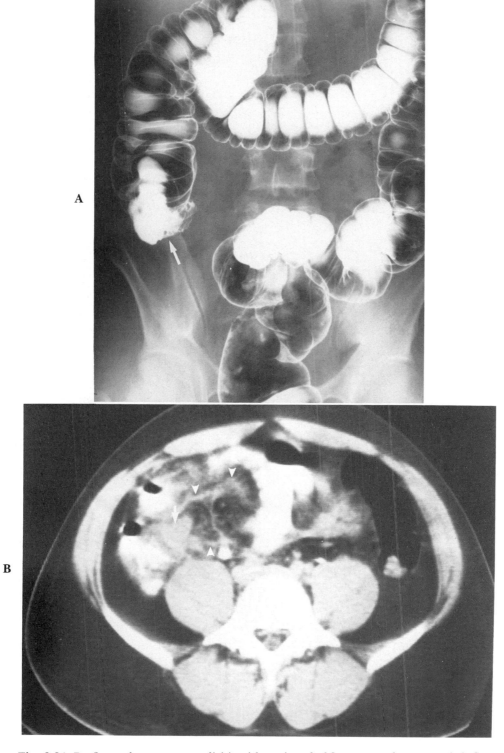

Fig. 6-31. Perforated, acute appendicitis with pericecal phlegmon and mesenteric inflammation. **A,** Barium enema shows flattening of the cecum and lack of visualization of the appendix *(arrow)*. **B,** Pericecal, ill-defined mass *(arrow)* and streaky densities are seen in the mesentery *(arrowheads)*.

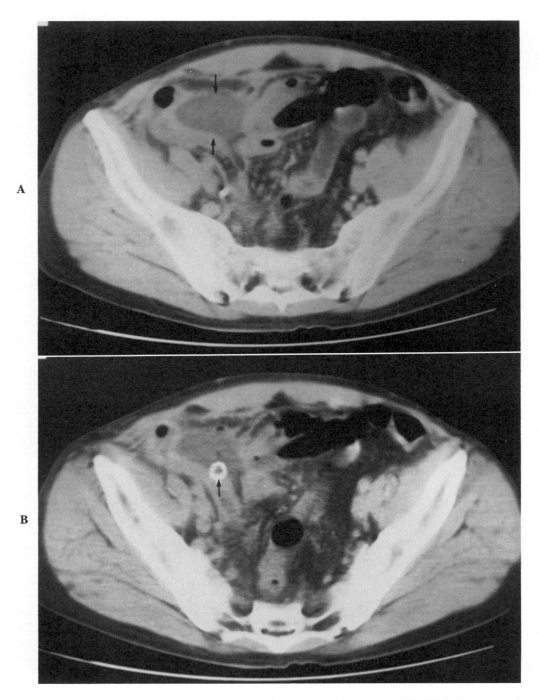

Fig. 6-32. Acute appendicitis with appendicolith and abscess. **A** and **B,** Right lower quadrant fluid collection *(arrows)* and ring-like calcification representing an appendicolith are seen *(arrow).*

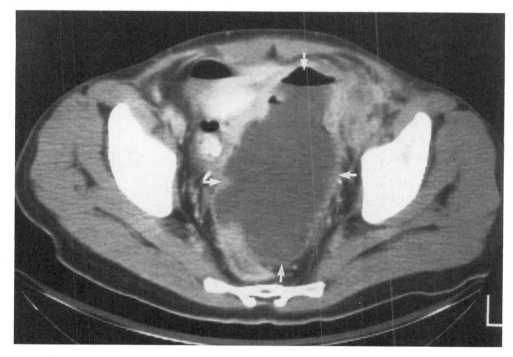

Fig. 6-33. Acute appendicitis and pelvic abscess in a 27-year-old man. CT demonstrates a very large, poorly defined, fluid collection containing air in the left pelvis *(arrows)*. A perforated, long pelvic appendix with a large abscess was found at surgery.

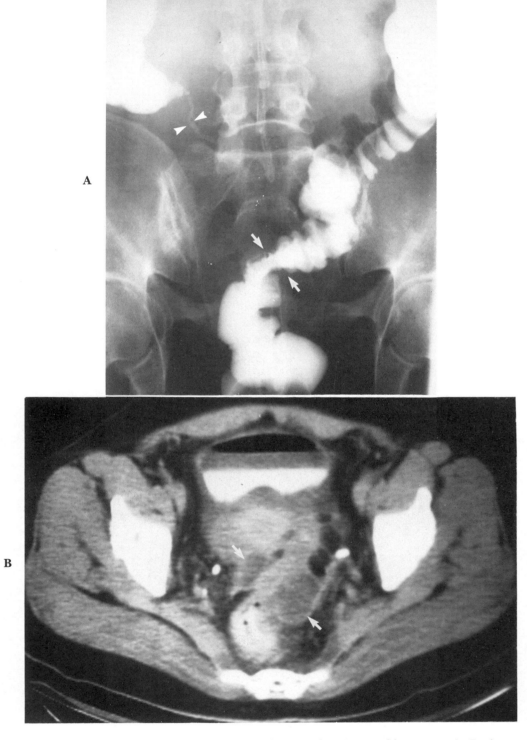

Fig. 6-34. Acute appendicitis with pelvic abscesses in 54-year-old woman. **A,** Barium enema shows slight asymmetrical narrowing of the sigmoid colon *(arrows)*. Note filling of the proximal appendix *(arrowheads)*. **B,** Several pockets of fluid are seen adjacent to the sigmoid colon *(arrows)*. A perforated appendicitis was found at surgery. CT findings mimic diverticulitis.

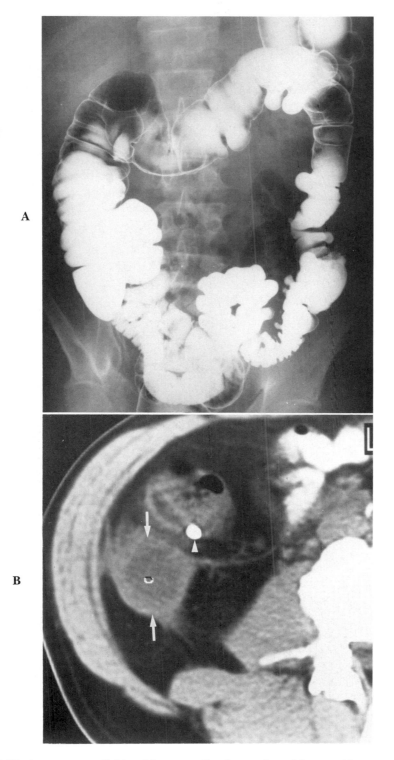

Fig. 6-35. Acute appendicitis with retrocolic abscess in a 58-year-old man. **A,** Barium enema showed no abnormalities. **B,** Encapsulated fluid collection was present posterior to the mid-ascending colon *(arrows)*. The barium-filled diverticulum is seen on the posterior wall of the colon *(arrowhead)*.

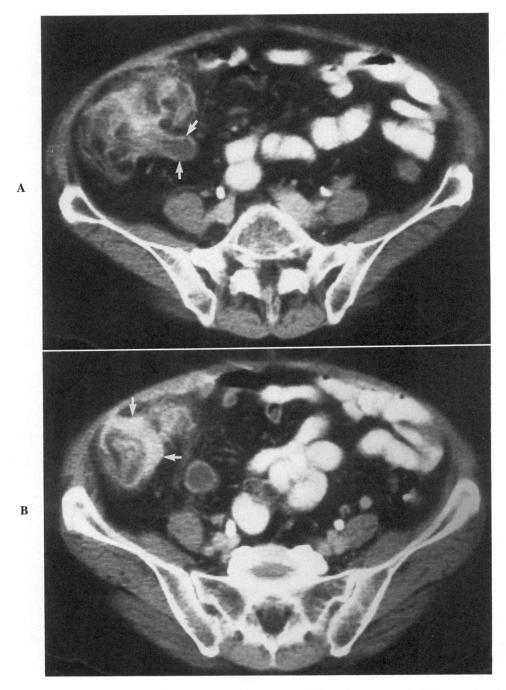

Fig. 6-36. Appendicitis with pericecal phlegmon and chronic mesenteric inflammation in a 70-year-old woman. **A** and **B,** CT demonstrates pericecal and mesenteric inflammation as well as thickening of the wall of the terminal ileum and cecum *(arrows).* Surgery confirmed these findings and a segmental resection was performed. CT and surgical findings mimic Crohn's disease.

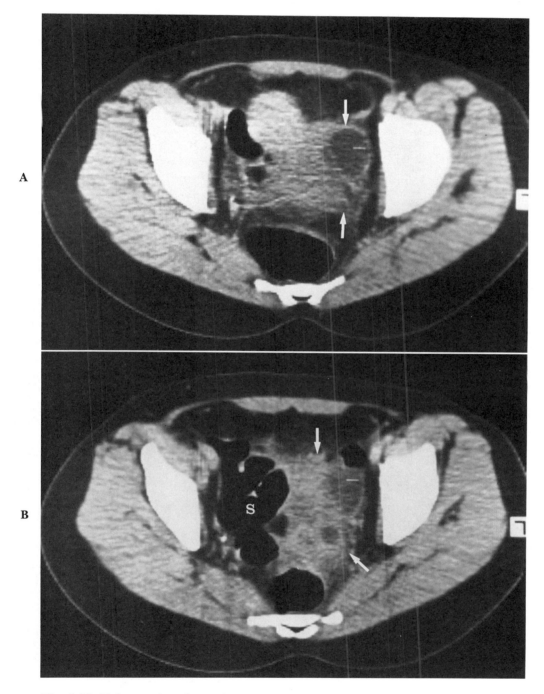

Fig. 6-37. Tubo-ovarian abscess in a 39-year-old woman. **A** and **B,** Poorly encapsulated fluid collections are seen in the left pelvis *(arrows)* adjacent to the sigmoid colon *(S).*

COLONIC NEOPLASM

Epithelial and mesenchymal tumors of the colon can be detected and evaluated by CT. Numerous reports published in the radiographic literature have described and analyzed the potential usefulness and advantages offered by CT when compared with barium enema or colonoscopic examination.[37-44] In addition to the colonic component, CT can detect pericolic invasion as well as distal metastases. Its accuracy depends mainly on the size of the tumor and on the technical quality of the examination. CT is not a primary diagnostic tool in the detection of colonic neoplasms but a valuable noninvasive complimentary method of evaluation.

Adenocarcinoma of the colon

During the routine examination for nonspecific abdominal complaints, CT can detect clinically unsuspected colon carcinoma. Its main clinical use, however, is in staging known lesions, in diagnosing early postoperative complications, and particularly in identifying residual, recurrent, and metastatic tumor on follow-up examinations.

Detection and appearance

CT sensitivity in detecting primary colon carcinoma is not known. On a clean colon with adequate technique, lesions larger than 1 to 2 cm in diameter can be demonstrated. Detection rates of 65%[37] and 100%[44] were reported in patients with known and generally large colonic and rectosigmoid lesions.

Adenocarcinoma appears as a localized, soft-tissue density that can be discreet and focal (Fig. 6-38) or that may show semicircular or circumferential increased thickness of the wall of the colon (Fig. 6-39). The tumor is usually homogeneous in density, although, particularly in large tumors, areas of decreased attenuation that represent zones of ischemia and necrosis may be present (Fig. 6-40). Primary mucinous adenocarcinoma usually has a lower density, and the metastatic lesions and lymph nodes rich in mucin have a similar low-density appearance. Psammomatous calcifications in primary colonic tumors are unusual; however, when they appear, they are diagnostic of mucinous adenocarcinoma (Fig. 6-41). The size of the tumor is variable, and its contour is usually lobulated and asymmetrical (Fig. 6-42). When the tumor is visualized longitudinally, an abrupt zone of transition, an overhanging edge, and an irregular rigid and narrow lumen may be seen (Fig. 6-42). On cross section, if there is circumferential infiltration, the tumor appears as a homogeneous symmetrical thickening of the bowel wall that resembles a doughnut (Fig. 6-43). Attenuation numbers are variable within the range of soft tissue, and contrast enhancement depends on the type of tumor, the amount and technique of iodine administration, and the time of scanning. Enhancement of about 10 to 30 H units should be expected with the higher values obtained after bolus injections. *Text continued p. 333.*

A

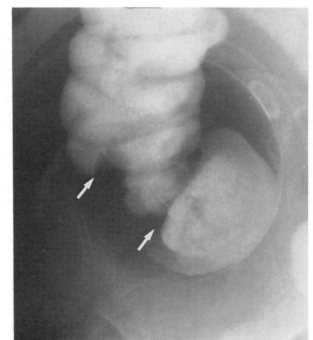

Fig. 6-38. Adenocarcinoma of the cecum in an 81-year-old woman. **A,** Barium enema shows a sessile lesion on the lateral wall of the cecum opposite to the ileocecal valve *(arrows).*

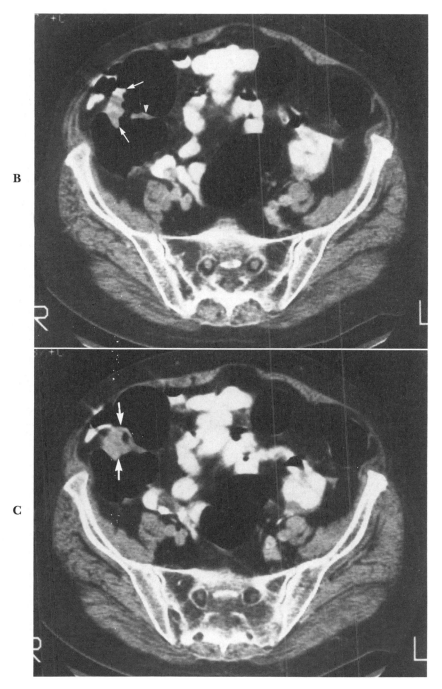

Fig. 6-38, cont'd. B and **C,** The cecum once distended with air, demonstrates a soft-tissue density lesion on the lateral wall *(arrows)* and a normal ileocecal valve medially *(arrowhead)*. The tumor is slightly lobulated but has a sharp, outer contour. Pathologic specimen showed tumor extension to the serosal adipose tissue and negative nodes.

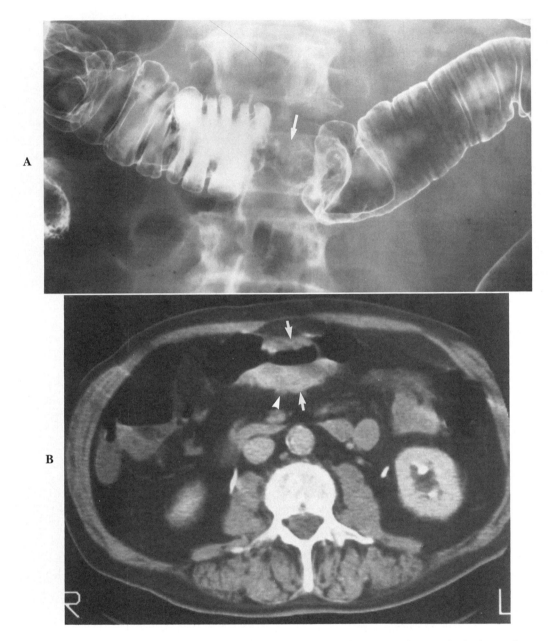

Fig. 6-39. Mucinous adenocarcinoma of the colon in a 72-year-old man. **A,** A circumferential, apple core tumor in the midtransverse colon *(arrow)* is seen. **B,** A circumferential soft-tissue density mass showing abrupt transition, luminal narrowing, and a slightly irregular outer contour *(arrows)* is visualized. A few nodular densities were seen in the pericolic fat *(arrowhead)*. Pathologic specimen showed tumor invasion into the pericolic adipose tissue and the replacement of four nodes by tumor.

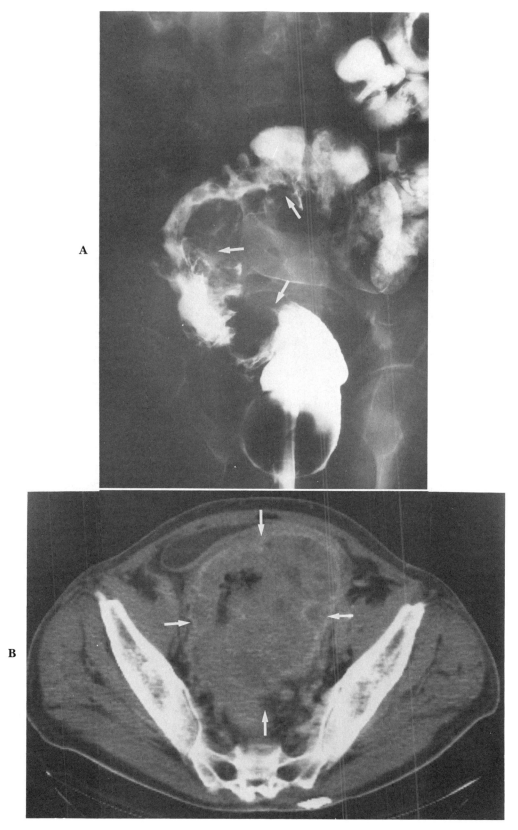

Fig. 6-40. Adenocarcinoma of the sigmoid colon in a 65-year-old man with a large pelvic mass. **A,** A long, infiltrating, malignant lesion is seen following barium enema *(arrows).* **B,** A large exophitic tumor and areas of necrosis (lower attenuation) are demonstrated by CT *(arrows).*

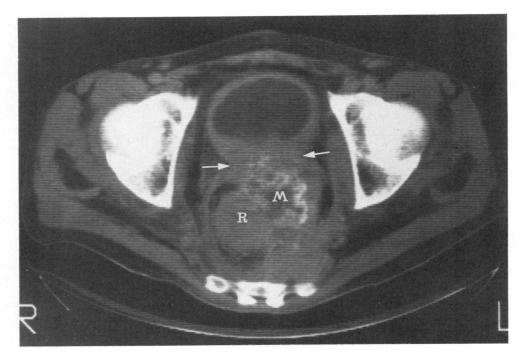

Fig. 6-41. Mucinous, calcified adenocarcinoma of the rectum in a 53-year-old man. CT shows calcifications within a soft-tissue mass *(M)* arising from the anterior left rectal wall *(R)*. Note the invasion of the posterior wall of the bladder *(arrows)* and thickening of the perirectal fascia. Findings were confirmed at surgery.

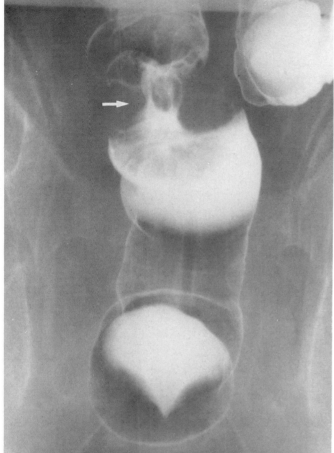

A

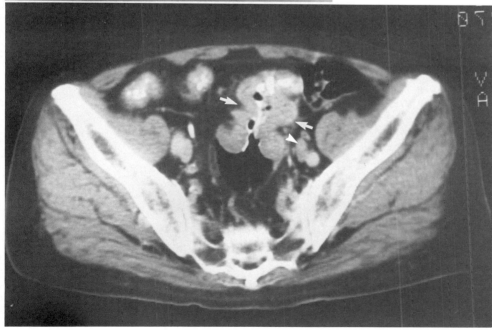

B

Fig. 6-42. A, Adenocarcinoma of the distal sigmoid colon appearing as an apple core lesion following barium enema *(arrow)*. **B,** CT demonstrates the thickness of the tumor, a lobulated, asymmetrical outer contour, and the distal overhanging edge *(arrows)*. Small nodules were seen in the adjacent fat *(arrowhead)*. Pathology showed tumor invasion of the pericolic fat and five positive nodes.

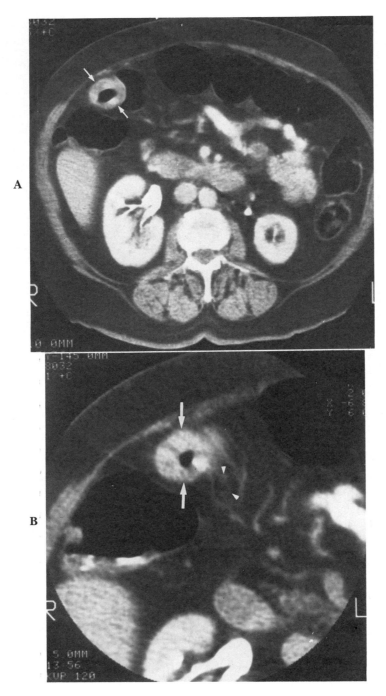

Fig. 6-43. A, Adenocarcinoma of the hepatic flexure appearing as a circumferential mass and resembling a doughnut *(arrows)*. **B,** A magnified view shows the lesion *(arrows)* and a few nodes in the adjacent pericolic fat *(arrowheads)*. Pathology showed slight serosal invasion and reactive hyperplasia in the pericolic nodes.

Linitis plastica or scirrhous carcinoma is a morphologic variety of adenocarcinoma characterized by a diffusely infiltrating and usually mucogenic anaplastic lesion.[41,45] Although it is commonly seen in the stomach, it may involve the colon, particularly the rectum and the sigmoid segment. The colonic lesions are either primary malignancies or metastases from other organs such as the stomach or breast. The bowel wall is greatly thickened measuring 2 to 3 cm, and the mucosal layer is smooth and grossly intact. Histologically mucosa shows a dense, chronic, and nonspecific inflammatory infiltrate, while the submucosa and muscularis is replaced by diffuse fibrosis and by malignant tumor cells containing mucin that resemble signet rings. Superficial mucosal biopsies are often nonspecific, and barium enema examination shows a long, narrow, and rigid segment with a smooth or serrated lumen without overhanging edges, intraluminal defects, or ulcerations. In individuals with repeated negative biopsies,[45] CT helps in establishing a correct diagnosis (Fig. 6-44) by demonstrating the significant thickening of the wall of the colon unexpected in an inflammatory lesion. Pericolic tumor invasion, lymphadenopathy, or distal metastases may also be present.

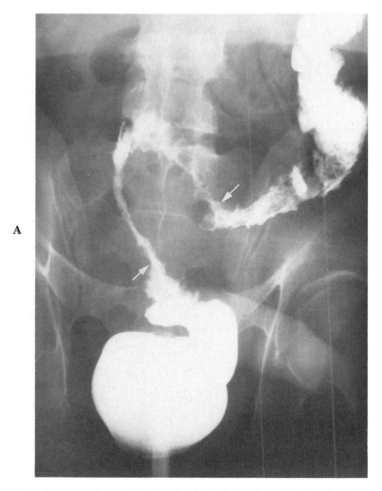

Fig. 6-44. Scirrhous carcinoma (linitis plastica) of the sigmoid colon in a 47-year-old man. **A,** Barium enema shows a long infiltrating lesion with rigidity and irregular luminal narrowing *(arrows)*.

Continued.

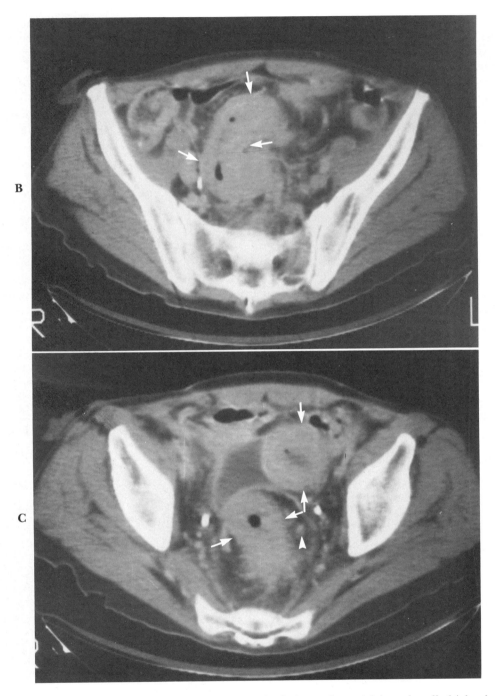

Fig. 6-44, cont'd. B and **C,** CT shows marked circumferential bowel wall thickening *(arrows)*, pericolic tumor invasion, and lymphadenopathy *(arrowhead)*. Findings were confirmed at surgery.

Cloacogenic and squamous cell carcinoma are anal cancers that arise from the transitional epithelium of the pectinate line or from the stratified squamous epithelium of the anal canal.[46-50] They represent about 1% to 2% of the malignant tumors of the large bowel and may be clinically deceptive, often resembling small abscesses, fissures, or fistulas. These are generally aggressive tumors showing early and deep mural invasion with perianal, lymphatic, and hematogeneous spread. At the time of diagnosis, 40% of squamous cell carcinomas are associated with regional lymph node metastases. The histologic differentiation is made only by biopsy. Barium enema demonstrates a localized infiltrating, plaquelike lesion starting at the anal orifice in squamous cell carcinoma and rising 2 to 3 cm above it in cloacogenic carcinoma. CT is valuable not only in identifying the primary lesions, but particularly in assessing the depth of involvement and the presence of local and distal metastases (Figs. 6-45 to 6-47).

CT differential diagnosis of carcinoma of the colon includes other primary colonic malignancies such as carcinoid tumor, lymphosarcoma, and leiomyosarcoma. When the primary lesion is not well seen and when localized, pericolic inflammatory changes are present, other benign conditions, such as, diverticulitis, appendicitis, and foreign body perforation, should be considered and ruled out (Fig. 6-48). CT features that suggest malignant rather than inflammatory disease are: (1) focal, lobulated, soft-tissue mass; (2) asymmetrical thickening of the bowel wall greater than 2 cm; (3) enhancement with intravenous contrast; and (4) associated regional and/or distal metastatic disease (Fig. 6-49).

Pitfalls in the CT diagnosis include fecal material, fluid-filled bowel loops, incomplete colonic distention, lack of pericolic fat in cachetic individuals, and technically poor examinations with artifacts. *Text continued p. 342.*

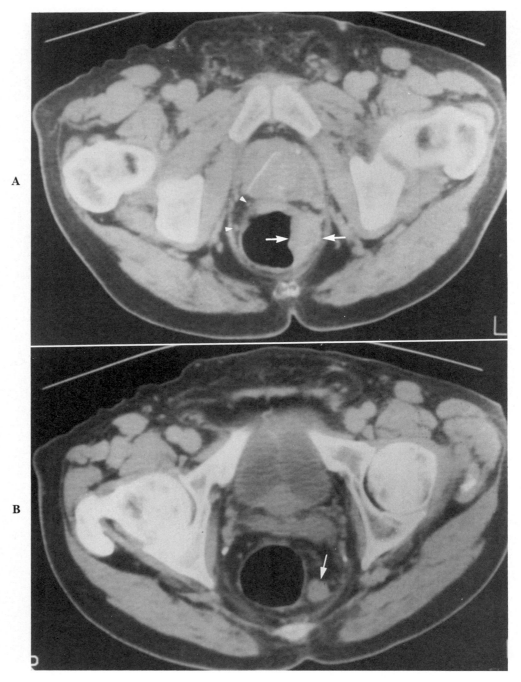

Fig. 6-45. A, Cloacogenic carcinoma infiltrating the left lateral wall of the distal rectum *(arrows).* Note thickening of the perirectal fascia and a few nodular densities in the perirectal fat *(arrowheads).* **B,** On a slightly superior level the rectum has a normal wall thickness but a perirectal large node is visualized *(arrow).* Lymphatic spread and nodes replaced by tumor were present at surgery.

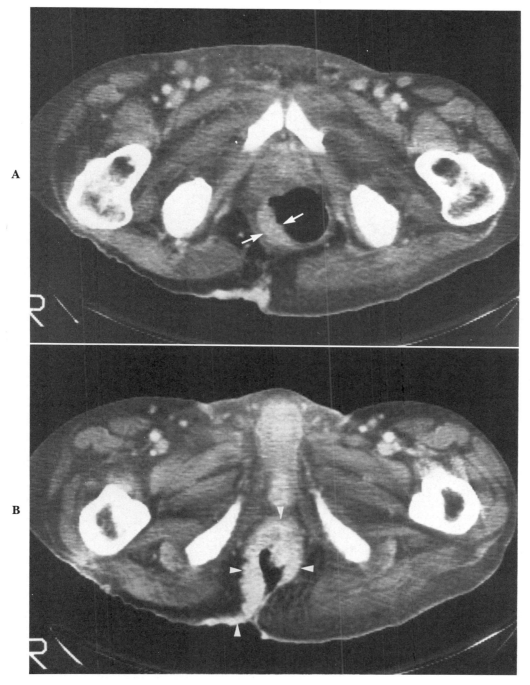

Fig. 6-46. Squamous cell carcinoma of the anal canal in a 76-year-old man. **A,** There is thickening of the right wall of the distal rectum *(arrows)* and inguinal nodes. **B,** A lower cut shows tumor extension to the anal verge and perianal skin *(arrowheads).*

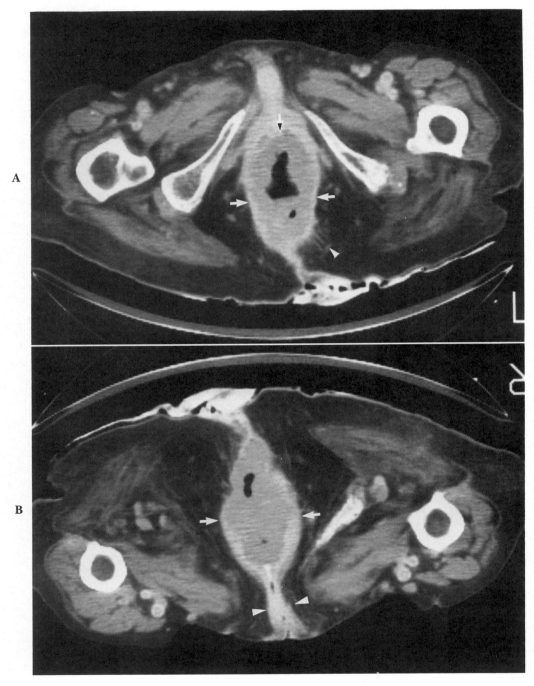

Fig. 6-47. A and **B,** Squamous cell carcinoma of the anal canal appearing as a lower attenuation, circumferential, infiltrating lesion *(arrows).* Note the extension of the tumor in the adjacent fat and perianal skin *(arrowhead).*

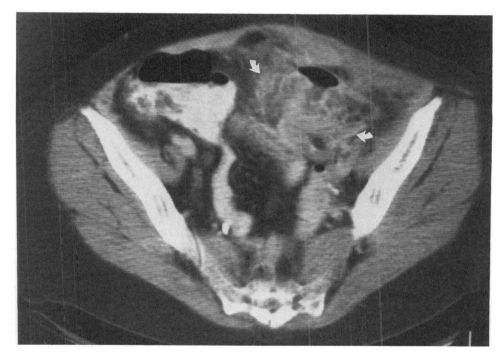

Fig. 6-48. Perforated sigmoid carcinoma in a 56-year-old woman with the clinical diagnosis of diverticulitis. Because of fever, tenderness, and peritoneal signs, the colon was not distended with air. Inflammatory changes were seen in the mesosigmoid *(curved arrows)* but the sigmoid tumor was not visualized. CT presentation mimics diverticulitis.

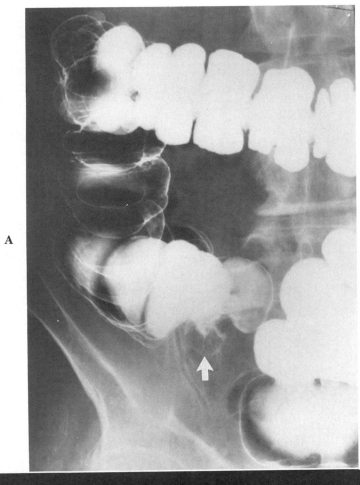

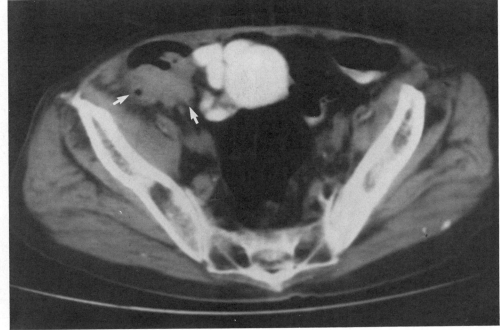

Fig. 6-49. CT differential diagnosis of two patients with similar clinical presentations and barium enema findings. **A** and **B,** Adenocarcinoma of the cecum. Barium enema shows an amputated cecum *(A),* and CT reveals a lobulated, well-defined, soft-tissue mass *(arrow)*. Pathology documented serosal invasion and positive nodes.

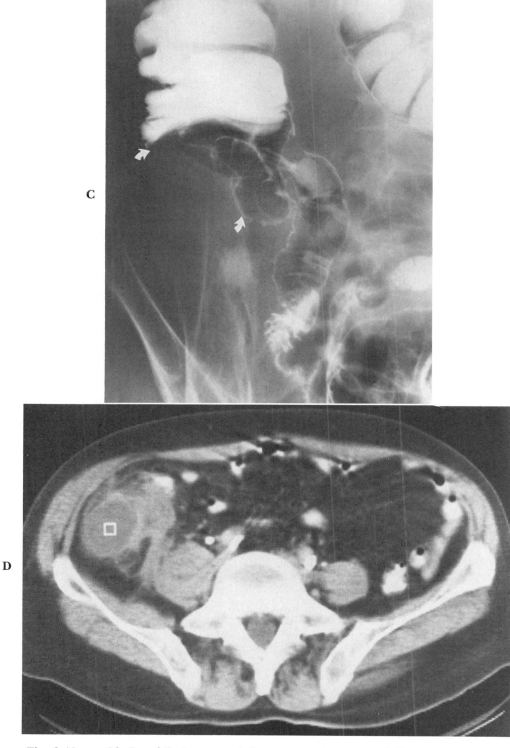

Fig. 6-49, cont'd. C and **D,** Intramural abscess secondary to cecal diverticulitis. Barium enema shows a large cecal filling defect *(C)*, and CT reveals an encapsulated fluid collection *(cursor)* and pericecal inflammatory reaction.

Staging

The need and accuracy of CT staging of primary colonic adenocarcinoma is still controversial and at this time only partially evaluated.[37-40,42-44] Most investigators have attempted to stage rectosigmoid lesions with insufficient data reported for the more proximal tumors. If the CT staging will prove to be a reliable and sensitive means of noninvasive evaluation, the usefulness of routine preoperative CT examination becomes obvious. Since the decision of type and degree of treatment is based largely on the extent of disease, certain categories of patients would benefit from this examination. Poor surgical candidates and patients harboring large invasive lesions with evidence of distant metastases will be spared unnecessary exploratory laparotomies. Alternate means of palliative therapy may be considered in these cases. There are data to suggest that improved survivals may be achieved if preoperative radiation is used for large invasive rectosigmoid tumors.[43,51] In addition, a baseline CT examination is very useful for evaluation of residual or recurrent disease after surgery.[37,44]

For accurate staging, optimal CT examinations should be performed. Since CT can not be expected to distinguish between mucosal, muscularis, and serosal invasion and since it is less accurate in determining adjacent lymph node metastases, Dukes staging system[52] is generally not used. Theoni and Moss have proposed an alternate method of CT classification of rectosigmoid cancer[44] that, if modified slightly, may be used to stage all colonic tumors (Table 6-2). Using this classification, they reported a staging accuracy of 92% in the evaluation of 39 patients with primary rectal or rectosigmoid carcinoma.[44] Similar high accuracy rates have been reported by others.[37,39,40] Van Waes, by using conventional CT supplemented by direct coronal and sagittal scans, has accurately staged 19 of 21 rectal carcinomas (90% accuracy rate) with two false-positive and two false-negative cases.[38] By using the TNM classification, excellent correlation with pathologic specimens has been reported in staging 11 cases of rectal carcinoma.[40]

Table 6-2. Staging of primary tumors of the colon by CT

Stage 1	Intraluminal polypoid mass without thickening of the bowel wall
Stage 2	Thickening of the bowel wall (>1 cm) without invasion of surrounding tissue
Stage 3	Slight invasion of adjacent surrounding tissues
Stage 4	Massive invasion of surrounding tissues, adjacent organs, and/or distant metastases

Modified from Thoeni, R.F., et al.: Detection and staging of primary rectal and rectosigmoid cancer by computed tomography, Radiology **141:**135-138, 1981.

The demonstration of soft-tissue densities and/or adjacent linear strands extending into the pericolic fat represents spread of tumor beyond the bowel wall (Figs. 6-50 and 6-51). An increase in the density of the pericolic fat with a delicate, linear reticular pattern and/or fluid collections are seen with sealed-off perforations (Fig. 6-48). In these cases there is serosal invasion and tumor nodules are usually present in the pericolic fat. The differentiation between pericolic tumor spread and sealed-off perforation with pericolic inflammation is sometimes difficult and should be made in the context of the clinical presentation.

Loss of fat planes between the tumor and an adjacent organ is suspicious but not pathognomonic for neoplastic invasion. Tumor invasion into the urinary bladder is recognized by visualizing the infiltration of the wall and the intraluminal component of the tumor mass (Figs. 6-52 and 6-53). The presence of air within the urinary bladder is characteristic of a fistulous tract, unless explained otherwise (Fig. 6-53). CT has proved to be the most sensitive means to diagnose colovesical fistulas, surpassing conventional techniques such as barium enema or cystography.[53]

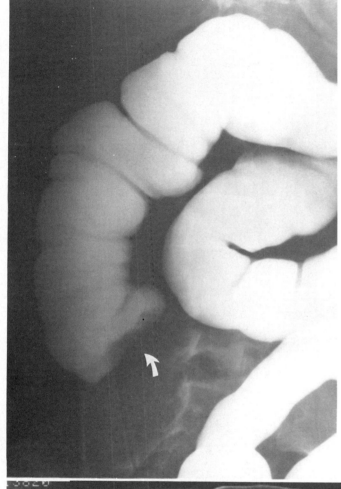

A

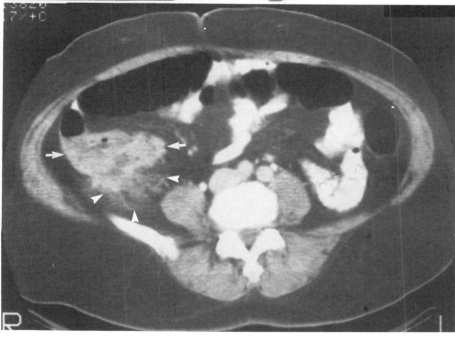

B

Fig. 6-50. Cecal adenocarcinoma in a 57-year-old woman with rectal bleeding. **A,** An amputated cecum seen following a barium enema *(curved arrow).* **B,** CT shows soft-tissue mass *(arrows)* and adjacent linear strands extending into the pericecal fat *(arrowheads).* This is a CT Stage 3 lesion. Serosal invasion and pericecal tumor infiltration were documented at surgery.

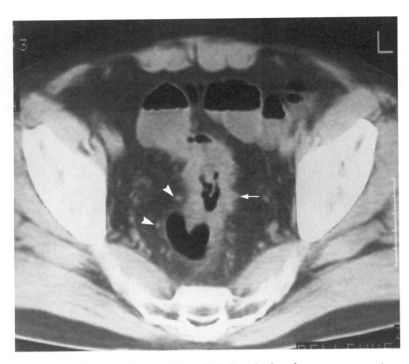

Fig. 6-51. Sigmoid adenocarcinoma with a slightly spiculated outer contour *(arrow).* Note the multiple nodular densities in the pericolic fat *(arrowheads).* This is a CT Stage 3 lesion. Pathology showed tumor penetration into the pericolic fat, adjacent lymphatics, blood vessels, and seven positive nodes.

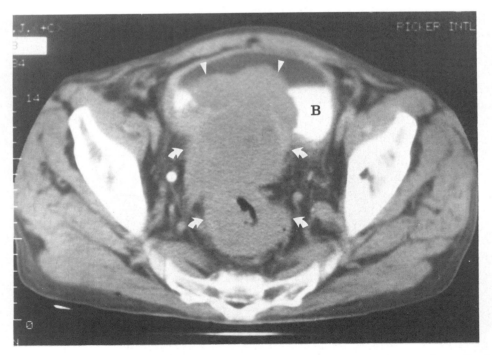

Fig. 6-52. Rectosigmoid carcinoma *(curved arrows)* with invasion of the posterior wall of the urinary bladder *(B)* and large intraluminal component *(arrowheads).* This is a CT Stage 4 lesion.

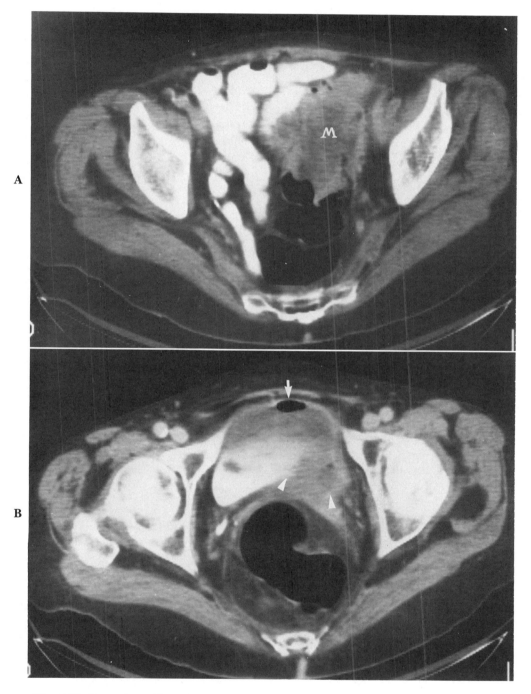

Fig. 6-53. Rectosigmoid carcinoma with invasion of the bladder and evidence of rectovesical fistula. **A,** A large, soft-tissue mass with a central area of lower attenuation *(M)* is visualized. **B,** There is invasion of the left posterior wall of the bladder *(arrowheads)* and intravesical air *(arrow)*.

A wide variety of CT abnormalities may be seen in patients with intraperitoneal metastases. Liver metastases are among the most common findings, appearing usually as multiple irregular areas of low attenuation that enhance slightly. Central zones of necrosis are common and stippled calcifications may be seen in patients with mucinous adenocarcinoma. Occasionally, metastatic liver tumors may exhibit a round, well-defined contour and a lower attenuation that can be misinterpreted as a benign cyst (Fig. 6-54). Ascites and/or small nodular densities scattered on the peritoneal surfaces are seen in patients with widespread peritoneal implants. Mesenteric and serosal implants or large cecal tumors may lead to small bowel obstruction (Fig. 6-55). Thickening of the greater omentum is seen in some patients, having homogeneous density or a smudged inhomogeneous appearance. It has been referred to as "omental cake" and it represents metastatic tumor infiltrating the omentum, enveloping and compressing the intraperitoneal contents (Fig. 6-56). A common site of tumor implant is the inferior peritoneal recess (Douglas' pouch), where a lobulated mass situated anterior to the rectum is often found (Fig. 6-57). Patients with primary colon carcinoma may develop ovarian metastases initially or on follow-up examination. This is a relatively common complication, appearing on CT as a cystic, pelvic, ovarian mass and usually exhibiting septations and some solid elements (Fig. 6-58). Depending on the time of the diagnosis, the ovarian tumors vary greatly in size and sometimes represent the only known metastatic lesion.

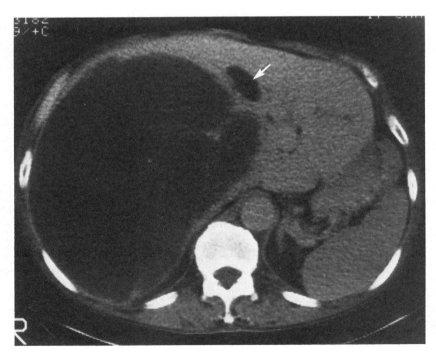

Fig. 6-54. Large metastatic hepatic adenocarcinoma from primary tumor in the hepatic flexure. The lesion has a low attenuation (24 H units), is well-defined, and slightly lobulated. A small secondary metastases is present in the left lobe *(arrow)*.

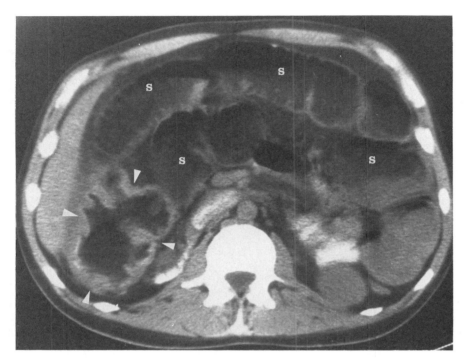

Fig. 6-55. Small bowel obstruction in a 37-year-old man with proved cecal adenocarcinoma. Massively distended, fluid-filled, small bowel loops are evident *(S)*. In addition, there is ascites, and a thickened irregular cecum is visualized *(arrowheads)*. (Courtesy Dr. R. Surapeneni, Veterans Administration Hospital, Brooklyn, New York.)

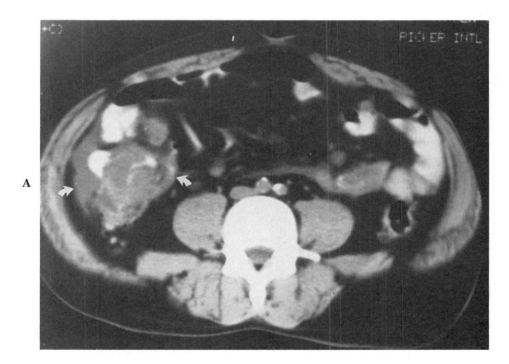

Fig. 6-56. Carcinoma of the cecum in 59-year-old man with widespread peritoneal metastases. **A,** A large, lobulated, soft-tissue mass is present in the cecum *(curved arrows)*.

Continued.

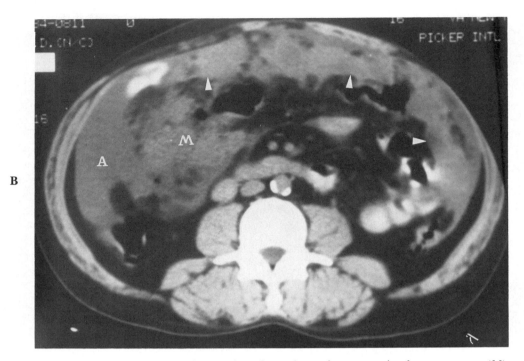

Fig. 6-56, cont'd. B, A superior section shows irregular tumor in the mesentery *(M)*, homogeneous thickening of the greater omentum ("omental cake") *(arrowheads)*, and ascites *(A)*. This is a CT Stage 4 lesion.

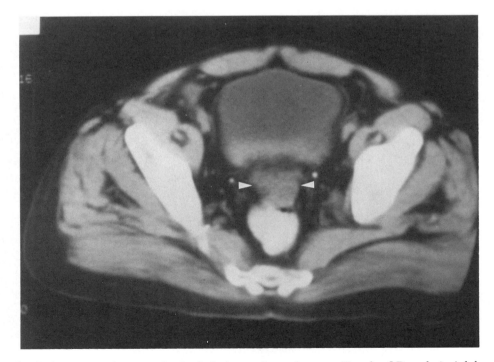

Fig. 6-57. Metastatic tumor in the inferior peritoneal recess (Pouch of Douglas). A lobulated, soft-tissue mass is present between the rectum and urinary bladder *(arrowheads)*.

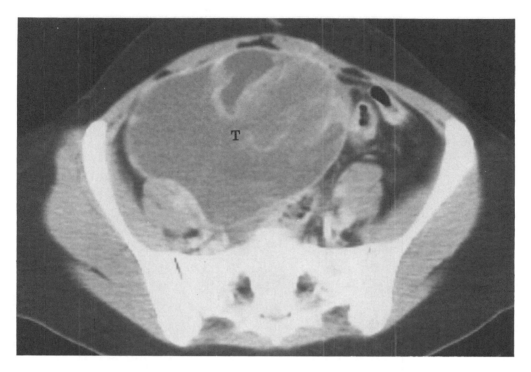

Fig. 6-58. Ovarian metastases from adenocarcinoma of the transverse colon. A large, ovarian, cystic mass with septations and solid nodular densities is demonstrated *(T)*.

There is no correlation established between the barium enema findings and the extramural extent of the neoplasm or presence of intraperitoneal metastases. This assessment can be made by CT. Among 80 patients with known primary colon carcinoma evaluated with CT by Mayes,[37] 25% had liver metastases, 15% had retroperitoneal nodes (see Fig. 6-69), 12.5% had hydronephrosis, and 10% had adrenal metastases. It should be underlined, however, that hepatic and/or intraperitoneal metastasis may be found at surgery in patients with negative CT examinations.

Although the results in our experience have been encouraging, at this time, several limitations are obvious in our attempts to stage colonic tumors. Given a focal lesion with a well-defined outer contour, the differentiation between a Stage 1 and Stage 2 tumor (Table 6-2) is difficult (Fig. 6-59). At the site where the tumor arises from the mucosa, the presence and degree of bowel wall thickening is hard to assess (Fig. 6-59). Although frank invasion in the pericolic fat is usually obvious (see Figs. 6-50 and 6-51), the demonstration of a perfectly sharp outer contour does not rule out serosal invasion (see Figs. 6-38 and 6-43). In addition the histology of a given tumor and the differentiation between a large adenomatous polyp, villous adenoma, and adenocarcinoma is unreliable (Fig. 6-60). Pericolic neoplastic adenopathy is hard to evaluate since small positive nodes may not be visualized and since the nodes demonstrated on CT may represent only hyperplastic nodes on pathologic examination (Fig. 6-43). It has been stated that nodes greater than 1.5 cm are metastatic[40]; however, in our experience most of the positive nodes are smaller than 1.5 cm in size (see Figs. 6-45 and 6-61). In addition, pericolic nodes can be confused with dilated collateral veins, which may be present in patients with portal hypertension (Fig. 6-62). When in doubt this differentiation can be made with a bolus injection. It is apparent that CT is more sensitive in staging large and advanced colonic tumors and that generally there is a tendency to downstage rather than upstage primary colonic malignancies.

In a recent study of 80 patients, Freeny et al. concludes that compared with the Duke's classification, CT has a poor accuracy in preoperative local staging of colorectal carcinoma.[43a] It correctly staged 47.5% of patients while downstaging 83.3% of the cases incorrectly staged.

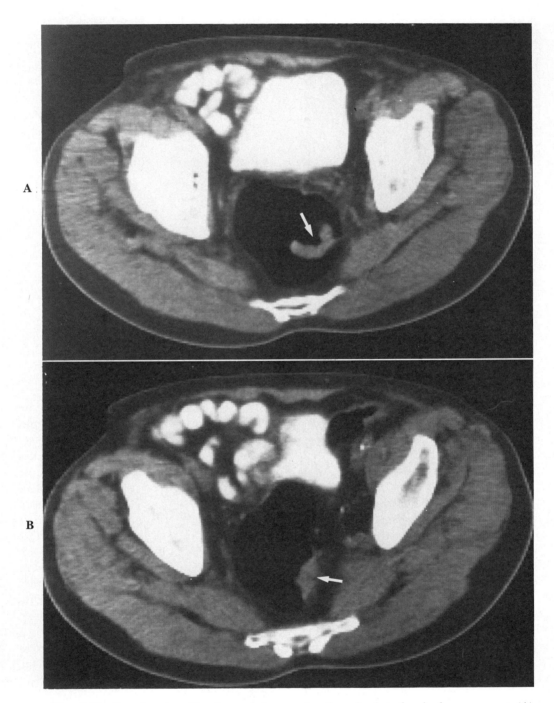

Fig. 6-59. Rectal polypoid adenocarcinoma showing the intraluminal component **(A)** *(arrow)* and thickening of the left rectal wall at the site of origin **(B)** *(arrow)*. Pathology showed only superficial mucosal involvement without intramural penetration. This is a Duke A lesion.

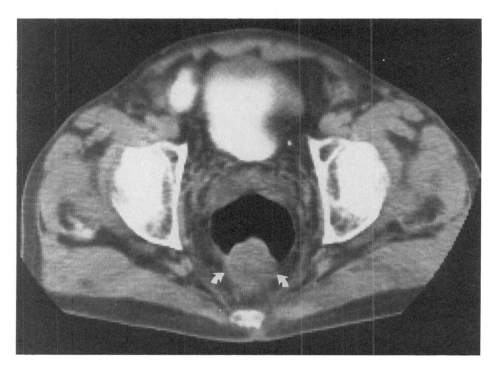

Fig. 6-60. Rectal villous adenoma appearing as a polypoid tumor with thickening of the posterior rectal wall *(curved arrows)*. CT appearance is indistinguishable from adenocarcinoma.

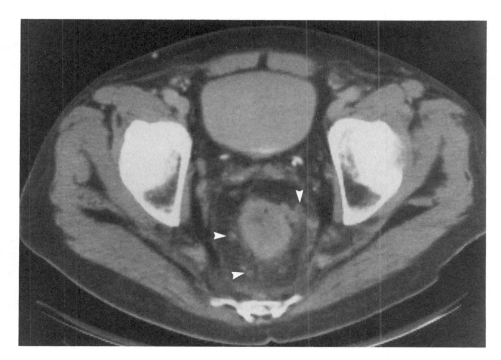

Fig. 6-61. Rectal adenocarcinoma with extension to the pericolic fat, lymphatic infiltration, and metastatic regional lymph nodes. Thickened perirectal fascia, linear strands, and multiple, small, perirectal nodular densities are seen *(arrowheads)*.

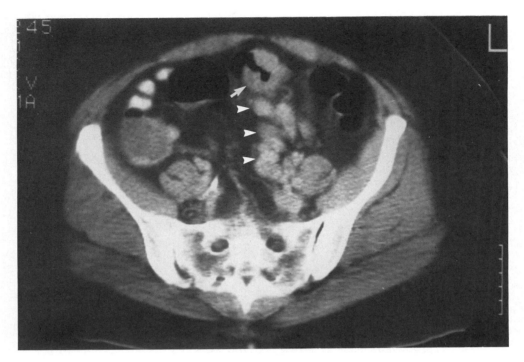

Fig. 6-62. Carcinoma of the sigmoid colon *(arrow)* with multiple nodular densities in the pelvis *(arrowheads)* that proved to be large varices. The patient had liver cirrhosis and portal hypertension.

Postoperative evaluation

CT plays an essential role in the follow-up evaluation of patients after surgical resection for primary carcinoma of the colon. It is used in the immediate postoperative period to diagnose surgical complications and has proved to be a sensitive method for detection of local and distant recurrent tumor. For a detailed analysis of the CT results, several recently published papers are available for review.[40,54-62]

Early postsurgical complications such as anastomotic perforations and the development of peritonitis, abscesses, and hematomas can be detected. In cases of anastomatic leakage, CT reveals the expected inflammation of the mesentery with increased haziness and streakiness in the pericolic fat and pericolic fluid collections (Fig. 6-63).

Postoperative examinations in asymptomatic patients after abdominoperineal resection have revealed essentially no CT abnormalities in one reported series,[59] while showing a high incidence of ill-defined, soft-tissue densities in the pelvis in other series.[54,55] The discrepancy is probably related to the time of the postoperative examination with most of the benign abnormalities detected early. These early postoperative findings represent unresolved hematomas, granulation, or fibrotic tissue. On follow-up examination they tend to diminish in size and acquire a sharper contour consistent with their benign nature.[54] Because of these findings, a baseline examination within 2 to 4 months after surgery followed by serial CT scans at about 6 month intervals is recommended to detect early asymptomatic recurrence.[54] A growing mass and/or a mass with an irregular indistinct contour is consistent with the development of recurrent tumor. If confusion exists about the nature of the visualized mass, percutaneous, CT-guided biopsy is indicated to secure the diagnosis.

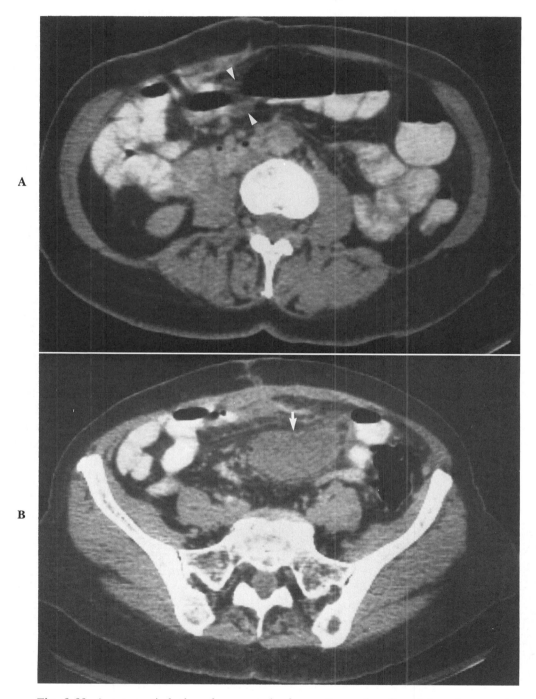

Fig. 6-63. Anastomotic leak and mesenteric abscess 5 months after right colectomy for carcinoma of the colon. **A,** There is slight thickening of the bowel wall at the anastomotic site *(arrowheads).* **B,** A slightly inferior cut shows a fluid collection in the mesentery that represents the abscess *(arrow).* A barium enema performed before CT examination did not reveal extravasation.

Recurrent carcinoma

Local recurrence after abdominoperineal resection for rectal carcinoma is as high as 30% to 50% despite the use of adjuvant radiotherapy.[56,58] Although 70% to 80% of these recur within 2 years after surgery, the tumor free interval may range from 3 months to 11 years.[57] Barium enema and colonoscopic examinations have limitations in their ability to diagnose recurrency because often the tumor grows in a submucosal or extramural location.

In a series of 51 patients with proven recurrent disease who were examined after anterior resections of rectosigmoid carcinoma, 72% had the tumor located at the anastomotic site while 28% had the tumor located in the perirectal region outside the bowel wall.[57] In addition, 20 patients had distal metastases as well. In this series among different diagnostic methods, the sensitivity to detect recurrent tumor was as follows: by rectoscopy 61%, by rising carcinoembryonic antigen (CEA) 76%, and by CT 78%. The extent of the extramural component of the mass as well as distal metastases could be best evaluated by CT. CT has a reported overall accuracy in detecting and staging recurrent rectosigmoid carcinoma of 78% to 95% with a false-positive rate under 5% and a very low false negative rate.[56,57,59] Similar results should be expected in the remainder of the colon.

At the anastomotic site recurrent tumor produces a localized asymmetrical thickening or a focal intramural mass (Figs 6-64 and 6-65). The findings are similar to primary lesions; however with recurrent tumors, there is a significantly higher incidence of extramural involvement.

Tumor adjacent to the anastomosis or in the pelvis after abdominoperineal resection appears as a globular homogeneous mass (Fig. 6-66) or as a well-defined mass with a central, low-density core surrounded by a thick soft-tissue rim. The CT appearance of distal metastatic tumor is often similar to the primary tumor (Fig. 6-67).

Common pitfalls in the CT diagnosis are unopacified small bowel loops, the prostatic gland in males, and a posterior and low location of the uterus in females (Fig. 6-68). Inflammatory and postsurgical fibrotic masses may mimic local recurrency as previously mentioned.

Patients evaluated for recurrent colonic carcinoma may develop a variety of intraabdominal metastases that can be detected by CT. Among them, liver metastases, ovarian metastases, serosal implants (Fig. 6-67), retroperitoneal and mesenteric nodes (Fig. 6-69), psoas muscle tumor deposits (Fig. 6-67), and ascites may be seen.

An excellent correlation between rising carcinoembryonic antigen and abnormalities detected during CT examination has been observed and reported.[60] In a series of 20 patients with rising carcinoembryonic antigen after surgery for carcinoma of colon, CT showed abnormalities consistent with metastatic disease in 19 patients.

CT represents the most efficient noninvasive method of evaluation for recurrent colonic carcinoma. The important role of percutaneous, CT-guided, needle biopsy in confirming the CT findings can not be over emphasized.[58]

Text continued p. 361.

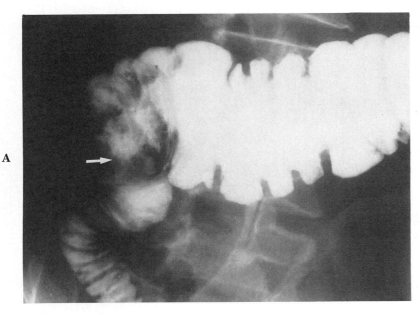

A

Fig. 6-64. Recurrent tumor at the anastomotic site 2 years following right hemicolectomy. **A,** Barium enema shows distortion of the anastomotic site but does not show obstruction or intrinsic defects *(arrow).*

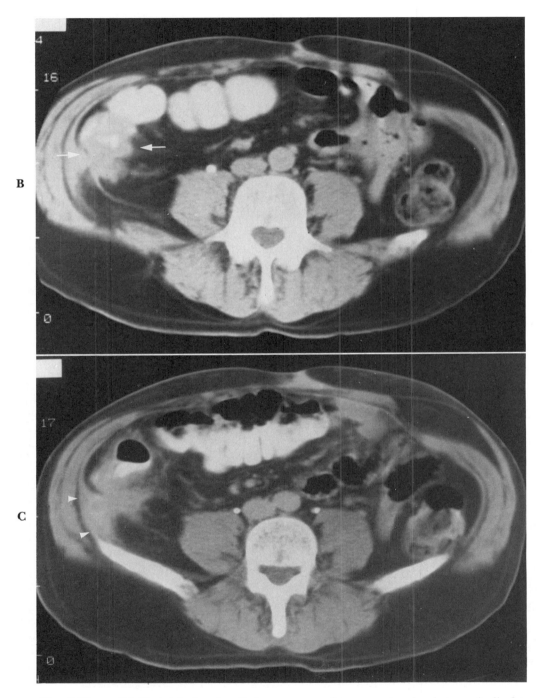

Fig. 6-64, cont'd. B, A lobulated, soft-tissue mass and tumor extension into pericolic fat are seen on CT *(arrows)*. **C,** The tumor extends into the mesenteric fat and infiltrates the parietal peritoneum on the lateral abdominal wall *(arrowheads)*. Findings were confirmed at surgery. (Courtesy Dr. R. Gordon, Veterans Administration Hospital, New York, New York.)

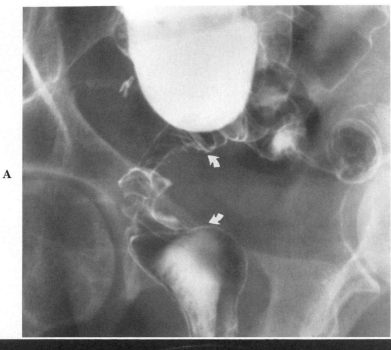

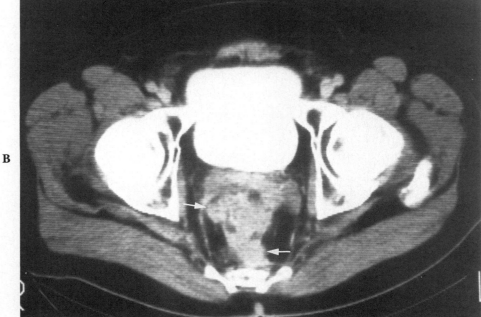

Fig. 6-65. Recurrent tumor at the anastomotic site 1 year after anterior resection of a Duke C rectosigmoid adenocarcinoma. **A,** At the anastomotic site there is narrowing and compression of the rectum by an adjacent mass *(curved arrows).* **B,** A lobulated, soft-tissue mass that extends laterally and posteriorly is demonstrated at the anastomotic site *(arrows).* The rectal lumen is not seen.

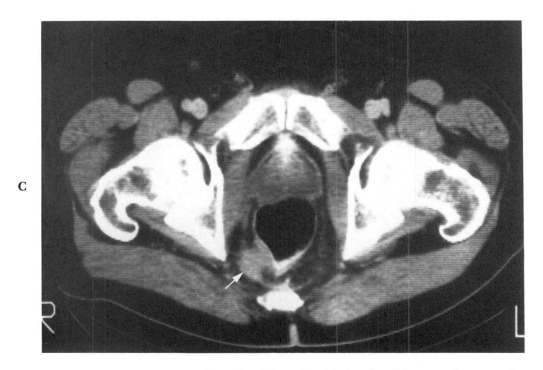

Fig. 6-65, cont'd. C, At an inferior level there is a lobulated, solid mass adjacent to the right and posterior rectal wall *(arrow)*.

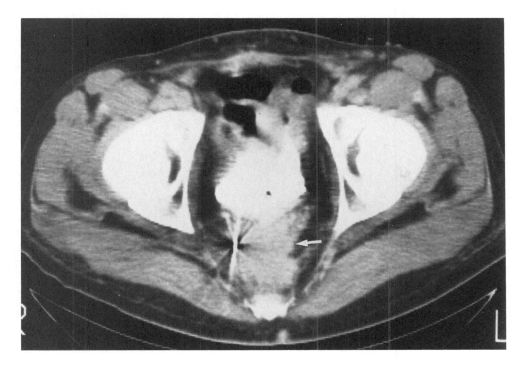

Fig. 6-66. Recurrent pelvic tumor following abdominoperineal resection. A lobulated, large, soft-tissue mass is present in the rectal bed adjacent to the surgical metalic clips *(arrow)*.

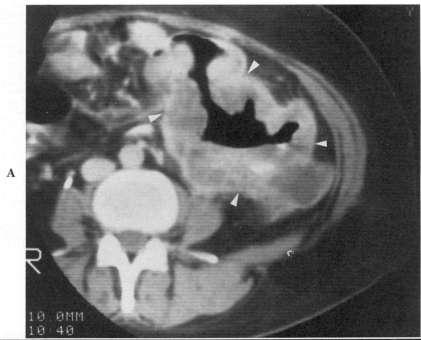

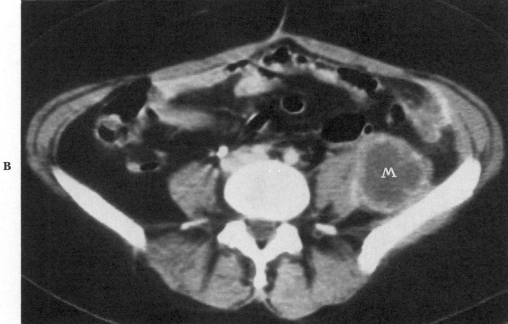

Fig. 6-67. Primary adenocarcinoma of the descending colon and recurrent intra-abdominal metastases 1 year later. **A,** The original CT shows a magnified view of the lesion in the descending colon. Note the large, lobulated mass of lower density and the irregular, rigid, air-filled lumen *(arrowheads)*. **B,** A follow-up CT scan in the upper pelvis shows a similar mass adjacent to the left psoas muscle *(M)*.

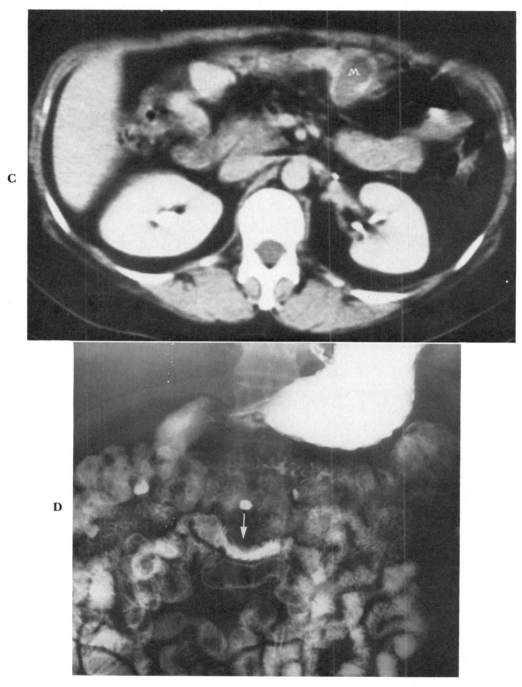

Fig. 6-67, cont'd. C, A similar low-density, soft-tissue mass is seen in the upper abdomen impinging on a small bowel loop. **D,** An upper gastrointestinal examination shows asymmetrical narrowing of a short small bowel segment consistent with serosal implant *(arrow)*. Metastatic lesions were proved by percutaneous needle biopsy.

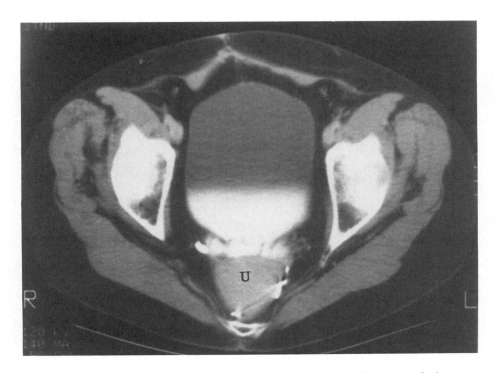

Fig. 6-68. Examination following abdominoperineal resection shows a soft-tissue mass representing the uterus *(U)* in a posterior position close to surgical clips. The CT finding may be mistaken as recurrent tumor.

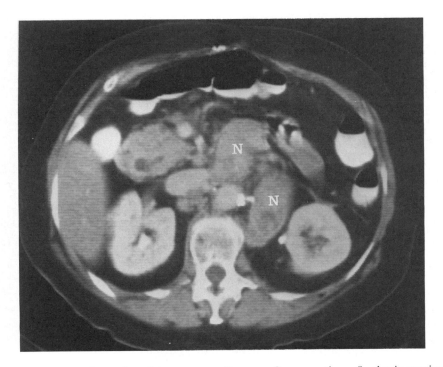

Fig. 6-69. Retroperitoneal nodal metastases 2 years after resection of colonic carcinoma. Large periaortic nodes are seen in the upper abdomen *(N)*.

Colonic polyps

CT has a low sensitivity of visualizing polyps and should not be used as a primary modality in these patients unless associated mesenteric abnormalities such as mesenteric desmoids in Gardner syndrome or metastases are suspected. Adenomatous or in-flammatory polyps can be visualized mostly when larger than 1 to 2 cm in size. To enhance their visualization CT images should be carefully scrutinized and photographed at wide windows (Fig. 6-70).

A

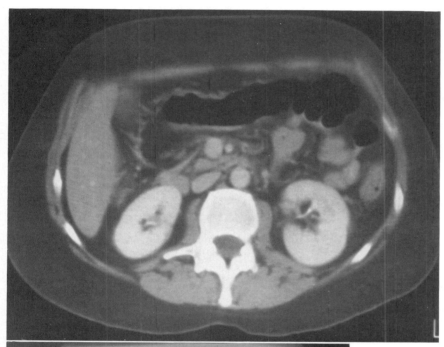

B

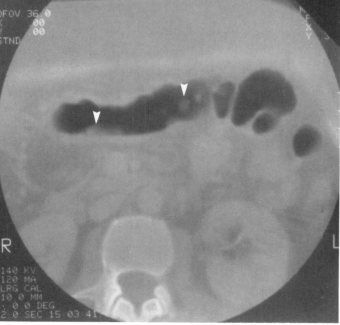

Fig. 6-70. Transverse colonic pseudopolyps in a patient with ulcerative colitis. **A,** An air-filled colon imaged at a window width of 500 H units and a window level of +35 H units does not show polyps. **B,** The same image obtained at a window width of 3000 H units and a window level of 125 H units reveals multiple colonic polyps *(arrowheads)*.

Colonic lipoma

Lipomas are benign, slow growing tumors found throughout the gastrointestinal tract but most commonly in the colon. At autopsy the incidence of colonic lipomas is about 0.25%. They occur anywhere in the colon, with a higher incidence in the cecum and ascending colon. At the time of the diagnosis most colonic lipomas are at least 2 to 3 cm in size and are clinically silent. Hemorrhage or colonic obstruction secondary to intussusception may occur occasionally. The tumor is located submucosally, may be sessile or pedunculated, and has a sharp surface and a round or ovoid shape. In the past the diagnosis was suspected during barium enema and colonoscopy, but confirmation was difficult unless deep biopsies were obtained. Since CT has proven to be extremely reliable in differentiating fat from other tissues, it represents an ideal noninvasive technique to diagnose colonic lipomas[63,64] (see Fig. 6-71). The CT demonstration of a sharply defined mass within the wall of the colon, having a homogeneous low density consistent with fat, is diagnostic. CT is the best imaging modality and is considered the definite method for diagnosing colonic lipomas.

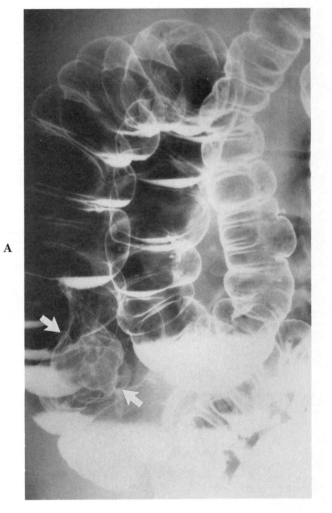

A

Fig. 6-71. Colonic lipoma. **A,** An air contrast barium examination demonstrates a pedunculated, oval, sharply defined filling defect in the ascending colon *(arrows).*

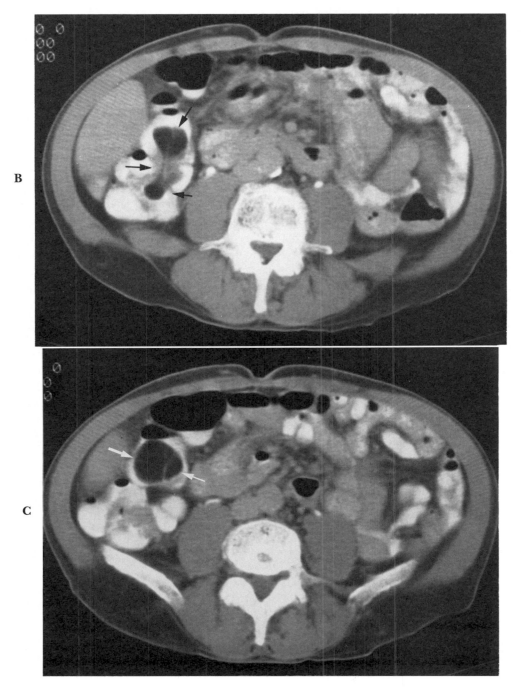

Fig. 6-71, cont'd. B and **C,** The tumor is visualized on CT sections at the level of the pedicle and proximal head **(B)** and more inferiorly at the level of its largest diameter **(C)** *(arrows).* Note that the lesion is sharply defined and has a negative attenuation value (−110 H units), which is characteristic of fat.

Colonic lymphoma

The colon may be primarily or secondarily involved by lymphoma. Among 275 patients with abdominal lymphoma reviewed by Megibow,[65] 9.5% had gastrointestinal tract involvement and 1.5% had colonic involvement. Colonic lymphoma occurs less commonly than gastric or small intestinal lymphoma and it is often advanced at the time of the diagnosis. About 50% of patients with gastrointestinal lymphoma have no symptoms related to the alimentary tract while in the other half anorexia, bleeding, or obstructive signs may be detected. Although the experience is still limited, there are no tissue characteristic differences reported among different types of non-Hodgkin's and Hodgkin's lymphomas on CT examination. Non-Hodgkin lymphoma and particularly the histiocytic form is more commonly encountered in the gastrointestinal tract. The colon may be affected at any level. Pathologically, lymphoma arises in lymphoid tissue of the lamina propria and grows submucosally, producing significant thickening of the bowel wall.[66] It is this characteristic that makes it particularly suitable to CT imaging. Large ulcerations, fistulas, and exophitic soft-tissue masses may be present, explaining different clinical manifestations.

The following CT features are considered highly suspicious for colonic lymphoma (Fig. 6-72):

1. Striking, mural, soft-tissue thickening measuring an average of 5 cm from lumen to serosa and as high as 12 cm in our experience. The mural mass may be circumferential and symmetrical or it may be focal, involving one side of the bowel wall. When it is circumferential, it encroaches and compromises the colonic lumen, producing a segmental smooth narrowing.
2. Homogeneous soft-tissue mass generally without areas of lower attenuation or calcifications.
3. Tumor of soft-tissue density range showing slight enhancement (about 10 to 20 H units) during the intravenous drip infusion or higher if bolus studies are performed.
4. Massive regional and distal mesenteric and retroperitoneal adenopathy.

Lymphadenopathy may be extensive, and solid organs may be involved (Fig. 6-73). The CT differential diagnosis of colonic lymphoma includes other primary or secondary malignancies, particularly adenocarcinoma and leiomyosarcoma. CT features are not specific and barium studies and endoscopic or percutaneous biopsies are required for histologic confirmation (Fig. 6-74).

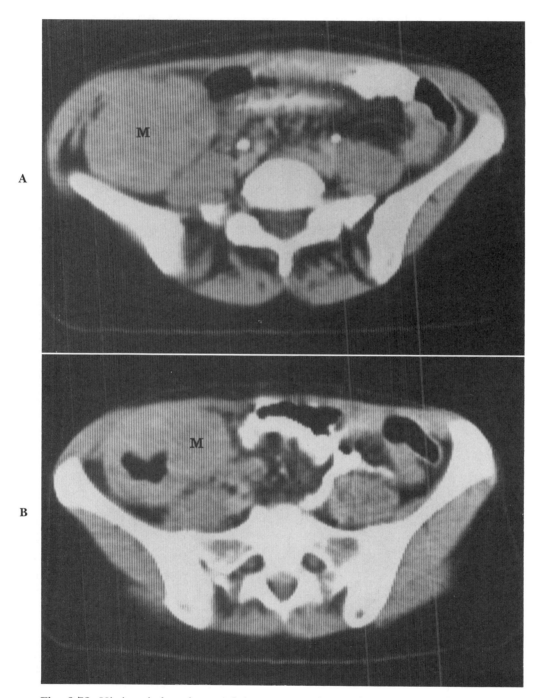

Fig. 6-72. Histiocytic lymphoma of the cecum and ascending colon. **A** and **B,** A large, homogeneous, and slightly lobulated soft-tissue mass is seen in the right colon *(M)*.

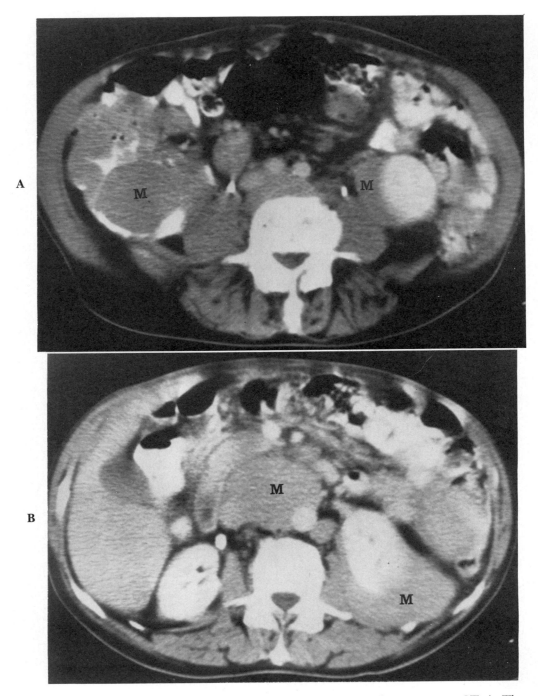

Fig. 6-73. Lymphosarcoma of the right colon appearing as a large mass on CT. **A,** The tumor has a lobulated and homogeneous appearance, and the colonic lumen is compromised *(M)*. **B,** Large, homogeneous, soft-tissue masses are seen in the retroperitoneum and posterior to the left kidney *(M)*.

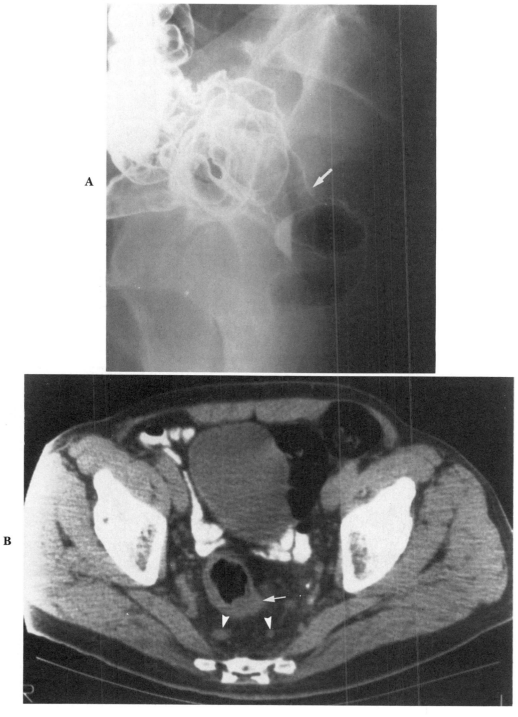

Fig. 6-74. Histiocytic lymphoma of the rectosigmoid colon. **A,** Barium enema shows a submucosal or extrinsic mass indenting the posterior rectal wall *(arrow)*. **B,** CT reveals asymmetrical rectal wall thickening *(arrow)* and perirectal nodular densities *(arrowheads)*. CT findings are indistinguishable from rectal carcinoma.

Colonic smooth muscle tumors

Leiomyoma and leiomyosarcoma are primary mesenchymal tumors that rarely develop in the colon and that constitute only about 3% of the smooth muscle tumors of the gastrointestinal tract.[67-70] They originate from the muscle coat and, when small, are totally intramural causing no symptoms and being diagnosed serendipitously. Their biological behavior and rate and pattern of growth differ, explaining the varied radiographic and clinical manifestations. Intraluminal growth produces a submucosal, sharply outlined defect (60%); subserosal extension leads usually to a large exophytic mass (35%) that may indent the intestinal lumen only slightly; dumb-bell tumors (5%) have combined intraluminal and extramural features.[68] At the time of the diagnosis, myomatous tumors are usually large with a reported average diameter of 4.5 cm for leiomyomas and 12 cm for gastrointestinal leiomyosarcomas.[69] The differentiation between a benign and malignant tumor is difficult histologically and often requires gross morphologic evaluation of the tumor. While other imaging modalities such as barium and angiographic studies have been useful, CT is helpful not only in detecting these tumors but in suggesting their benign or malignant nature.[69]

On CT examination leiomyoma usually appears as a small to moderate size (2 to 5 cm), spherical or ellipsoid, sharply outlined soft-tissue mass (Fig. 6-75). It has a homogeneous appearance, and it enhances uniformly and significantly. Depending on the amount and rate of contrast injection, the enhancement ranges between 30 to 60 H units and may be as high as 1 to 1.5 times its baseline value, reaching its peak about 10 seconds after injection.[69]

Leiomyosarcomas on the other hand are generally large tumors, lobulated and irregular in outline, and predominantly exophitic (Fig. 6-76). They may show evidence of local infiltration of adjacent vessels and organs. These lesions are nonhomogeneous, showing irregular and blotchy enhancement and central zones of low density, surrounded by a thick lobulated rim of tumor tissue (Fig. 6-76). The central zone of necrosis may lead to liquefaction and the development of a thick-walled fluid-containing cystic mass that may be confused with a benign cyst. The presence of air or positive contrast material within the confines of the tumor usually signifies the existence of a large ulceration communicating with the bowel lumen. Dystrophic calcifications may be present in the mass. Metastases appear as multiple, round, well-defined masses of variable density present in the liver and/or peritoneal cavity. Their ominous significance even when associated with a relatively benign looking primary tumor is obvious.

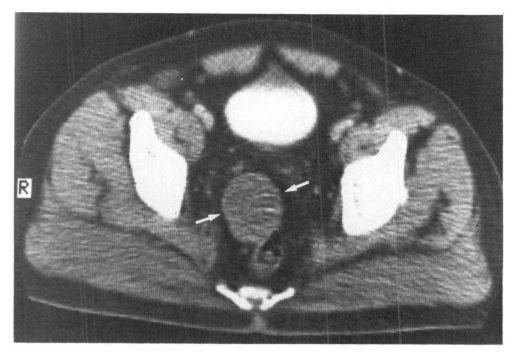

Fig. 6-75. Rectal leiomyoma appearing as a small, homogeneous, well-defined mass anterior to the rectal wall *(arrows)*. The mass was displacing seminal vesicles anteriorly, suggesting a rectal rather than prostatic origin.

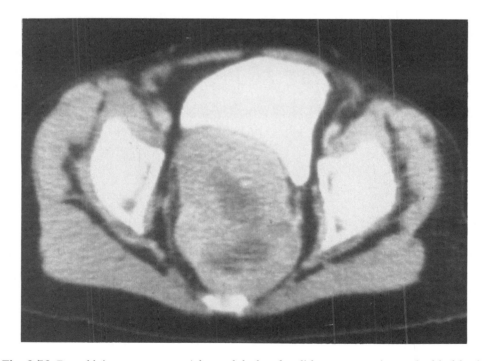

Fig. 6-76. Rectal leiomyosarcoma. A large, lobulated, solid mass posterior to the bladder is seen in the pelvis. Note the areas of irregular lower densities within the mass that represent necrosis.

MISCELLANEOUS LESIONS

CT has been found useful in the diagnosis and evaluation of a variety of colonic lesions other than those that are inflammatory or neoplastic in nature. While in some pathologic entities its contribution is negligible or marginal, in others CT has already been proven important in suspecting or diagnosing primary or secondary colonic pathology.

Colonic intussusception

Colonic intussusception implies an invagination of the terminal ileum or of a part of the colon into the lumen of the immediately distal colon. Although barium enema remains the primary technique in diagnosing colonic intussusceptions, the CT diagnosis of this entity has been recently reported in the literature.[71-75] In adults colonic intussusceptions are caused by an intraluminal mass, usually large polyps, villous adenoma, polypoid carcinoma, or lymphosarcoma. The apposition of several tissue layers of varying densities at the same level within the confines of the colon is characteristic and explains the potential usefulness of CT to detect this condition. At the pathologic site the core of the lesion is represented by the collpased intussusceptum, containing residual fluid, air, or fecal material. Adjacent intraluminal mesentery that contains fat is usually present and covered by an outer mantle of soft-tissue density representing the wall of the colonic intussuscipiens. The CT image should be expected to vary depending on the cause and degree of intussusception, the time of the examination in its evolution, and the angle of the incident CT beam relative to the longitudinal and transverse axes of the colonic segment examined.[74] The presence of a complex mass composed of layers of fat and soft-tissue density (Fig. 6-77), a mixed density core, and a homogeneous peripheral mantle is sufficiently characteristic to allow CT recognition. Proximal small bowel obstruction and signs of intestinal ischemia or ascites may be seen when complications develop. This CT appearance should not be confused with mesenteric or omental masses, abscesses, or nonhomogeneous, necrotic, colonic tumors. If the CT diagnosis is only tentative, barium enema examination is recommended for confirmation. The cause of the intussusception is more difficult to identify during the CT examination.

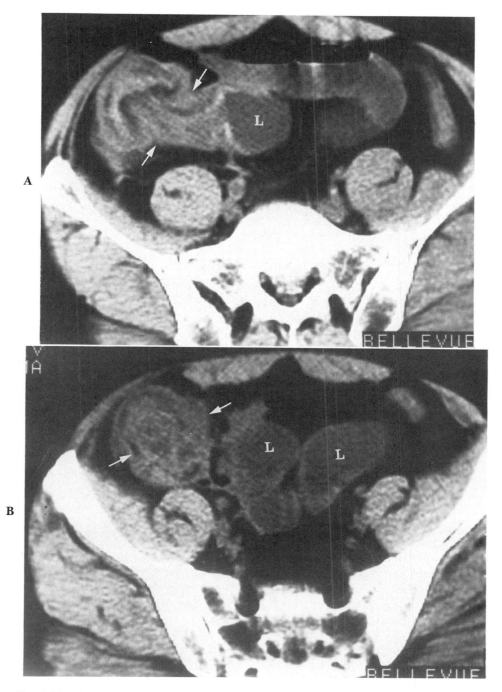

Fig. 6-77. Ileocolic intussusception. The patient is a 56-year-old man with intramural, small bowel hemorrhage secondary to anticoagulant therapy. **A,** CT shows fluid-filled, distended ileal loops *(L)* and a collapsed, thick-walled, distal ileum invaginating into the colon *(arrows).* **B,** A complex mass composed of layers of varying densities and a mixed density core is seen in the right colon *(arrows).* Note the distended, fluid-filled distal ileum *(L).*

Appendicular mucocele and pseudomyxoma peritonei

The slow and continuous accumulation of mucin in the appendix leads to the development of a cystic mass known as a mucocele. Although initially considered a benign complication of appendicular obstruction, it has been found in some instances to represent a true neoplasm, such as, mucinous cystadenoma or cystadenocarcinoma.[76,77] The cystic mass is variable in size, usually round, and sharply defined. On barium enema studies it appears as a smooth indentation on the medial and inferior wall of the cecum. Curvilinear calcifications in the wall of the cyst may be present. CT examination reveals a thin-walled cystic structure with homogeneous low-attenuation contents attached to or adjacent to the cecum in the right lower quadrant (Figs. 6-78 and 6-79).

Pseudomyxoma peritonei ("jelly belly," "gelatinous ascites") is a clinical entity in which a slow, insidious accumulation of large amounts of intraperitoneal gelatinous material leads eventually to massive abdominal distention. It is believed to occur secondary to rupture of a mucinous adenocarcinoma, usually of the appendix or ovary. However, it has been rarely associated with malignancy of the colon, stomach, uterus, pancreas, common bile duct, and omphalomesenteric or urachal duct.[78,79] Patients are generally in good health, experiencing slowly progressive abdominal distention, recurrent abdominal pain, and episodes of intestinal obstruction. The clinical entity may develop years after the primary surgical procedure, or it may manifest initially without the benefit of a pertinent history. Repeated surgical evacuation of mucinous ascites is common with 5-year survival rates of about 50% reported.[78]

The conventional radiographic features of pseudomyxoma peritonei are nonspecific and usually indicative of massive ascites. Ill-defined, large, asymmetrical soft-tissue masses displacing and compressing abdominal organs and containing several annular or semicircular calcifications are considered highly suggestive.[79,80] These faint curvilinear or mottled calcifications, originally described by Pugh[80] are rarely seen, but when present, are helpful in the differential diagnosis.

CT has considerably improved our ability to diagnose this entity. Although the CT findings are not always pathognomonic, several features observed and reported recently[81-86] should allow a correct preoperative diagnosis in most cases (Figs. 6-78 and 6-79).

1. Ascites of varying amounts, sometimes filling the entire peritoneal cavity, may be present. The fluid is often loculated in different compartments; septations are present; and scalloping of the lateral margin of the liver as a result of the pressure from adjacent peritoneal implants is seen.[81,84]
2. Several thin-wall cystic masses of different sizes with or without associated ascites may be present at different levels in the peritoneal cavity.[82,83]
3. With large amounts of mucinous ascites the mesenteric structures and small bowel loops are compressed posteriorly.[81] Conversely, in the ordinary transudative ascites the small bowel is floating in the intraperitoneal fluid.
4. Thickening of the greater omentum (omental cake) similar to other forms of intraperitoneal metastases may be present.
5. Occasional curvilinear calcifications may be recognized.[85,86]

Pseudomyxoma peritonei is an indolent form of peritoneal carcinomatosis in which distal hematogeneous metastases, lymphadenopathy, or liver metastases, although reported,[83] are very unusual. In addition to the recognition and extent of involvement, CT may help in identifying the primary site of origin by demonstrating cystic appendicular or ovarian tumors (Fig. 6-78) or low attenuation lesions in other intra-abdominal organs such as the pancreas.[84] CT guided aspiration and biopsy can rapidly establish the diagnosis. Depending on the CT presentation, the differential diagnosis includes peritoneal metastases from other primary sites, pancreatitis with pseudocysts, pyogenic peritonitis, and widespread echinococcal disease. Visualization of bubbles of air within one or several loculated fluid collections is indicative of intra-abdominal abscess that may develop in this entity secondary to a perforated viscus.[85]

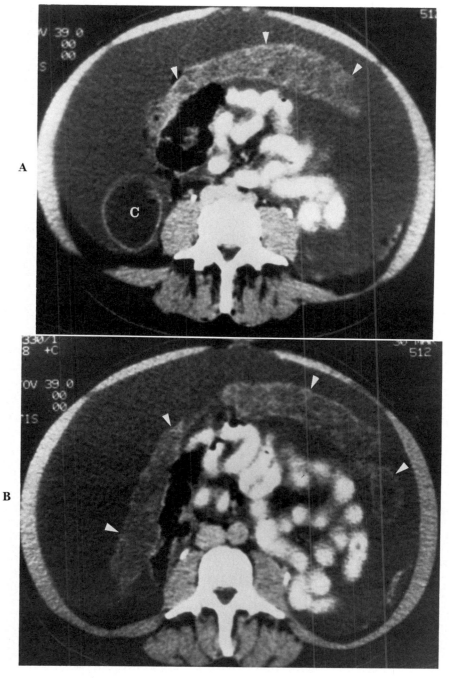

Fig. 6-78. Mucocele of the appendix with associated pseudomyxoma peritonei. **A** and **B,** thin-walled, cystic mass with homogeneous low-density content is seen in the right lower abdomen *(C)*. There is associated massive ascites and nonhomogeneous thickening of the greater omentum ("omental cake") *(arrowheads)*. The mesentery, small bowel loops, and colon are compressed centrally and displaced posteriorly.

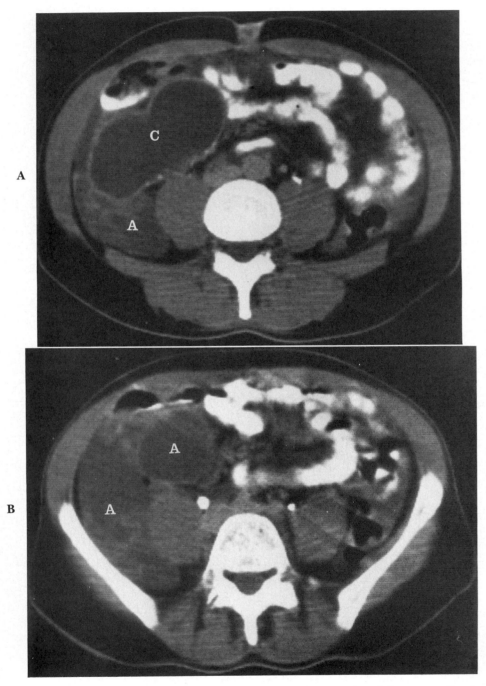

Fig. 6-79. Pseudomyxoma peritoneal secondary to a mucocele of the appendix. **A,** A mucocele is visualized as a large, cystic, low-density mass with minute calcifications in the wall *(C)*. Ascites is present in the right lower quadrant *(A)*. **B,** Partially loculated fluid collections are noted in the right lower abdomen and pelvis *(A)*. (Courtesy Dr. S. Goldfine, Maimonides Hospital, Brooklyn, New York.)

Pneumatosis coli

Intramural colonic air is seen rarely and can usually be demonstrated by conventional radiographic techniques. It develops as a complication of a variety of underlying disorders:

1. Intestinal ischemia or infarction
2. Intestinal obstruction or ileus
3. Colonoscopy and biopsy
4. Barium enema
5. Colitis
6. Post-surgical bowel anastomosis
7. Collagen disease, especially scleroderma
8. Chronic obstructive lung disease
9. Steroid therapy

In the context of a proper clinical presentation, intramural air may represent the first radiographic manifestation of intestinal ischemia and necrosis. The air may be located submucosally or subserosally and in most instances it occurs as a consequence of loss of mucosal integrity and raised intraluminal pressure.[87] CT can visualize intramural air[88-90] and has been found more sensitive than plain abdominal films when properly performed. To enhance visualization, the colonic lumen should be distended and preferably filled with a positive contrast agent and close scrutiny of images using lung window settings should be performed.[89] Under these circumstances CT can delineate better the location and extent of pneumatosis coli and help in the etiologic diagnosis by revealing associated colonic and mesenteric abnormalities.

The CT diagnosis is based on the detection of air circumferentially distributed around the bowel lumen and paralleling the bowel wall (Fig. 6-80). The air appears as cystic, or curvilinear collections, has no fluid levels, and should be seen on the posterior aspect of the bowel wall in the supine position. In cases of bowel ischemia and gangrene, the wall is thickened and shows contrast enhancement. In addition, gas in the peripheral branches or the main trunk of the mesenteric vein, intrahepatic portal air, free air in the peritoneal cavity, or thrombosis with obstruction of the mesenteric artery or vein may be seen. Although regarded as an ominous sign, the presence of air in the portal system may rarely be seen in benign conditions and not always associated with intestinal ischemic necrosis.[90] Potentially confusing images that lead to false-positive interpretations may result when gas is trapped between pieces of stool or within multiple adjacent diverticula.[88] The intraluminal and dependent location of these air collections helps in the establishment of a correct diagnosis.

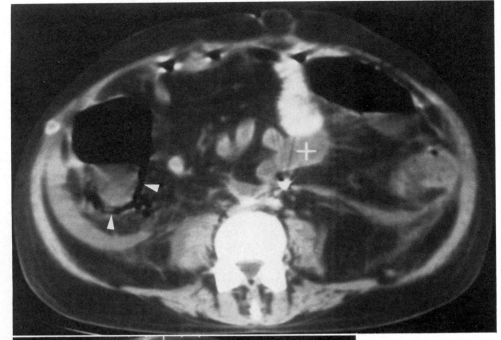

A

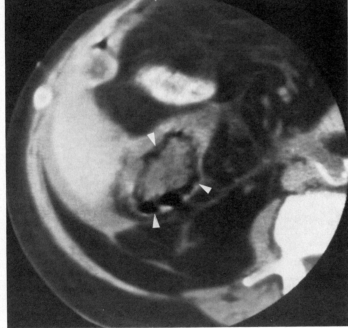

B

Fig. 6-80. Pneumatosis coli of the right colon secondary to colonic infarction after repair of abdominal aortic aneurysm. **A** and **B,** There is circumferential distribution of intramural air parelleling the colonic wall *(arrowheads).* There are no fluid levels and the curvilinear air is located on the posterior aspect of the bowel wall.

Sigmoid volvulus

Sigmoid volvulus develops when a severe twist of the two limbs of the sigmoid colon and of the mesosigmoid occurs. The degree of torsion varies, but in most symptomatic individuals it is about 360 degrees. Patients become distended, exhibiting abdominal pain and signs of intestinal obstruction.

Delay in diagnosis and treatment may lead to colonic ischemia, necrosis, perforation, and peritonitis. Plain abdominal films and barium enema can promptly and reliably diagnose sigmoid volvulus by recognizing radiographic features well described in the literature.[91,92] CT appears to be able to detect intestinal volvulus.[93,94] The experience is

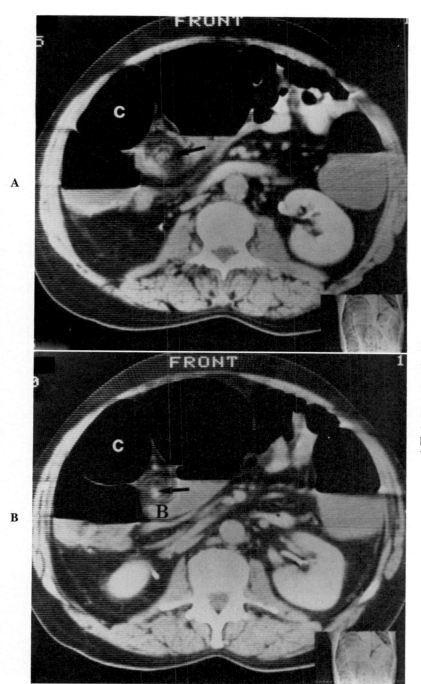

Fig. 6-81. CT diagnosis of sigmoid volvulus. **A** and **B,** The whirl sign is demonstrated with its central core representing the tightly twisted mesentery *(arrow)*. The distended proximal colon *(C)* and the tapered sigmoid (beak sign) *(B)* are seen leading into the volvulus. (Courtesy Dr. M. Shaff, Vanderbilt University Medical Center, Nashville, Tennessee.)

however still very limited and its sensitivity is unknown. CT should be expected to show distention of the proximal colon and a massively distended sigmoid. At the point of torsion a central soft-tissue mass enveloped in fatty tissue, containing semi-circular densities, and known as the "whirl sign"[93] is visualized (Fig. 6-81). The whirl is formed by the twisted afferent and efferent intestinal limbs and by the tightly torsioned mesentery. The smoothly tapered limbs of the sigmoid are similar in shape to the beak sign seen during barium enema examination. The recognition of this sign helps in the prompt diagnosis of volvulus in cases unsuspected clinically in which CT examinations are performed for other unrelated reasons.

Anorectal giant condyloma acuminatum (Buschke-Löwenstein tumor)

Giant condyloma acuminatum is a variant of venereal wart, having a similar cause and similar histologic features but distinguished by its large size and local infiltration of adjacent structures. It is caused by a virus, and it occurs predominantly in the genital and perianal areas, rarely involving the rectum. The tumor grows slowly, tends to invade the surrounding tissues, and causes fistulous tracks, inflammation, fibrosis, and hemorrhage.[95,97] The biologic potential of condyloma acuminatum to undergo malignant degeneration is recognized.[97] These lesions are considered precancerous; however, the neoplastic degeneration is observed rarely. The presence of malignancy in this inherently invasive lesion can be established only on histologic examination. Some of the tumors are benign, while others show a complex histologic pattern with areas of benign condyloma intermixed with zones of epithelial dysplasia, verrucous (low-grade) carcinoma, and well-differentiated squamous cell carcinoma.

Conventional radiologic studies are very limited in assessing the presence and degree of involvement of the giant anorectal condyloma. Excellent pathological correlation can be achieved with CT, which documents the location and extent of rectal, perirectal, and perineal involvement and helps in the preoperative staging and extent of surgical resection.[98] The CT diagnosis is based on the demonstration of several papilomatous perianal skin lesions, obliteration of the subcutaneous fat, and varying degrees of perineal, perirectal, and rectal tumor infiltration (Fig. 6-82). If not adequately treated, the process leads eventually to severe rectal luminal narrowing, perirectal fascial thickening, and asymmetrical tumor infiltration with obliteration of the normal fat planes (Fig. 6-82). Although CT accurately documents the morphology of the lesion it does not discriminate between different histologic types of soft tissue infiltration.[98]

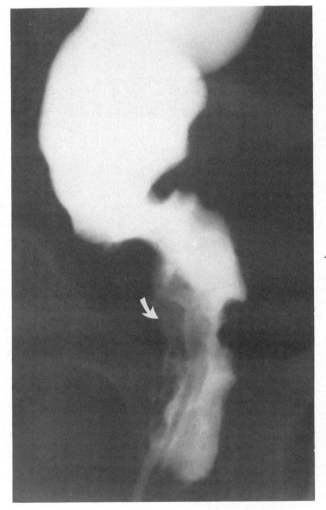

A

Fig. 6-82. Giant condyloma acuminatum (Buschke-Löwenstein tumor). **A,** Barium enema shows tumor infiltration with asymmetrical narrowing and nodular defects in the rectum *(curved arrow)*.

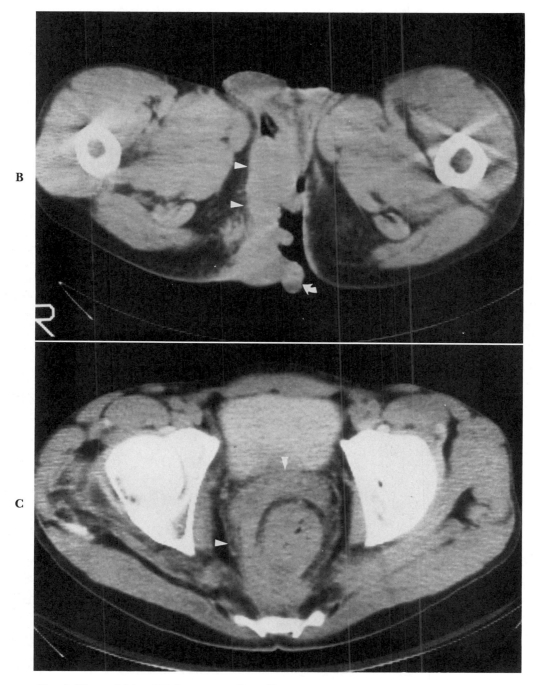

Fig. 6-82, cont'd. B, CT shows several papillomatous skin lesions *(curved arrow)* and tumor infiltration with obliteration of the perineal subcutaneous fat *(arrowheads)*. **C,** Thickening of the rectal wall and tumor invasion into the perirectal fat tissue is demonstrated *(arrowheads)*.

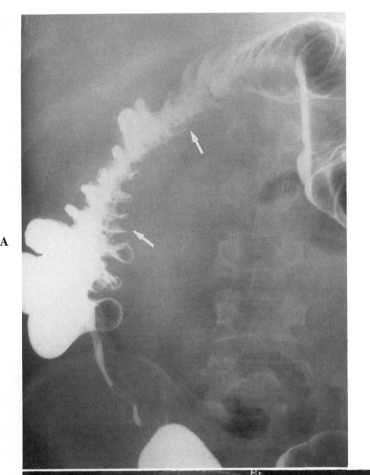

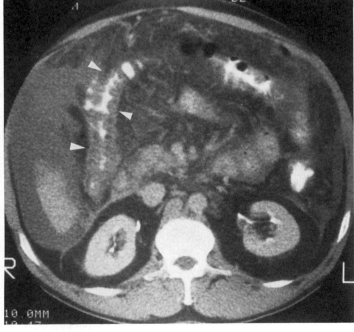

Colonic edema

Segmental or diffuse intestinal edema can occur in a variety of conditions, including inflammatory disease, allergic reactions, protein-losing enteropathies, nephrosis, and hepatic cirrhosis. Most cases of noninflammatory colonic edema are seen in patients with cirrhosis secondary to portal hypertension and hypoalbuminemia. Its pathogenesis and different types of radiographic manifestations have been thoroughly described in the literature.[99,100] The right colon or the entire colon may be affected, showing on barium enema studies an irregular serrated contour, distortion of the haustral pattern, incomplete distensibility, and severe mucosal thickening. CT shows a partially collapsed colon, asymmetrical haustrations, and circumferential bowel wall thickening (Fig. 6-83). In addition, CT documents the presence of ascites, a cirrhotic liver, and venous collateral circulation consistent with portal hypertension. These important associated findings helps differentiate colonic edema from other segmental or diffuse inflammatory conditions that induce circumferential colonic wall thickening.

Fig. 6-83. Colonic edema in a patient with cirrhosis and portal hypertension. **A,** Barium enema demonstrates right-sided involvement with narrowing, serrated contour, and a distorted haustral pattern *(arrows)*. **B,** CT shows a collapsed colon and circumferential wall thickening *(arrowheads)*. In addition, ascites and enlarged collateral veins are seen in the mesentery.

Colon involvement in pancreatitis

Paracolic inflammatory masses and abscesses of different origins may secondarily affect the colon. This complication, however, is most commonly seen associated with acute hemorrhagic pancreatitis. Extravasated pancreatic enzymes visualized on CT as fluid collections are frequently located in the lesser sac and in the anterior pararenal space, particularly on the left. In addition, as described by Meyers et al.,[101] inflammatory exudate and activated enzymes spread via the mesocolon into the transverse colon and phrenocolic ligament (Fig. 6-84). Any segment of the transverse colon may be affected, although the splenic flexure is the most common site. The radiographic manifestations include colonic atonia appearing as a dilation of the transverse colon (colon cut-off sign), functional spasm at the splenic flexure, and, when more severe, organic inflammatory lesions leading to permanent fibrotic strictures.[101-103] Although con-

ventional barium enema studies demonstrate segmental inflammatory lesions and strictures, they are limited in establishing the cause of these abnormalities. On CT the presence and location of the extravasated fluid collections are clearly demonstrated. Fluid in the left anterior pararenal space can be seen encasing the splenic flexure, and phlegmons in the mesocolon adjacent and posterior to the transverse colon can be seen,[104] (Fig. 6-85). In these cases follow-up CT examinations are indicated to assess the evolution of these abnormal collections and to rule out complications such as abscess formation or intestinal perforation. In addition, CT documents the development of a stricture that appears as a segmental smooth narrowing with circumferential symmetrical wall thickening (Fig. 6-85). Associated residual pancreatic and peripancreatic inflammatory reaction is usually present to allow a specific etiologic diagnosis.

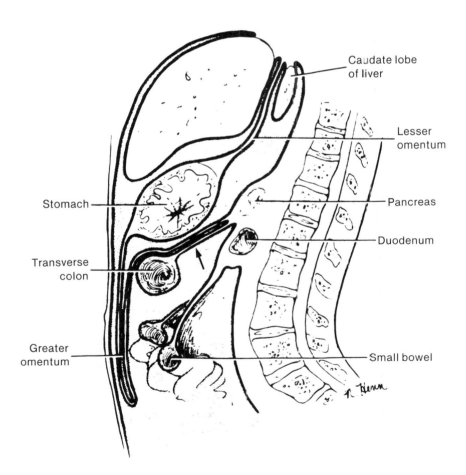

Fig. 6-84. Diagram showing the peritoneal and mesenteric reflections in the upper abdomen. Peripancreatic inflammatory exudate can spread to the transverse colon via the mesocolon *(arrow)*.

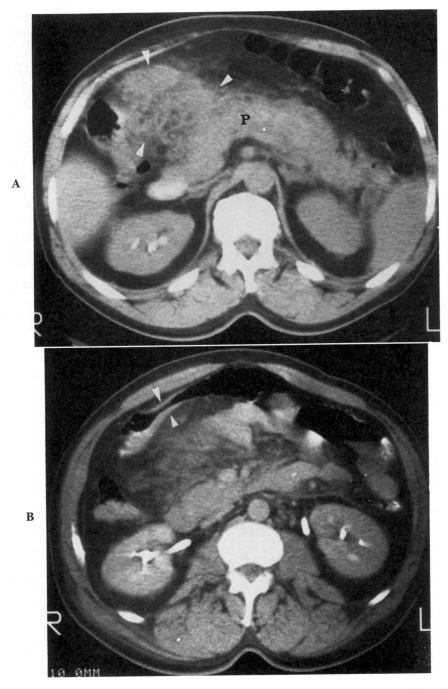

Fig. 6-85. Colon involvement in pancreatitis. **A,** Examination reveals an enlarged pancreas *(P)* and an inflammatory mass (phlegmon) in the right anterior abdomen within the mesocolon *(arrowheads)*. **B,** There is smooth narrowing of the proximal transverse colon with circumferential wall thickening *(arrowheads)*.

REFERENCES

1. Aronberg, D.J., Lee, J.K.T., Sagel, S.S., et al.: Techniques in computed body tomography, New York, 1983, Raven Press.

2. Mitchell, D.G., Bjorgvinsson, E., terMeulen, D., et al.: Gastrografin versus dilute barium for colonic CT examination: a blind, randomized study, J. Comput. Assist. Tomogr. 9:451-453, 1981.

3. Megibow, A.J., Zerhouni, E., Hulnick, D.H., et al.: Air contrast techniques in gastrointestinal computed tomography, Scientific Exhibit, American Roentgen Ray Society, 1985.

4. Megibow, A.J., Zerhouni, E.A., Hulnick, D.H., et al.: Air insufflation of the colon as an adjunct to computed tomography of the pelvis, J. Comput. Assist. Tomogr. 4:797-800, 1984.

5. Fagelman, D., Warhit, J.M., Rieter, J.D., et al.: Case report: CT diagnosis of fecaloma, J. Comput. Assist. Tomogr. 8:559-561, 1984.

6. Cunningham's Textbook of anatomy, ed. 11, London, 1972, Oxford University Press.

7. Grabbe, E., Lierse, W., Winkler, R.: The perirectal fascia: morphology and use in staging of rectal carcinoma, Radiology 149:241-246, 1983.

8. Tisnado, J., Amendola, M.A., Walsh, J.W., et al.: Computed tomography of perineum, AJR 136:475-481, 1981.

9. Fisher, J.K.: Normal colon wall thickness on CT, Radiology 145:415-418, 1982.

10. Fisher, J.K.: Abnormal colonic wall thickening on computed tomography, J. Comput. Assist. Tomogr. 7:90-97, 1983.

11. Gore, R.M., Marn, C.S., Kirby, D.F., et al.: CT findings in ulcerative, granulomatous and indeterminate colitis, AJR 143:403-404, 1984.

12. Goodman, P.C., and Federle, M.P.: Pseudomembranous colitis, J. Comput. Assist. Tomogr. 4:403-404, 1980.

13. Megibow, A.J., Streiter, M.L., Balthazar, E.J., et al.: Pseudomembranous colitis: diagnosis by computed tomography, J. Comput. Assist. Tomogr. 8:281-283, 1984.

14. Brunner, D., Feifarek, C., McNeely, D., et al.: CT of pseudomembranous colitis, Gastrointest. Radiol. 9:73-75, 1984.

15. Frick, M.P., Maile, C.W., Crass, J.R., et al.: Computed tomography of neutropenic colitis, AJR 143:763-765, 1984.

16. Balthazar, E.J., Megibow, A.J., Fazzini, E., et al.: Cytomegalovirus colitis in AIDS: radiographic findings in 11 patients, Radiology 155:585-589, 1985.

17. Jones, B., Fishman, E.K., and Siegelmann, S.S.: Ischemic colitis demonstrated by computed tomography, J. Comput. Assist. Tomogr. 6:1120-1123, 1982.

18. Federle, M.P., Chun, G., Jeffrey, R.B., et al.: Computed tomographic findings in bowel infarction, AJR 142:91-95, 1984.

19. Skinner, D.B., Zarins, C.K., and Moossa, A.R.: Mesenteric vascular disease, Am. J. Surg. 128:835-839, 1974.

20. Ottinger, L.W., and Austen, W.G.: A study of 136 patients with mesenteric infarction, Surg. Gynecol. Obstet. 116:474-478, 1963.

21. Doubleday, L.C., and Bernardino, M.E.: CT findings in the perirectal area following radiation therapy, J. Comput. Assist. Tomogr. 4:634-638, 1980.

22. Fishman, E.K., Zinreich, E.S., Jones, B., et al.: Computed tomographic diagnosis of radiation ileitis, Gastrointest. Radiol. 9:149-152, 1984.

23. Goldberg, H.J., Gore, R.M., Margulis, A.R., et al.: Computed tomography in the evaluation of Crohn's disease, AJR 140:277-282, 1983.

24. Frager, D.H., Goldman, M., and Beneventano, T.C.: Computed tomography in Crohn's disease, J. Comput. Assist. Tomogr. 7:819-824, 1983.

25. Kerber, G.W., Greenberg, M., and Rubin, J.M.: Computed tomography evaluation of local and extraintestinal complications of Crohn's disease, Gastrointest. Radiol. 9:43-48, 1984.

26. Berliner, L., Redmond, P., Purow, E., et al.: Computed tomography in Crohn's disease, Am. J. Gastroenterol. 77:548-553, 1982.

27. Megibow, A.J., Bosniak, M.S., Ambos, M.A., et al.: Case report: Crohn's disease causing hydronephrosis, J. Comput. Assist. Tomogr. 5:909-911, 1981.

28. Schnur, M.J., and Weiner, S.N.: The "string sign" on computerized tomography, Gastrointest. Radiol. 7:43-46, 1982.

29. Siskind, B.N., Burrell, M.I., Klein, M.L., et al.: Case report: toxic dilatation in Crohn's disease with CT correlation, J. Comput. Assist. Tomogr. 9:193-195, 1985.

30. Hulnick, M.A., Megibow, A.J., Balthazar, E.J., et al.: Computed tomography in the evaluation of diverticulitis, Radiology 152:491-495, 1984.

31. Lieberman, J.M., and Haaga, J.R.: Computed tomography of diverticulitis, J. Comput. Assist. Tomogr. 7:431-433, 1983.

32. Goldman, S.M., Fishman, E.K., Gatewood, O.M.B., et al.: CT demonstration of colovesical fistulae secondary to diverticulitis, J. Comput. Assist. Tomogr. 8:462-468, 1984.

33. Jones, B., Fishman, E.K., and Siegelman, S.S.: Computed tomography and appendiceal abscess: special applicability in the elderly, J. Comput. Assist. Tomogr. 7:434-438, 1983.

34. Fish, B., Smulewicz, J.J., and Barek, L.: Role of computed tomography in diagnosis of appendiceal disorders, N.Y. State J. Med. 81:900-904, 1981.

35. Gale, M.E., Birnbaum, S., Gerzof, S.G., et al.: CT appearance of appendicitis and its local complications, J. Comput. Assist. Tomogr. 9:34-37, 1985.

36. Hoffer, F.A., Ablow, R.C., Gryboski, J.D., et al.: Primary appendicits with an appendico-tubo-ovarian fistula, AJR 138:742-743, 1982.

37. Mayes, G.B., and Zornoza, J.: Computed tomography of colon carcinoma, AJR 135:43-46, 1980.

38. van Waes, P.F., Koehler, P.R., and Feldberg, M.A.: Management of rectal carcinoma: impact of computed tomography, AJR 140:1137-1142, 1983.

39. Dixon, A.K., Fry, I.K., Morson, B.C., et al.: Preoperative computed tomography of carcinoma of the rectum, Br. J. Radiol. 54:655-659, 1981.

40. Zaunbauer, W., Haertel, M., and Fuchs, W.A.: Computed tomography in carcinoma of the rectum, Gastrointest. Radiol. 6:79-84, 1981.

41. Oliver, T.W., Somogyi, J., and Gaffney, E.F.: Primary linitis plastica of the rectum, AJR 140:79-80, 1983.

42. Hamlin, D.J., Burener, F.A., and Sischy, B.: New technique to stage early rectal carcinoma by computed tomography, Radiology 141:539-540, 1981.

43. Meyer, J.E., Dosoretz, D.E., Gunderson, L.L., et al.: CT evaluation of locally advanced carcinoma of the distal colon and rectum, J. Comput. Assist. Tomogr. 7:265-267, 1983.

43a. Freeny, P.C., Marks, W.M., Ryan, J.A., et al.: Colorectal carcinoma evaluation with CT: preoperative staging and detection of postoperative recurrence, Radiology 158: 347-353, 1986.

44. Thoeni, R.F., Moss, A.A., Schnyder, P., et al.: Detection and staging of primary rectal and rectosigmoid cancer by computed tomography, Radiology 141:135-138, 1981.

45. Balthazar, E.J., Rosenberg, A.D., and Davidian, M.M.: Primary and metastatic scirrhous carcinoma of the rectum, AJR 132:711-715, 1979.

46. Khan, M.H., and Barron, J.: Cloacogenic carcinoma: a study of six cases and review of literature, Am. J. Gastroenterol. 77:137-140, 1982.

47. Kyaw, M.M., Gallagher, T., and Mains, J.O.: Cloacogenic carcinoma of the anorectal junction: roentgenologic diagnosis, AJR 115:384-391, 1972.

48. Beahrs, O.H.: Management of cancer of the anus, AJR 133:791-795, 1979.

49. Beahrs, O.H., and Wilson, S.M.: Carcinoma of the anus, Ann. Surg. 184:422-428, 1976.

50. Dillard, B.M., Spratt, J.S., Ackerman, L.V., et al.: Epidermoid cancer of anal margin and canal: review of 79 cases, Arch. Surg. 86:772-776, 1963.

51. Roswit, B., Higgins, G.A., Jr., and Keeh, R.J.: Preoperative irradiation for carcinoma of the rectum and retrosigmoid colon: report of a national Veterans Administration randomized study, Cancer 35:1597-1602, 1975.

52. Dukes, C.E.: The classification of cancer of the rectum, J. Pathol. Bacteriol. 35:323-332, 1932.

53. Goldman, S.M., Fishman, E.K., Gatewood, O.M.B., et al.: CT in the diagnosis of enterovesical fistulae, AJR 144: 1229-1233, 1985.

54. Kelvin, F.M., Korobkin, M., Heaston, D.K., et al.: The pelvis after surgery for rectal carcinoma: serial CT observations with emphasis on nonneoplastic features, AJR 41: 959-964, 1983.

55. Reznek, R.H., White, F.E., Young, J.W.R., et al.: The appearances on computed tomography after abdominoperineal resection for carcinoma of the rectum: a comparison between the normal appearances and those of recurrence, Br. J. Radiol. 56:237-240, 1983.

56. Moss, A.A., Theoni, R.F., Schnyder, P., et al.: Value of computed tomography in the detection and staging of recurrent rectal carcinomas, J. Comput. Assist. Tomogr. 5: 870-874, 1981.

57. Grabbe, E., and Winkler, R.: Local recurrence after sphincter-saving resection for rectal and rectosigmoid carcinoma: value of various diagnostic methods, Radiology 155:305-310, 1985.

58. Butch, R.J., Wittenberg, J., Mueller, R.R., et al.: Presacral masses after abdominoperineal resection for colorectal carcinoma: the need for needle biopsy, AJR 144:309-312, 1985.

59. Lee, J.K.T., Stanley, R.J., Sagel, S.S., et al.: CT appearance of the rectal carcinoma, Radiology 141:737-741, 1985.

60. Shirkhoda, A., Staab, E.V., Bunce, L.A., et al.: Computed tomography in recurrent or metastatic colon cancer: relation to rising serum carcinoembryonic antigen, J. Comput. Assist. Tomogr. 8:704-708, 1984.

61. Husband, J.E., Hodson, N.J., and Parsons, C.A.: The use of computed tomography in recurrent rectal tumors, Radiology 134:677-682, 1980.

62. Ellert, J., and Kreel, L.: The value of CT in malignant colonic tumors, CT 4:225-240, 1980.

63. Megibow, A.J., Redmond, P.E., Bosniak, M.A., et al.: Diagnosis of gastrointestinal lipomas by CT, AJR 133:743-745, 1979.

64. Heiken, J.P., Forde, K.A., and Gold, R.P.: Body computed tomography: computed tomography as a definitive method for diagnosing gastrointestinal lipoma, Radiology 142: 409-414, 1982.

65. Megibow, A.J., Balthazar, E.J., Naidich, D.P., et al.: Computed tomography of gastrointestinal lymphoma, AJR 141:541-547, 1983.

66. Dawson, M.P., Coines, J.S., and Morson, B.C.: Primary malignant lymphoid tumors of the intestinal tract: report of 37 cases with factors influencing prognosis, Br. J. Surg. 49:80-89, 1961.

67. Balthazar, E.J.: Gastrointestinal leiomyosarcoma, unusual sites: esophagus, colon, porta hepatis, Gastrointest. Radiol. 6:295-303, 1981.

68. Baker, H.L., and Good, C.A.: Smooth muscle tumors of the alimentary tract, AJR 74:246-255, 1955.

69. Megibow, A.J., Balthazar, E.J., Hulnick, D.H., et al.: CT evaluation of gastrointestinal leiomyomas and leiomyosarcomas, AJR 144:727-731, 1985.

70. Clark, R.A., and Alexander, E.S.: Computed tomography of gastrointestinal leiomyosarcoma, Gastrointest. Radiol. 7:127-129, 1982.

71. Styles, R.A., and Larsen, D.R.: Case report: CT appearance of adult intussusception, J. Comput. Assist. Tomogr. 7:331-333, 1983.

72. Donovan, A.T., and Goldman, S.M.: Computed tomography of ileocecal intussusception: mechanism and appearance, J. Comput. Assist. Tomogr. 6:630-632, 1982.

73. Parienty, R.A., Lepreux, J.F., and Gruson, B.: Sonographic and CT features of ileocolic intussusception, AJR 136: 608-610, 1981.

74. Iko, B.O., Teal, J.S., Suryananarayana, S.M., et al.: Computed tomography of adult colonic intussusception: clinical and experimental studies, AJR 143:769-772, 1984.

75. Curcio, C.M., Feinstein, R.S., Humphrey, R.L., et al.: Computed tomography of entero-enteric intussusception, J. Comput. Assist. Tomogr. 6:969-974, 1982.

76. Higa, E., Rosai, J., Pizzimbono, C.A., et al.: Mucosal hyperplasia, mucinous cystadenoma and mucinous cystadenocarcinoma of the appendix: a reevaluation of appendiceal mucocele, Cancer 32:1525-1541, 1973.

77. Gibbs, N.M.: Mucinous cystadenoma and cystadenocarcinoma of the vermiform appendix with particular reference to mucocele and pseudomyxoma peritonei, J. Clin. Pathol. 26:413-421, 1973.

78. Fernandez, R.N., and Daly, R.M.: Pseudomyxoma peritonei, Arch. Surg. 115:409-413, 1980.

79. Balthazar, E.J., and Javors, B.R.: Pseudomyxoma peritonei: clinical and radiographic features: the radiology corner, Am. J. Gastroenterol. 68:501-509, 1977.

80. Pugh, D.G.: Roentgenologic aspect of pseudomyxoma peritonei, Radiology 139:320-322, 1942.

81. Seshul, M.B., and Coulam, C.M.: Pseudomyxoma peritonei: computed tomography and sonography, AJR 136: 803-806, 1981.

82. Novetsky, G.J., Berlin, L., Epstein, A.J., et al.: Case report: pseudomyxoma peritonei, J. Comput. Assist. Tomogr. 6: 398-399, 1982.

83. Mayes, G.B., Chuang, V.P., and Fisher, R.G.: Case reports: CT of pseudomyxoma peritonei, AJR **136**:807-808, 1981.

84. Gustafson, K.D., Karnaze, G.C., Hattery, R.R., et al.: Case report: pseudomyxoma peritonei associated with mucinous adenocarcinoma of the pancreas: CT findings and CT-guided biopsy, J. Comput. Assist. Tomogr. **8**:335-338, 1984.

85. Fishman, E.K., Jones, B., Magid, D., et al.: Intraabdominal abscesses in pseudomyxoma peritonei: the value of computed tomography, J. Comput. Assist. Tomogr. **7**:449-453, 1983.

86. Goldberg, M.E., Frick, M., Maile, C., et al.: Case of the day, AJR **144**:1290-1295, 1985.

87. Meyers, M.A., Grahremani, G.G., Clements, J.L., et al.: Pneumatosis intestinalis, Gastrointest. Radiol. **2**:91-105, 1977.

88. Kelvin, F.M., Korobkin, M., Rauch, R.F., et al.: Computed tomography of pneumatosis intestinalis, J. Comput. Assist. Tomogr. **8**:276-280, 1984.

89. Connor, R., Jones, B., Fishman, E.K., et al.: Pneumatosis intestinalis: role of computed tomography in diagnosis and management, J. Comput. Assist. Tomogr. **8**:269-275, 1984.

90. Fisher, J.K.: Clinical image: computed tomography of colonic pneumatosis intestinalis and mesenteric and portal venous air, J. Comput. Assist. Tomogr. **8**:573-574, 1984.

91. Balthazar, E.J.: Sigmoid volvulus. In Marshak, R.L., Lindner, A.E., Maklansky, D., editors: Radiology of the colon, Philadelphia, 1980, W.A. Saunders Co.

92. Figiel, L.S., and Figiel, S.J.: Sigmoid volvulus variations in roentgen pattern, AJR **81**:690-693, 1959.

93. Fisher, J.K.: Computed tomography diagnosis of volvulus in intestinalis malrotation, Radiology **140**:145-146, 1981.

94. Shaff, M.I., Himmelfarb, E., Sacks, G.A., et al.: The whirl sign: a CT finding in volvulus of the large bowel, J. Comput. Assist. Tomogr. **9**:410-412, 1985.

95. Shah, I.C., and Hertz, R.E.: Giant condyloma acuminatum of the anorectum: report of two cases, Dis. Colon Rectum **15**:207-210, 1971.

96. Knoblich, R., and Failing, J.R., Jr.: Giant condyloma acuminatum (Buschke-Löwenstein tumor) of the rectum, Am. J. Clin. Pathol. **48**:389-395, 1967.

97. Friedberg, M.J., and Serlin, O.: Condyloma acuminatum: its association with malignancy, Dis. Colon Rectum **6**:352-355, 1963.

98. Balthazar, E.J., Streiter, M., and Megibow, A.J.: Anorectal giant condyloma acuminatum (Buschke-Löwenstein tumor): CT and radiographic manifestations, Radiology **150**:651-653, 1984.

99. Marshak, R.H., Khilnani, M., Eliasoph, J., et al.: Intestinal edema, AJR **101**:379-387, 1967.

100. Balthazar, E.J., and Gade, M.F.: Gastrointestinal edema in cirrhotics: radiographic manifestations and pathogenesis with emphasis on colonic involvement, Gastrointest. Radiol. **1**:215-223, 1976.

101. Meyers, M.A., and Evans, J.A.: Effects of pancreatitis in the small bowel and colon: spread along mesenteric planes, AJR **119**:151-165, 1973.

102. Balthazar, E.J., and Lutzker, S.: Radiological signs of acute pancreatitis, CRC Crit. Rev. Clin. Radiol. Nucl. Med. **7**:199-242, 1976.

103. Schwartz, S., and Nadelhoft, J.: Simulation of colonic obstruction at the splenic flexure by pancreatitis: roentgen conditions of bowel, AJR Radium Ther. Nucl. Med. **78**:607, 1957.

104. Strax, R., Toombs, B.D., and Rauschkolb, E.N.: Correlation of barium enema and CT in acute pancreatitis, AJR **136**:1219-1220, 1981.

Chapter Seven

PERCUTANEOUS DRAINAGE OF ABDOMINAL ABSCESSES AND FLUID COLLECTIONS

Harvey V. Steinberg
Michael E. Bernardino

Computed tomography has been shown to be the diagnostic modality of choice in detecting abdominal abscesses and fluid collections, as well as in determining their full extent and precise relationships to normal anatomical structures.[1,2] A logical extension of this belief is the use of CT to guide percutaneous abscess and fluid collection drainage (PAFD). The efficacy of percutaneous drainage has been both documented and lauded in the radiologic and surgical literature.[1,3,4,5] Thus CT assisted percutaneous drainage has become a widely accepted therapeutic procedure in the medical community. This chapter discusses the current status of percutaneous drainage of abdominal abscesses and fluid collections with respect to procedural concepts, methodology, and results.

PATIENT SELECTION

CT provides the anatomical detail and information so critical in determining the capability of percutaneous abscess and fluid collections to be drained. Gerzof et al.[1] have proposed criteria to help define those patients who are amenable to percutaneous drainage: (1) a well-defined unilocular cavity; (2) a safe drainage route; (3) concurring evaluation by surgical and radiologic services; and (4) immediate operative capability in case of failure or complication. Using these criteria, Gerzof et al. concluded that approximately 90% of abdominal abscesses and fluid collections can be drained percutaneously.[1]

However, these initial criteria were very rigid. vanWaes et al.[6] have reported a 64% success rate in percutaneously draining 14 cases that did not meet the previously described criteria. Multiloculated abscesses and multiple abscesses have been incriminated by some as a contraindication to percutaneous drainage. In evaluating such cases, one should be aware that a lesion initially thought to represent two distinct cavities may in fact represent a single, unusually shaped cavity that may either suggest or actually demonstrate direct communication on appropriate CT slices. By injecting either air or water-soluble contrast material into the collection, communication may be confirmed.[7] Furthermore, if a multiloculated abscess exists, the appropriate placement of one or more catheters may be all that is needed to achieve successful drainage. Multiple catheters may also be required in draining multiple distinct abscess cavities. In general, we believe that if successful percutaneous drainage appears obtainable with the use of two catheters or less, it should be attempted. We will also consider placement of more than two catheters in a patient with multiple collections or loculations if the patient is a poor operative risk or if such a procedure would be beneficial as a temporary measure.

Interloop abscesses have also been thought by many to represent a contraindication to percutaneous drainage. In those cases where a safe pathway cannot be mapped out, percutaneous drainage should not be attempted. However, a safe approach without traversing bowel can often be planned using CT guidance, since these abscesses tend to displace bowel as they enlarge. If a safe route of entry can be formulated, there is no reason not to attempt percutaneous drainage.

Abscesses that form fistulae to the gastrointestinal and genitourinary tract have a significantly lower rate of successful drainage. Although concomitant decompression of the involved system will increase the success rate in these cases, the clinician and patient should be aware that the likelihood of a cure through percutaneous drainage is not as high as in other cases. Thus the alternatives should be seriously discussed before percutaneous drainage is performed.

Abscesses containing viscous fluid, debris, or necrotic material also have a lesser likelihood of cure by percutaneous drainage. Irrigation by normal saline and/or acetylcysteine (Mucomyst) increases the probability of cure, but once again the overall success rate is somewhat decreased. However, even in those cases where surgery is ultimately required, very often the initial percutaneous drainage is helpful to the surgeon.

Many consider coagulopathies (either primary or secondary) to be a contraindication to percutaneous drainage. However, in a life or death situation, a percutaneous drainage procedure seems a safer alternative than surgery. Of course every effort should be made to correct the coagulopathy before attempting a percutaneous drainage procedure.

One of the only true contraindications to percutaneous drainage of intra-abdominal abscesses or fluid collections is lack of a safe drainage pathway. In these cases, surgical intervention is suggested. With CT guidance and flexibility in patient positioning, this occurrence is indeed rare.

Finally, the importance of making the distinction between an abscess or fluid collection from a phlegmon must be stressed. Phlegmon, most commonly seen in association with the pancreas in pancreatitis, consists predominantly of inflamed granulation tissue. Thus its consistency is such that it is not amenable to drainage by either a percutaneous or surgical approach.

PATIENT PREPARATION

Before a diagnostic aspiration or percutaneous drainage procedure is performed, antibiotics are administered intravenously. It is believed that the antibiotics may help decrease the chance of hematogenous spread of infection and prevent overwhelming sepsis at the time of catheter placement and manipulation. Broad-spectrum antibiotics provide adequate coverage from a multitude of organisms. If a specific organism is suspected clinically, the appropriate antibiotic is added to the regimen. After obtaining culture and sensitivity results from acquired specimens, any necessary modifications of antibiotic treatment can be instituted.

Preparations for percutaneous drainage procedures are very similar to those employed in percutaneous needle biopsies. A radiopaque marker, such as a catheter, is taped onto the patient's skin in a cephalocaudad axis over the abdomen just before scanning. At this point, the patient is instructed to hold his or her breath in the same manner for the diagnostic CT scan and the percutaneous aspiration and/or drainage procedure. Variations in breathing techniques result in a change in the location or relationship of the fluid collection to surrounding organs.

Following a diagnostic CT scan, time and care must be taken in choosing the site of entry for the percutaneous drainage procedure. The shortest straight line distance from the skin to the abscess or fluid collection that does not traverse bowel or other organs is the entry site of choice. Furthermore, an approach allowing for subsequent dependent drainage is desirable. Once the CT slice demonstrating the optimum site of entry is chosen, approach measurements can be made on the CT console using a radiopaque marker, the patient's skin, and the intra-abdominal collection as reference points. Using this method, the entry site of choice has been pinpointed and can now be marked on the patient's skin. In addition, the optimal angulation and depth penetration required to reach the intra-abdominal collection can be determined.

Intravenous sedation and analgesia may be given at this point. Any drug allergies of the patient are elicited before administration. We routinely use an initial dose of 2 to 5 mg diazepam (Valium) as well as an initial dose of 2 to 4 mg morphine, although many other antianxiety and analgesic drugs can be used with similar efficacy. One can appropriately titrate the dosage of these drugs during the procedure as seen fit. Periodic monitoring of vital signs and maintainance of an ongoing rapport with the patient during the procedure are mandatory.

DIAGNOSTIC ASPIRATION

Using sterile technique, the skin is cleansed and sterile drapes are placed. The skin and subcutaneous tissues are locally anesthetized. A small horizontal incision (approximately 4 to 5 mm), slightly more generous than that used for percutaneous biopsies, is used. Blunt dissection using a hemostat is important to help create a tract with the least amount of resistance for the eventual placement of a percutaneous catheter.

Although some authors recommend the use of smaller bore needles, for example, 22-gauge, such needles will only be helpful in obtaining thin, nonviscous material. Furthermore, we believe that in experienced hands the use of an 18-gauge needle in these cases is quite safe. Thus we advocate the use of an 18-gauge Teflon sheath needle for diagnostic aspiration (Figs. 7-1 and 7-2).

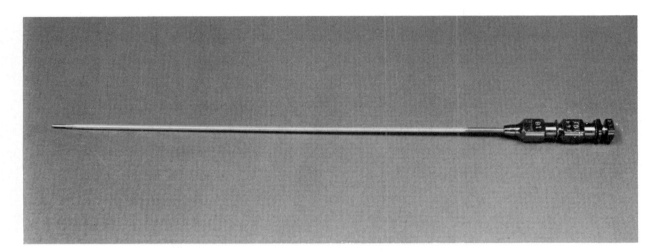

Fig. 7-1. Eighteen-gauge Teflon sheath needle used for the initial aspiration.

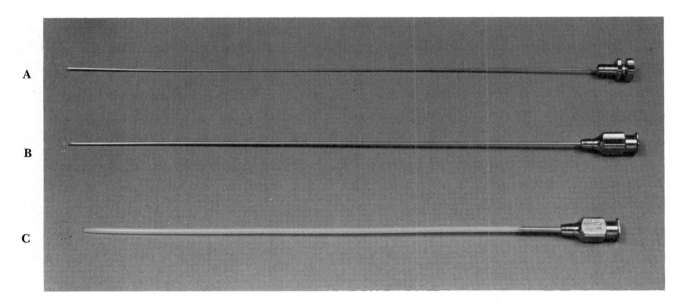

Fig. 7-2. The sheath needle contains an inner cannula **A,** which is removed initially after the sheath **C,** is inserted into the collection. The sheath is then slid over the metal stylet **B.**

The needle is inserted into the intra-abdominal collection at the premeasured depth and angulation. The stylet is removed, and a cap is placed over the external aperture of the sheath. Location of the sheath is verified by CT before aspiration. After confirming satisfactory sheath placement, a small amount of aspirate is obtained and sent for Gram stain and culture. Aspiration of a significant amount of the lesion's contents should be avoided since this may partially collapse the cavity and change the relationship of the collection to neighboring structures, making placement of a drainage catheter much more difficult.[8]

Diagnostic needle aspiration achieves four purposes: (1) it confirms the presence of a collection; (2) it determines whether the collection is infected; (3) it determines if the material is liquified enough to be drained[9]; and (4) it aids the radiologist in choosing the catheter size best suited for drainage by revealing the consistency and viscosity of the collection (Fig. 7-3).

If no fluid is obtained with an 18-gauge sheath needle in an adequate position, biopsy specimens may be obtained and sent for bacteriologic, cytologic, and pathologic examination. In only rare cases where collections are unusually viscous will a small catheter be successful in evacuating a collection that an 18-gauge needle was unable to obtain.[9]

False-negative diagnoses of abscess or fluid collections after needle aspiration can occasionally result from sampling of the supernatant portion of a layered fluid collection. A sample containing only clear supernatant component may yield a falsely negative finding on Gram stain examination, and it is thus important to direct a needle or cannula sheath into the dependent sediment for an accurate diagnosis.[9]

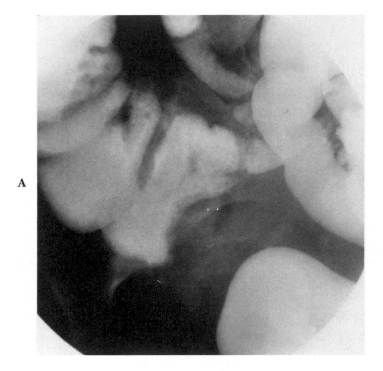

Fig. 7-3. Fifty-eight-year-old female patient with mild, right lower quadrant pain, slight weight loss, and intermittent low-grade fever. A barium enema was performed first, since the provisional diagnosis was appendicitis. **A,** An extrinsic defect on the cecum was appreciated without significant peri-inflammatory change. **B,** A CT scan revealed a low-density collection involving the right lower quadrant and extending into the pelvis. The possibilities included abscess or neoplasm originating in either the abdomen or pelvis.

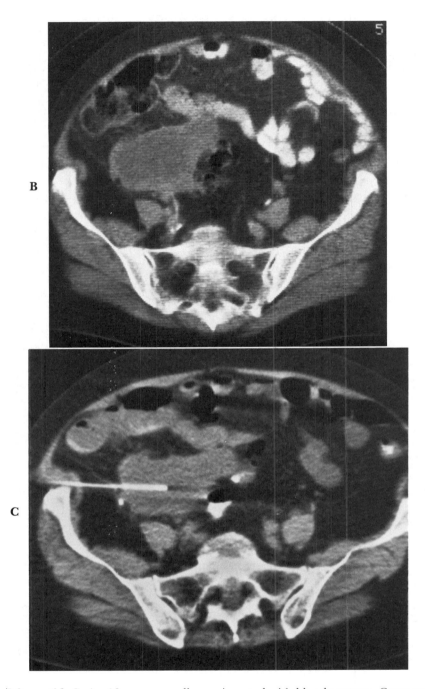

Fig. 7-3, cont'd. C, An 18-gauge needle was inserted with bloody return. Gram stain was negative. The surgical staff decided it was best to operate and at surgery removed a twisted ovarian cyst that had ruptured. This case illustrates the valuable information that can be obtained from an aspiration, even in those cases where a drainage procedure is not performed.

GENERAL DRAINAGE TECHNIQUES

After the initial diagnostic aspiration is complete there are two basic methods used for drainage procedures. These methods are the modified Seldinger technique and the Trocar catheter technique, both of which have been described in the literature.[1,3,8] A discussion of these methods follows.

Modified Seldinger technique

After diagnostic aspiration, a 0.038 inch J-tip guidewire is passed through the sheath. An effort is made to direct the guidewire such that the drainage catheter will eventually lie in as dependent a position as possible. The sheath is removed and dilation of the tract is achieved with appropriate angiodilators while the position of the guidewire is carefully maintained. Finally, the appropriate catheter is threaded over the guidewire and inserted to the appropriate depth. The guidewire is removed and the position of the catheter confirmed using CT or fluoroscopy.

Trocar catheter technique

The Trocar catheter technique is used in cases where the abscess or fluid collection is more easily accessible and in cases where the collection is somewhat larger or more superficial. After the initial aspiration with an 18-gauge Teflon sheath is performed, the sheath is removed. A Trocar catheter, containing within it a pointed stylet that fits through a metal stiffening cannula, is passed into the collection following the same pathway into the same depth as used in the diagnostic aspiration. When the desired depth is reached, the stylet is removed and the catheter is advanced over the stylet. At this point the stylet is removed and the external aperture of the catheter is capped. The position of the catheter is then documented using CT.

Final catheter placement

Once a catheter is placed into the collection, the remainder of the procedure is similar whether one has used the modified Seldinger technique or the Trocar method. Further manipulation under CT or fluoroscopic guidance may occasionally be needed to achieve optimal catheter placement. It is important that all sideholes of the drain are seen within the collection when the catheter is in its final position. A three-way stopcock is attached externally to the catheter. This in turn is attached to a drainage bag. By using this method, a closed system can be maintained whereby the collection can be drained directly into the drainage bag so that the precise quantity and quality of the collection aspirated can be readily observed. As much of the collection as possible is aspirated through the syringe and injected directly into the drainage bag by manipulating the three-way stopcock. Thereafter, the system is left to drain by gravity.

The skin and entry site are cleansed and an antibiotic ointment applied locally. After the skin is treated with any of a number of commercial preparations used to minimize skin irritation a dressing is carefully applied. An appropriately sized Molnar disk is used to secure the catheter to the patient's skin. Further security can be ensured by suturing the disk to the patient's skin. All external connections of the system are fastened and taped. In addition, the tape can serve as a mesentery, anchoring the catheter to the patient's body wall.

Immediate gentle irrigation of the cavity with normal saline is performed after catheter placement and after evacuation of all freely drainable material. This irrigation must be under low pressure or septicemia may be induced. Effective irrigation may require copious amounts of saline, sometimes totaling several hundred ml. An endpoint is reached when the irrigant returns are clear. Irrigation immediately after catheter placement helps serve three purposes: (1) it helps debride the cavity; (2) it helps prevent subsequent occlusion of the catheter by particulate debris and/or necrotic tissue; and (3) it can help break up loculations and septations that would otherwise result in either incomplete drainage or necessitate the use of multiple catheters to achieve a cure.[9]

Dilute, water-soluble contrast material, gently injected under fluoroscopic control into the cavity by way of the drainage tube, can (1) document catheter position, (2) determine whether the abscess cavity or fluid collection was inadequately drained, (3) ascertain whether multiple loculations communicate, (4) outline the presence of any fistulous tract, and (5) serve as a baseline in monitoring the progressive collapse and dissolution of the cavity.

After the drainage procedure the patient is returned to the room on a stretcher. The immediate post-drainage orders should include frequent monitoring of the patient's vital signs over the ensuing 4 to 6 hours. Strict bedrest over the following 4 to 6 hours is also recommended. Nurses are advised to measure and chart drainage quantities per shift. Intravenous antibiotic therapy is continued.

CATHETER SYSTEMS

In choosing the appropriate catheter to drain an abscess or fluid collection, the smallest bore catheter that can ensure adequate drainage is chosen. Factors that influence catheter selection include the size of the collection and, more importantly, the viscosity of the fluid. This may be determined at the initial diagnostic aspiration. There are three basic types of catheters currently used in percutaneous drainages. They are pigtail angiographic catheters, Trocar catheters, and sump catheters.

Pigtail angiographic catheters (Fig. 7-4, *A*)

Placement of a pigtail catheter into a fluid collection requires the use of the modified Seldinger technique outlined earlier. The curled pigtail shape of the distal end of the catheter helps prevent perforation through the wall of the cavity while simultaneously protecting against dislodgement. This catheter, however, is limited in its use by its relatively small sideholes. Thus pigtail catheters should not be used to drain larger more tenacious collections. The use of pigtail catheters is best reserved for draining smaller, less viscous abscesses and fluid collections.

Trocar catheters (Fig. 7-4, *B*)

The placement of Trocar catheter systems into intra-abdominal collections can be accomplished by using either the Trocar method or the modified Seldinger technique. The latter technique requires the removal of the inner Trocar portion; removal of the metal stylet is optional when feeding the catheter over the guidewire. The major advantage Trocar catheters have over pigtail angiocatheters is the larger caliber of their sideholes. Trocar catheters are available in a variety of sizes ranging from 8 French to 16 French. The somewhat limited flexibility and slight configuration of Trocar systems represent their only drawbacks.

Sump catheters (Fig. 7-4, *C* and 7-5)

Large bore (12 French to 14 French), double lumen, sump catheters can be inserted either with the Trocar or modified Seldinger technique. The catheter has a large caliber lumen accompanied by multiple large sizes that help ensure good drainage even in the presence of viscous material or particulate matter. The sump system (second lumen) allows for the ingress of room air at ambient pressure, which, in theory, helps prevent the occlusion of the sideholes and secondary collapse of the cavity wall around the catheter. These catheters are available with distal curve, which, as mentioned earlier, aids in both the safety and security of the system. Considering the aforementioned advantages of sump catheters, it should come as no surprise that this system is the one preferred by most radiologists when draining larger, more viscous, intra-abdominal abscesses or fluid collections.

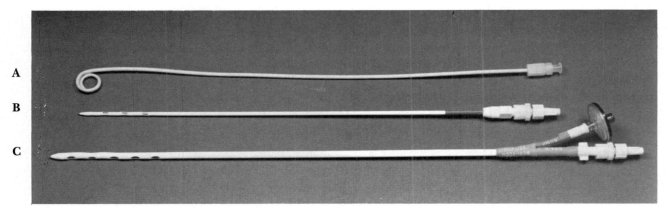

Fig. 7-4. A, An 8.3 French pigtail catheter. **B,** An 8.3 French Trocar catheter. **C,** A 14 French vanSonnenberg (sump) catheter.

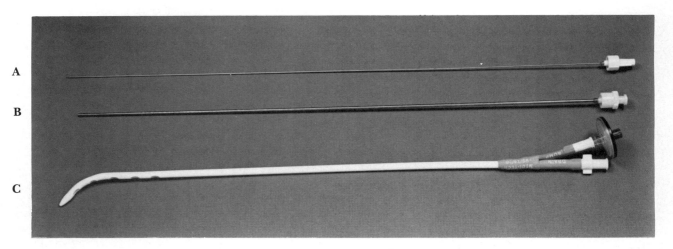

Fig. 7-5. A disassembled 14 French vanSonnenberg catheter. **A,** Metal stylet, **B,** intertrocar portion, and **C,** 14 French catheter with distal curve.

CATHETER MANAGEMENT
Catheter maintenance

It is important for the radiologist to realize that his or her role is not completed when the patient leaves the department with a percutaneous drainage tube in place. The radiologist should visit the patient a minimum of once a day. This gives the radiologist a chance to follow the patient's progress and allows facilitation of appropriate measures that may help ensure and/or expedite successful drainage procedure.

Although strict bedrest is recommended for the patient for the first several hours following the drainage procedure, mobilization of the patient thereafter is encouraged. Body movement and respiratory motion help promote continuous catheter drainage.

Delayed irrigation of the catheter with approximately 10 to 20 ml of normal saline is a simple bedside procedure that may be helpful in draining those more tenacious, debris-laden collections. The frequency with which these irrigations should be performed is dictated by the nature and consistency of the free flowing drainage material as well as that of the irrigant returns. Multiple daily irrigations may be required to afford optimal drainage and catheter patency.

The use of the mucolytic and proteolytic agent acetylcysteine as an adjunct in draining more viscous collections is somewhat controversial. Its chemical structure is such that it has been shown to promote the reduction of larger, more viscous molecules to smaller, less viscous ones under certain precisely defined conditions (pH and incubation time being the most important variables).[10] vanWaes[6] et al. have reported cases in which acetylcysteine has liquified abscesses whose contents were previously too viscous to drain. Sheffner's data[10] however, reveal that acetylcysteine's value is limited by the chemical composition of its target. When acetylcysteine was tested on solutions containing material similar to that found in prurient collections, it was found that the decrease in viscosity was no greater than that seen with similar tests using only normal saline.[10,11] We believe that the efficacy of acetylcysteine must be further studied and that its role at the present time is unclear.

Catheter removal

Several endpoints must be reached before the drainage catheter is removed. General improvement in the patient's clinical status should be established. The patient should be afebrile for a minimum of 48 hours. In addition, marked diminution in catheter output should be observed. If minimal drainage still exists, its consistency should be of a serosanguinous nature. A final CT scan to document resolution of the cavity as well as to rule out the presence of other disease in the abdomen should be performed. We also recommend a final sinogram before catheter removal to further document collapse of the cavity and, more importantly, to rule out any fistulous communications or sinus tracts that might not be appreciated on CT. If all of these parameters are satisfied, the catheter is removed.

SPECIAL CONSIDERATIONS

Although the basic precepts for percutaneous drainage procedures apply to any intra-abdominal abscesses or fluid collection, specific considerations must be made with respect to the exact anatomic location of the lesion. A discussion of several distinct anatomic areas that warrant specific attention as a result of their unique location follows.

Subphrenic collections (Figs. 7-6 and 7-7)

The subphrenic space represents a technically demanding area from which to obtain safe percutaneous access because of its relationship to the diaphragm. The contour of the diaphragm is such that the posterior attachments of the diaphragm are more caudal than the anterior attachments. By keeping this fact in mind and by implementing a caudiocranial angulation technique (triangulation)[12] in placing these catheters percutaneously, inadvertent puncture of the pleural space with subsequent development of a pneumothorax or empyema is minimized. The modified Seldinger technique is recommended to further minimize complications. In our experience, the anterior or middle axillary lines usually serve as the best entry points when dealing with right subphrenic collections, and the middle or posterior axillary lines serve as better landmarks for the left subphrenic collections since they tend to be situated somewhat more posteriorly. Appropriate positioning of the patient in either the oblique or decubitus position can also be helpful in determining the safest and most easily accessible route.

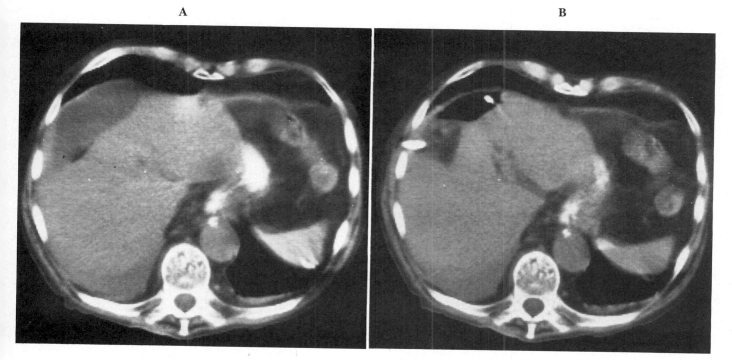

A   **B**

Fig. 7-6. Patient following cholecystectomy developed a right subphrenic abscess that was drained surgically. Several weeks later the patient complained of fever and mild, right upper quadrant pain. **A,** A diagnostic CT scan revealed a subphrenic fluid collection. Aspiration revealed turbid, bilious fluid. Gram stain was positive for *Escherichia coli* disease. An 8.3 French Trocar catheter was inserted using the triangulation method. **B,** This collection was fully drained with subsequent CT images revealing only a small amount of air that had been introduced into the space by way of the catheter.

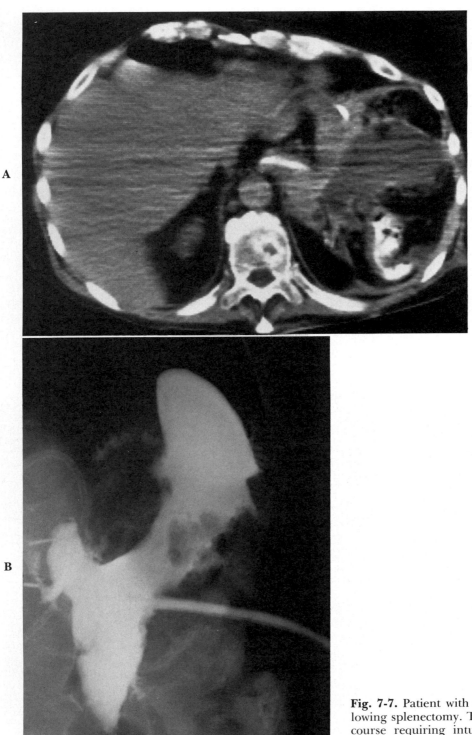

Fig. 7-7. Patient with chronic lymphocytic leukemia following splenectomy. The patient experienced a downhill course requiring intubation. **A,** Because of persistent fever, a CT scan was performed revealing a left subphrenic collection. Artifact is noted secondary to respiratory motion. A 14 French vanSonnenberg catheter was inserted after several milliliters of viscous material was aspirated with an 18-gauge sheath needle. **B,** A subsequent "abscessogram" helped outline the cavity.

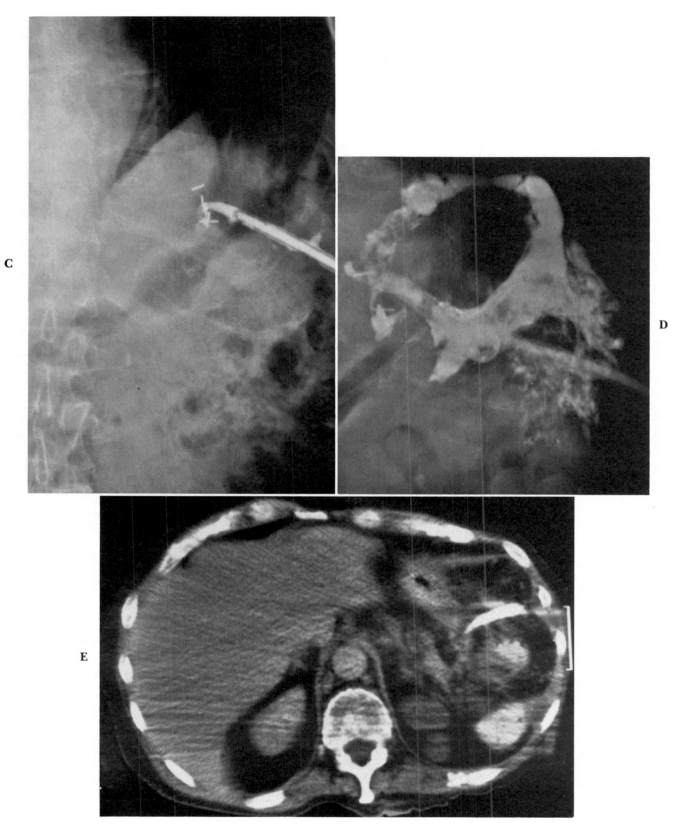

Fig. 7-7, cont'd. C, Although it took several months to fully collapse, follow-up "abscessograms" documented the gradual diminution of the cavity, until it resolved, **D. E,** Repeat CT scan confirmed the abscess resolution.

Lesser sac collections (Fig. 7-8)

In draining collections of the lesser sac, a left lateral approach traversing the gastrolienal ligament is usually used. By placing the patient in a right posterior oblique or right lateral decubitus position the stomach will move anteriorly, frequently resulting in easier access to the collection. Care should be taken to avoid penetrating the spleen, stomach, splenic flexure, and the abundant blood vessels in this region. For this reason, the modified Seldinger technique is once again recommended to minimize complications unless the collection extends adjacent to the abdominal wall.

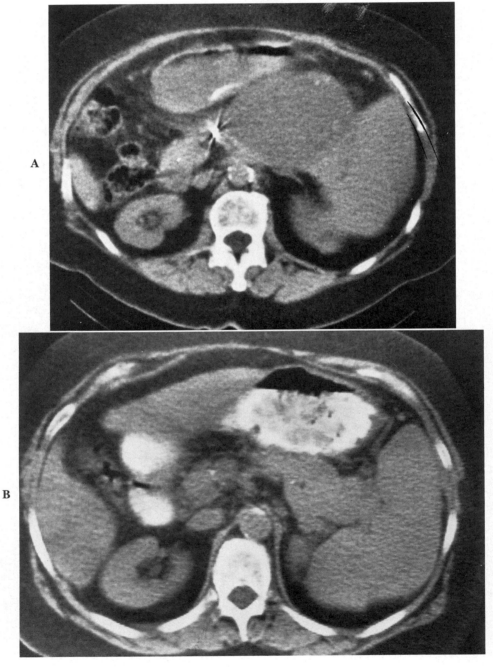

Fig. 7-8. Postoperatively this patient developed fever and leukocytosis. **A,** A CT scan revealed a lesser sac collection that proved to be an abscess. **B,** This collection was percutaneously drained with a follow-up scan revealing no evidence of disease.

Subhepatic collections (Fig. 7-9)

These collections are usually best approached posterolaterally using a caudocranial angulation technique identical to that used in draining subphrenic collections.

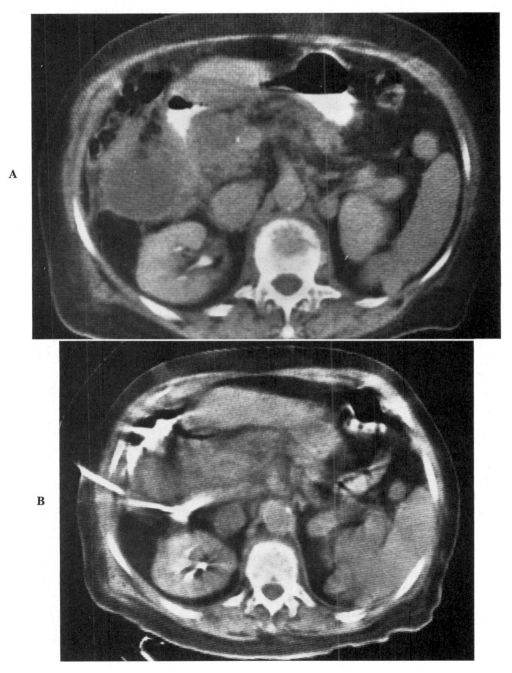

Fig. 7-9. Immunosuppressed patient with persistent, right-sided abdominal pain. **A,** CT scan revealed a collection in the subhepatic space. **B,** This abscess was successfully drained percutaneously.

Paracolic, pericolic, and pelvic collections
(Figs. 7-10 to 7-13)

The full extent and involvement of any of the potential peritoneal spaces must be determined so that the most efficacious drainage route can be chosen. Care should be exercised to avoid bowel, blood vessels, and nerve bundles so plentiful in these anatomic locations. The CT scan may give back valuable, previously unknown information as to the cause of the abscess or fluid collection (i.e., appendicitis or diverticulitis). Tubo-ovarian abscesses are best treated medically with antibiotics alone and followed by serial ultrasound examinations.

Text continued p. 408.

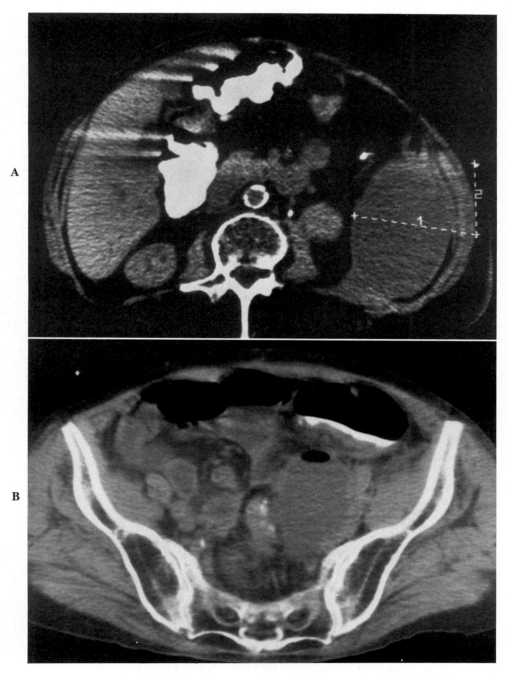

Fig. 7-10. Patient with a history of ovarian carcinoma following chemotherapy and radiation therapy. The patient complained of fever, leukocytosis, and left flank pain. CT revealed two separate collections—one in the left flank **A,** and one in the left pelvis that contained air, **B.**

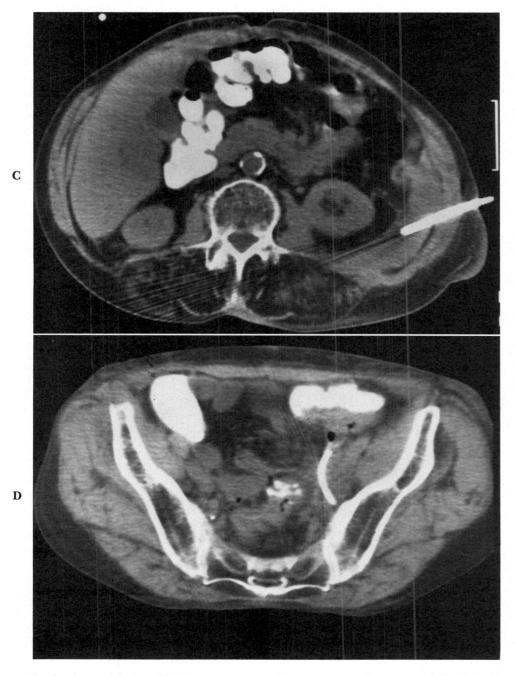

Fig. 7-10, cont'd. C and **D,** Two separate catheters were used to successfully drain the abscesses, and only minimal inflammatory thickening of the left posterior perirenal space was noted after the drainage procedures.

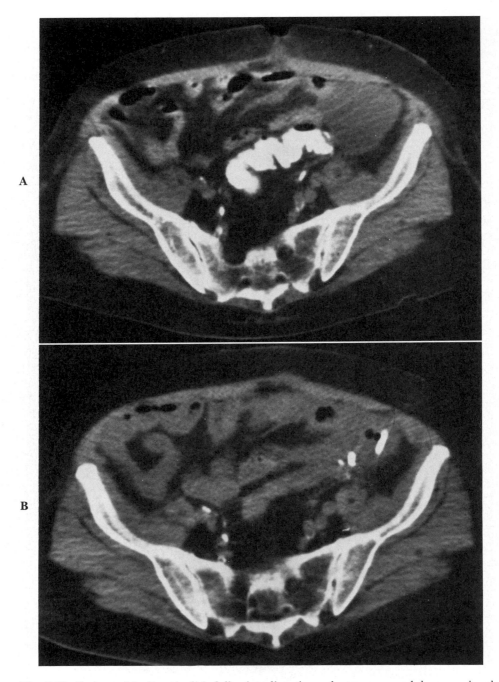

Fig. 7-11. Patient with diverticulitis following diverting colostomy several days previously. The patient was still experiencing nocturnal temperature spikes. **A,** A CT scan revealed a fluid collection juxtaposed to the bowel in the left lower quadrant. **B,** Infected material was aspirated and subsequently drained. **C,** A baseline sinogram was performed. **D,** After drainage had ceased, a repeat sinogram verified complete resolution of the cavity, and the catheter was removed. **E,** A follow-up CT scan showed no evidence of recurrence.

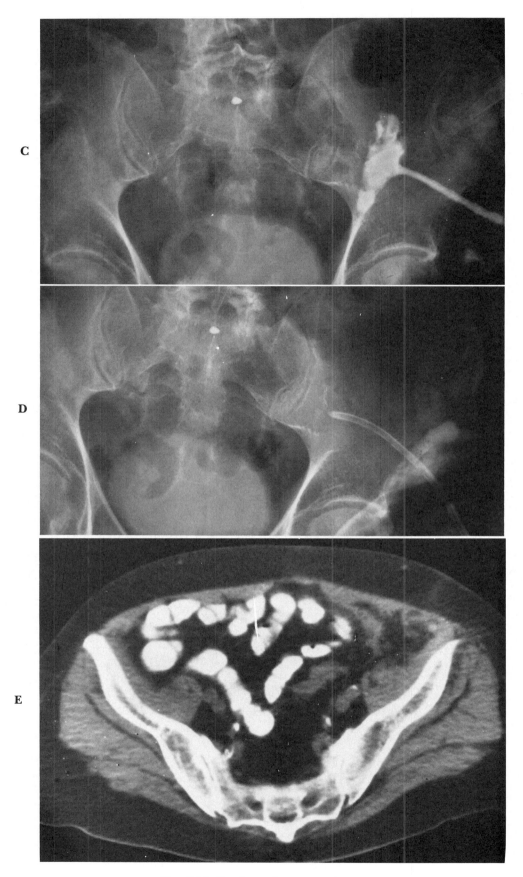

Fig. 7-11. For legend see opposite page.

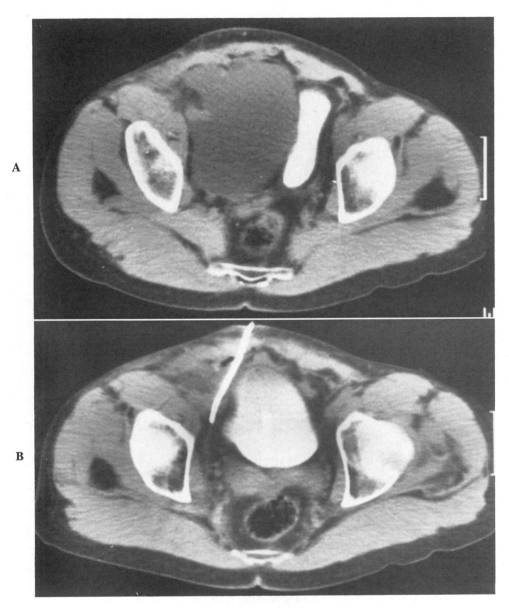

Fig. 7-12. Patient 2 weeks following renal transplant. Ultrasound revealed a large fluid collection situated between the transplant kidney and the bladder. **A,** CT revealed a fluid collection compressing the contrast-filled bladder to the left. Aspiration and laboratory results confirmed this to be a urinoma. **B,** A drainage catheter placed percutaneously using CT guidance resulted in complete resolution of this collection.

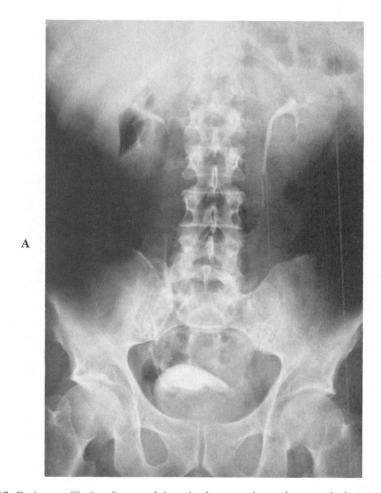

A

Fig. 7-13. Patient suffering from pelvic pain, hematuria, and a drop in hematocrit following pelvic trauma several days previously. No fractures were seen on plain films of the pelvis. An intravenous urogram (IVP) revealed the upper urinary tract to be within normal limits. However, the bladder was elevated and its contour was noted as irregular, **A.** *Continued.*

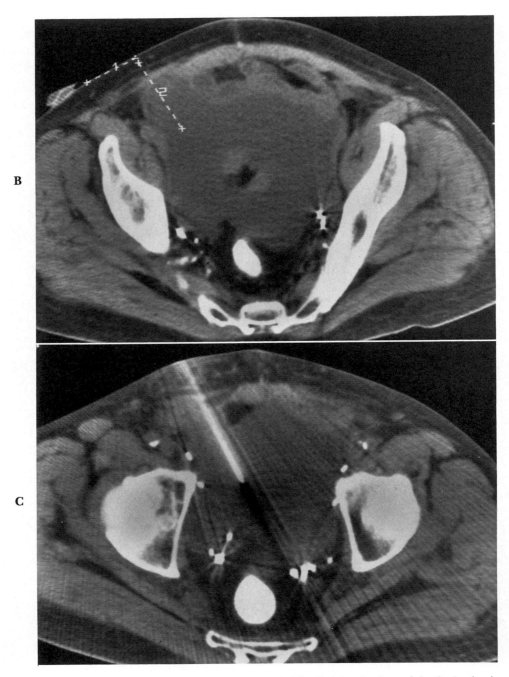

Fig. 7-13, cont'd. B, CT scan revealed a large fluid collection in the pelvis. **C,** Aspiration with an 18-gauge sheath needle resulted in bloody return.

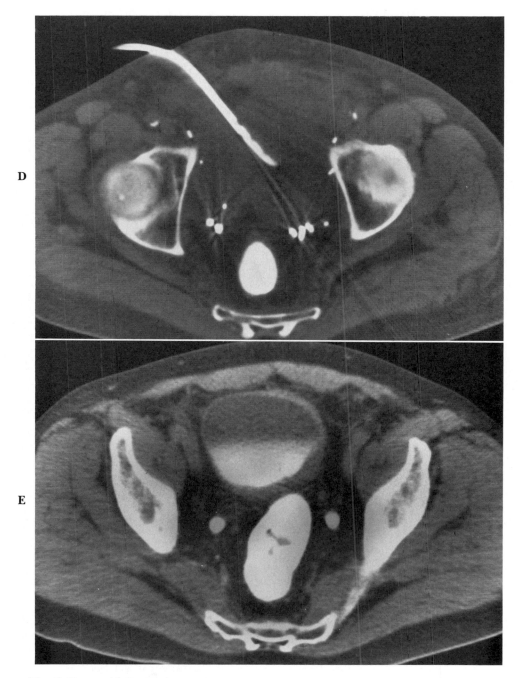

Fig. 7-13, cont'd. D, A 14 French vanSonnenberg catheter with a distal curve was percutaneously placed into this hematoma. Complete resolution of the hematoma was accomplished in less than 48 hours. **E,** A follow-up CT scan was normal.

Retroperitoneal collections (Figs. 7-14 to 7-16)

Retroperitoneal collections are best drained using an extraperitoneal approach. Once again, delineation of the full extent of these collections is paramount for optimal drainage. For example, the pararenal spaces extend from the level of the diaphragm into the pelvis. Thus collections of sig-

nificant length may require two (or more) strategically placed catheters. This double catheter technique facilitates passive drainage, helps prevent loculations, and permits irrigation through one catheter with simultaneous aspiration through the second catheter.[13]   *Text continued p. 414.*

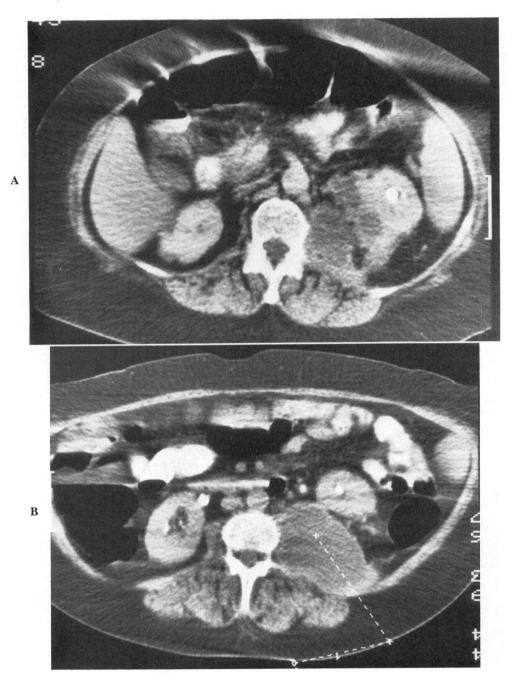

Fig. 7-14. Patient with fever, left costovertebral tenderness, and a urine culture positive for gram-negative rods. **A,** CT revealed a left perinephric abscess extending into the left psoas muscle. After placing a radiopaque marker on the patient's back, an optimal site was chosen for drainage. **B,** The distance from the marker, as well as the depth and angulation required to reach the abscess, was calculated on the CT console.

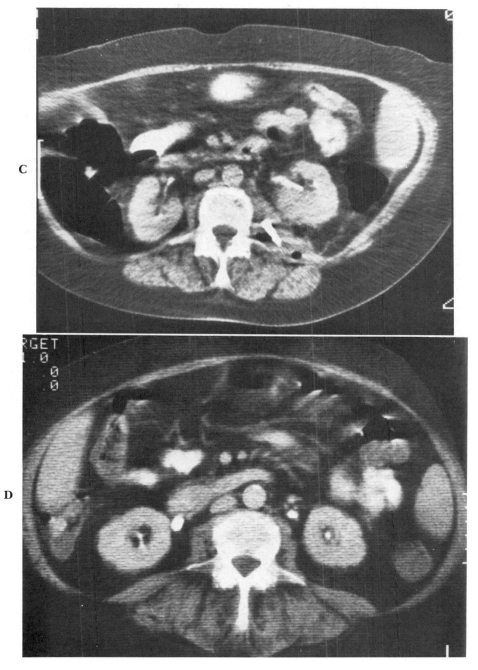

Fig. 7-14, cont'd. A small amount of thick purulent material was aspirated through an 18-gauge sheath needle and removed. **C,** A 14 French vanSonnenberg catheter was inserted into the collection, and complete drainage and collapse of the cavity was accomplished. The patient was afebrile without tenderness or pain within 4 hours. The catheter was removed after 48 hours since there was no drainage and no evidence of any residual collection seen on follow-up CT scans. **D,** A CT scan performed several months later showed no evidence of residual or recurrent disease.

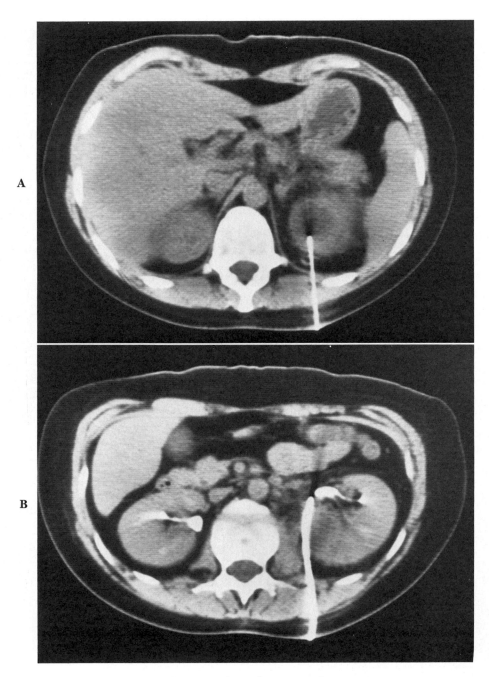

Fig. 7-15. For legend see opposite page.

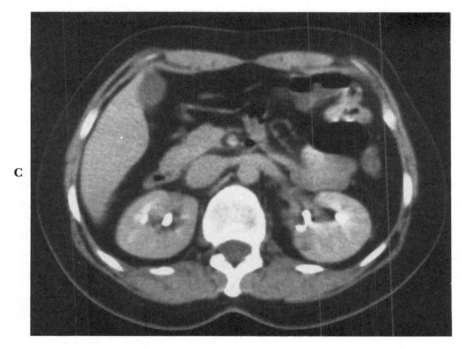

Fig. 7-15. Patient with left flank pain and fever. **A,** A CT scan revealed a low-density collection involving the upper pole of the left kidney. Aspiration revealed purulent material. **B,** A 14 French drainage catheter was placed into the collection and the abscess successfully drained. The patient defervesced within 24 hours. **C,** A repeat CT scan several weeks later revealed no evidence of abscess.

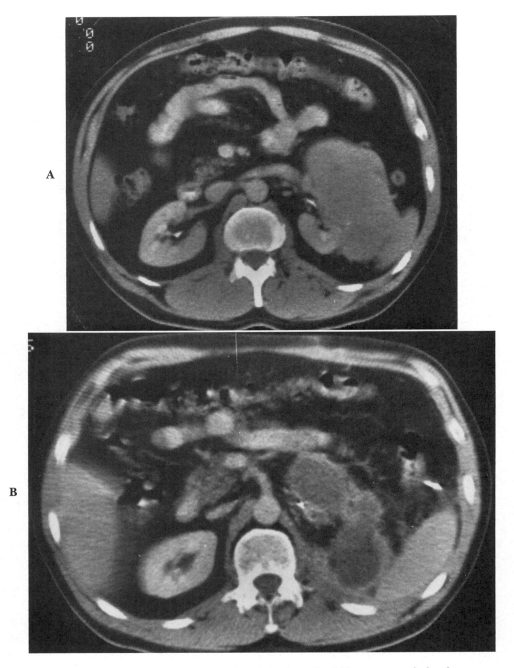

Fig. 7-16. Patient with hematuria and weight loss. **A,** CT scan revealed a large mass involving the left kidney. A left nephrectomy was performed, and pathology confirmed the presence of a hypernephroma. Several weeks following surgery the patient began spiking intermittent fevers. **B,** A CT scan revealed a collection occupying the left renal fossa.

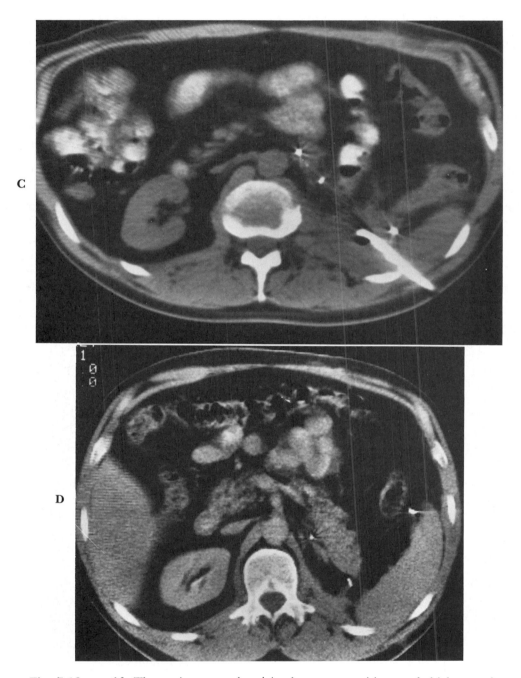

Fig. 7-16, cont'd. The patient was placed in the prone position, and thick, tenacious purulent material was aspirated. A 14 French drainage catheter was placed into the collection. **C,** A CT scan taken after drainage had diminished revealed a remaining pocket of material that was easily drained by withdrawing the catheter several centimeters. **D,** Follow-up CT scan revealed only post-drainage inflammatory changes.

Pancreatic collections

Pseudocysts (Figs. 7-17 to 7-19). There is some degree of controversy with respect to the best time to drain pseudocysts. We advocate observation of pseudocysts for 6 weeks, allowing for either spontaneous resolution or maturation of the cyst wall. Although most pseudocysts are confined to the pancreatic bed, extension into the lesser sac and pararenal spaces is not uncommon. Extension of pancreatic pseudocysts into the perirenal space, mesentery, kidney, spleen, liver, colon, pelvis, and mediastinum are more rarely observed occurrences.

Percutaneous external drainage of pancreatic pseudocysts has been reported with variable success in the literature. While some groups[1,14] have reported a 100% success rate without any recurrence, others have noted recurrence rates of 30% to 80%.[15,16] Failure in most cases appears secondary to either persistent communication of the pseudocyst with the pancreatic duct or fistulae. Thus many believe that surgical gastrocystostomy is the preferred method for pancreatic pseudocyst drainage.[17] Recently, two new promising approaches for percutaneous drainage of pancreatic pseudocysts have been suggested in an effort to more definitively treat them without surgery. They both use a transgastric approach that results in the formation of a gastrocystostomy without the risks of surgery. The method described by Ho and Taylor[18] results in external drainage while the method proposed by Bernardino and Amerson[19] accomplishes internal drainage of the pseudocyst.

Text continued p. 420.

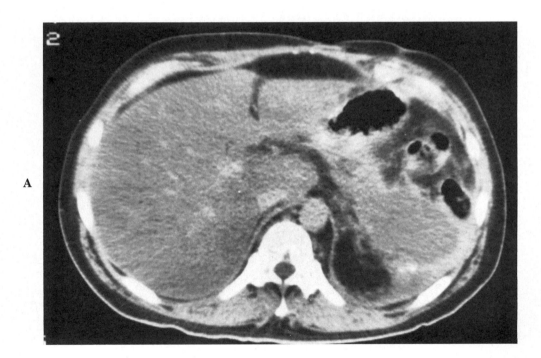

Fig. 7-17. Patient with a history of pancreatic pseudocysts. **A,** A CT scan revealed a fluid collection with a ring around it, arising from the pancreatic tail and extending into the left renal space.

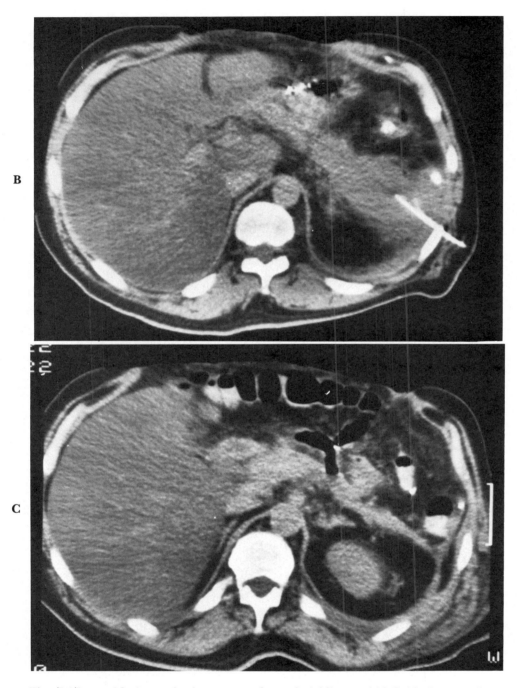

Fig. 7-17, cont'd. An aspiration was performed yielding turbid fluid. Gram stain was positive for gram-positive and gram-negative organisms. **B,** An 8.3 French Trocar catheter was placed into the collection with successful evacuation of its infected pseudocyst. **C,** A CT scan following drainage revealed only minimal inflammatory thickening of the left pararenal fascia.

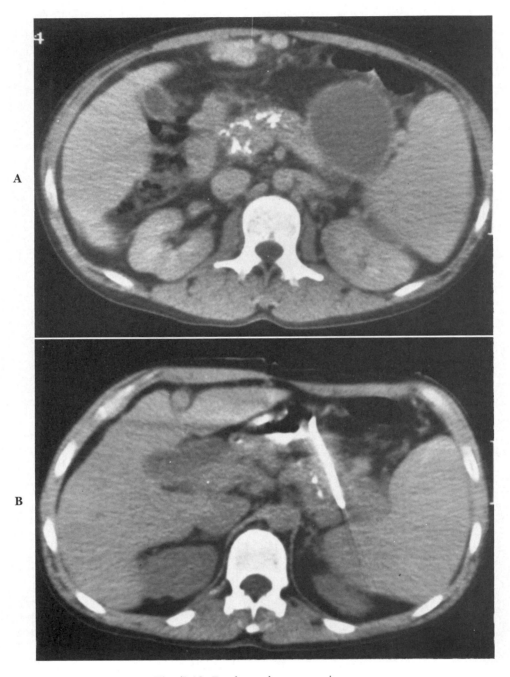

Fig. 7-18. For legend see opposite page.

C

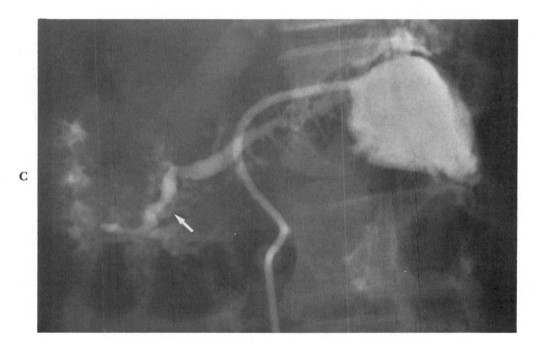

Fig. 7-18. Patient with a mature pseudocyst, **A,** and a history of chronic pancreatitis. A drainage catheter was inserted, resulting in almost complete collapse of the cavity, **B.** However, persistent drainage ensued. A sinogram revealed communication of the pseudocyst with the pancreatic duct. In addition, a persistent filling defect was noted within the pancreatic duct (**C,** *arrow*). The patient eventually underwent a pancreatectomy at which time a stone was found lodged within the pancreatic duct.

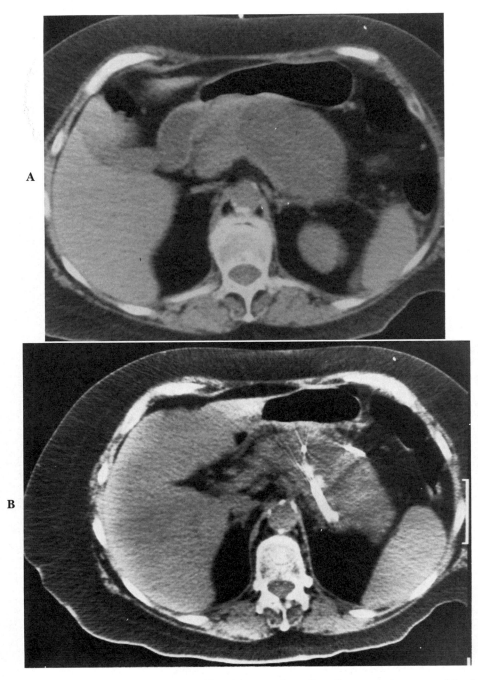

Fig. 7-19. Obese, elderly patient with a history of cardiac disease and pancreatitis. **A,** A CT scan 3 months following the patient's last bout of pancreatitis revealed two mature pseudocysts directly posterior to the stomach. The patient began developing increasing abdominal pain and nausea. Because of the patient's risk factors, surgical gastrocystostomy was deferred. Instead, a gastrocystostomy was performed percutaneously. **B,** Under CT guidance, a 10 French double Malecot catheter was placed through both the anterior and posterior gastric walls into the larger pancreatic pseudocyst, using the modified Seldinger technique.

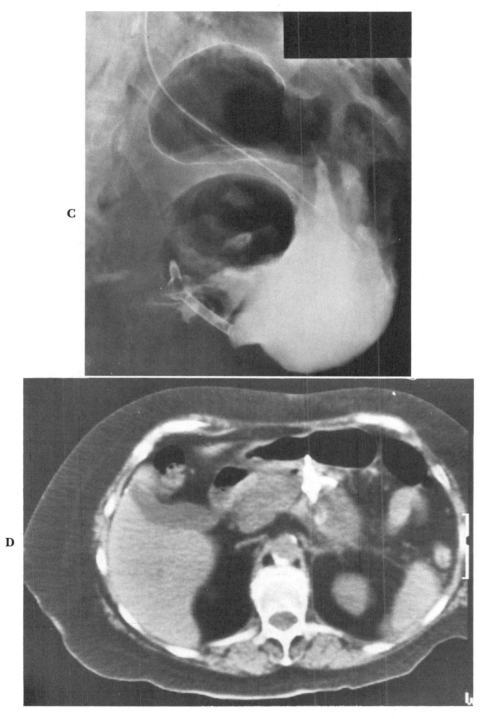

Fig. 7-19, cont'd. Proper positioning was achieved with silk suture tied around the gastric stent so that it could be retrieved and manipulated. The patient's symptoms subsided almost immediately after the procedure. The patient received nothing by mouth and had nasogastric suction for 48 hours in an effort to allow the anterior gastric wall time to heal. **C,** A gastrointestinal series (Gastrografin) at 48 hours demonstrated no leakage of contrast material with significant evacuation of the pseudocyst. At 72 hours the patient was fed. She was discharged within 1 week of the procedure. **D,** A CT scan at 8 weeks revealed total resolution of the pseudocyst. The stent was removed endoscopically.

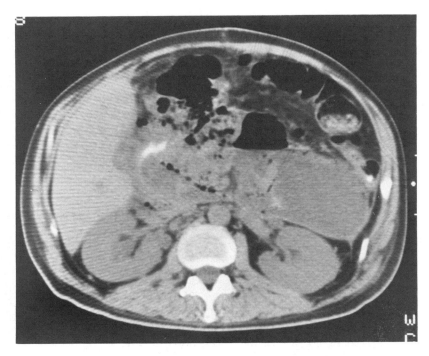

Fig. 7-20. Patient with pancreatic abscess. Although there was a fluid-like collection only in the area of the pancreatic tail, the entire pancreas was involved. Mottled, inhomogeneous densities, as well as air bubbles, were noted within the pancreatic head and body. Percutaneous drainage of this abscess was only partially successful. Intraoperatively the pancreatic head and body revealed only necrotic tissue with no normal pancreatic tissue or drainable fluid collections found. A total pancreatectomy was performed.

Abscesses (Fig. 7-20). The reported experience with percutaneous catheter drainages of pancreatic abscesses is somewhat limited.[5,14] The reported success in the literature as well as our own experience is somewhat lower than that reported for other intra-abdominal abscesses. This is probably secondary to the fact that pancreatic abscesses tend to diffusely infiltrate the gland, not loculating into a well-defined cavity. In addition, they often contain tissue debris and are thus more difficult to completely drain. Multiple catheter systems and irrigation can sometimes overcome these difficulties.

RESULTS OF PERCUTANEOUS ABSCESS AND FLUID DRAINAGE

Several large series have been published with respect to the efficacy of percutaneous abscess and fluid drainage, demonstrating a success rate between 84% and 89%.[1,3,9,20] Failures have been reported most commonly in lesions that are: (1) phlegmonous in nature; (2) multiple or multiloculated; (3) associated with fistulous communication; and (4) highly viscous. Recurrence rates of up to 8% have been reported.[1,3,9,20] Recurrences are most frequently associated with persistent fistulous communications or leaks secondary to the postsurgical breakdown of anastomotic sites. Premature removal of a drainage catheter and underlying tumors resulting in superimposed infection are less common causes of recurrence.

Complication rates varying from 4% to 15% have been reported.[1,3,9,20] Complications include transient septicemia, catheter backbleed, peritoneal spillage, fistulous or sinus communications, pneumothorax, and empyema. Laceration of mesenteric vessels and death, although extremely rare, have been reported.

CONCLUSIONS

The data available show that percutaneous drainage of abdominal abscesses and fluid collections compares favorably with surgical intervention. Table 7-1 demonstrates lower rates of morbidity, mortality, failures, recurrences, complications, and shorter drainage times for percutaneous drainage versus surgery. Furthermore, percutaneous drainage: (1) avoids the inherent risks of surgery and anesthesia; (2) minimizes the occurrence of postoperative complications such as atelectasis, pneumonia, and pulmonary embolism; (3) saves considerable time and expense; (4) makes for easier nursing care; and (5) is met with greater patient acceptance.

Surgical intervention is clearly indicated for those collections without a safe drainage route or in those cases where percutaneous drainage has failed. However, percutaneous drainage is the treatment of choice for the majority of intra-abdominal abscesses and fluid collections.

Table 7-1. Abscess drainage: percutaneous versus surgical*

	Percutaneous drainage	Surgical drainage
Success rate	84% to 89%	57% to 70%
Complication rate	4% to 15%	11% to 49%
Recurrence rate	Up to 8%	14% to 49%
Mortality rate	Up to 11%	11% to 43%
Mean duration of catheter	2 to 3 weeks	3 to 5 weeks

*References 1, 3, 9, 14, 20, 21, and 22.

REFERENCES

1. Gerzof, G., Robbins, A.H., Johnson, W.C., et al.: Percutaneous catheter drainage of abdominal abscesses: a five-year experience, N. Engl. J. Med. **305:**653-657, 1981.
2. Haaga, J.R., Alfidi, R.J., Havrilla, T.R., et al.: CT detection and aspiration of abdominal abscesses, AJR **128:**465-474, 1977.
3. Haaga, J.R., and Weinstein, A.J.: CT guided percutaneous aspiration and drainage of abscesses, AJR **135:**1187-1194, 1980.
4. Welch, C.E., and Mult, R.A.: Abdominal surgery, N. Engl. J. Med. **308:**753-760, 1983.
5. Gerzof, G., Robbins, A.H., Burkett, D.H., et al.: Percutaneous catheter drainage of abdominal abscesses guided by ultrasound and computed tomography, AJR **133:**1-18, 1979.
6. vanWaes, P.F., Felberg, M.A., Mali W.P., et al.: Management of loculated abscesses that are difficult to drain: a new approach, Radiology **147:**157-163, 1983.
7. Bernardino, M.E., Berkman, W.A., Plemmons, M., et al.: Percutaneous drainage of multiseptated hepatic abscesses, J. Comput. Assist. Tomogr. **8:**38-41, 1984.
8. Gerzof, S.G., Spira, A.R., and Robbins, A.H.: Percutaneous abscess drainage, Semin. Roentgenol. **16:**62-71, 1981.
9. Mueller, P.R., vanSonnenberg, E., and Ferrucci, J.T.: Percutaneous drainage of 250 abdominal abscesses and fluid collections. Part II: procedural concepts, Radiology **151:**344-347.
10. Sheffner, A.L.: The reduction in vitro in viscosity of mucoprotein solutions by a new mucolytic agent, N-acetylcysteine, Ann. N.Y. Acad. Sci. **1:**298-310, 1963.
11. Dawson, S.L., Mueller, P.R., and Ferrucci, J.T.: Mucomyst for abscesses: a clinical comment, Radiology **151:**342, 1982.
12. Gerzof, S.G.: Triangulation: indirect CT guidance for abscess drainage, AJR **137:**1088, 1981.
13. Sones, P.J.: Percutaneous drainage of abdominal abscesses, AJR **142:**35-39. 1984.
14. Karlson, K.B., Martin, E.C., Frankuchen, E.I., et al.: Percutaneous drainage of pancreatic pseudocysts and abscesses, Radiology **142:**619-624, 1982.
15. Crass, R.A., and Way, L.W.: Acute and chronic pancreatic pseudocysts are different, Am. J. Surg. **142:**660-663, 1981.
16. Lieberman, R.P., Crummy, A.B., and Matallana, R.H.: Invasive procedures in pancreatic disease, Semin. Ultrasound **1:**192-208, 1980.
17. Bradley, E.L., and Austin, H.: Multiple pancreatic pseudocysts: the principle of internal cystocystostomy in surgical management, Surgery **92:**111-116, 1982.
18. Ho, C.S., and Taylor, B.: Percutaneous transgastric drainage of percutaneous pseudocysts, AJR **143:**623-625, 1984.
19. Bernardino, M.E., and Amerson, J.R.: Percutaneous gastrocystostomy: a new approach to pancreatic pseudocyst drainage, AJR **143:**1096-1097, 1984.
20. Johnson, W.C., Gerzof, S.G., Robbins, A.H., et al.: Treatment of abdominal abscesses: comparative evaluation of operative drainage vs. percutaneous catheter drainage guided by computed tomography or ultrasound, Ann. Surg. **194:**510-520, 1981.
21. DeCosse, J.J., Poulin, T.L., Fox, P.S., et al.: Subphrenic abscesses, Surg. Gynecol. Obstet. **138:**841-846, 1974.
22. Bonfiels-Roberts, E.A., Barone, J.E., and Nealon, T.F.: Treatment of subphrenic abscesses, Surg. Clin. North Am. **55:**1361-1366, 1975.

Chapter Eight

RADIOLOGIC-PATHOLOGIC CORRELATION IN COMPUTED TOMOGRAPHY OF SELECTED GASTROINTESTINAL DISEASES

Louis Engelholm
Jean DeToeuf
Fabienne Rickaert
Marc Zalcman

The following atlas is presented to assist the reader in understanding the gross pathologic correlation of radiologic findings that are present on computed tomograms of gastrointestinal lesions. The atlas correlates findings on in vivo computed tomograms, barium radiography, plain radiographs of air insufflated resected specimens, computed tomograms of air insufflated resected specimens, surgical pathologic specimens, and microscopic sections. Each group of figures represents images from a single patient.

TECHNIQUES

The resection specimens were air insufflated and both proximal and distal ends were clamped. The plain radiographs were then obtained utilizing low kv and ma levels (40 kv, 25 ma), using mamographic film. This allowed for precise correlation with the CT slices.

The CT scans were performed with thin sections and a small field of view using high mas, allowing a more detailed radiograph than possible in vivo.

The gross pathologic specimens were sectioned in the axial plane to provide improved correlation with the CT images.

CT EVALUATION OF BOWEL WALL THICKENING

Air insufflation allows one to evaluate the following parameters on computed tomograms:

1. *The inner border* (luminal surface).
2. *The wall,* which may be thickened either asymmetrically, diffusely, or circumferentially. Furthermore, the thickening may be homogeneous or inhomogeneous (double halo sign). One may observe diverticuli, intramural fistulae, or sinus tracts.
3. *The outer border* (serosa).
4. *Mesentery.* Mesenteric infiltration may occur in diverticulitis, Crohn's disease, or pancreatitis resulting from edema, cellulitis, microabscess, or mesenteric fistulae. Mesenteric infiltration in neoplastic conditions is usually denser than in inflammation. Lymph nodes may be present in both inflammatory and neoplastic conditions.

There is a wide overlap of radiographic findings making precise differentiation of benign from malignant disease impossible in every case. Therefore the radiologist must integrate the varying degree of abnormality reflected in each of these four parameters and offer a differential diagnosis based on the character and predominance of given radiologic findings.

DIVERTICULITIS (Figs. 8-1 and 8-2)

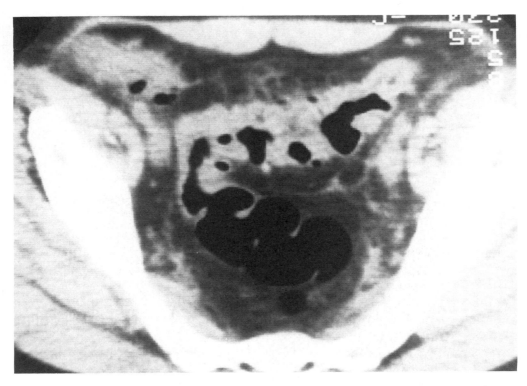

Fig. 8-1. CT scan performed with the patient in a prone position following rectal air insufflation, reveals changes of colonic diverticulosis. The hazy infiltration of the pericolic fat suggests diverticulitis.

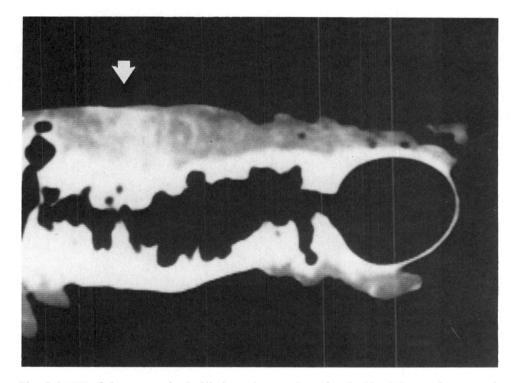

Fig. 8-2. CT of the resected, air-filled specimen oriented as in Fig. 8-1 reveals a smooth inner border and a wall diffusely thickened and penetrated by multiple air-filled diverticuli. There is uniform thickening of the serosa and a focal region of mesenteric infiltration representing an area of pericolic cellulitis *(arrow)*.

DIVERTICULITIS WITH INTRAMURAL
MASS (Figs. 8-3 to 8-6)

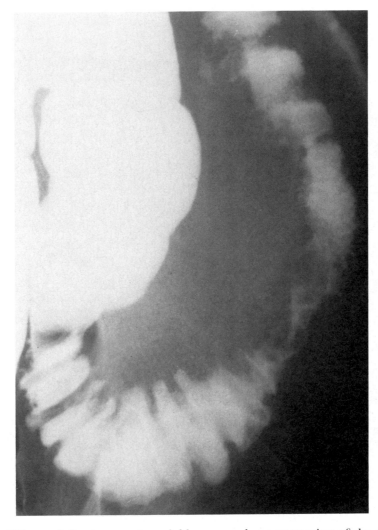

Fig. 8-3. CT scan following a water-soluble enema shows narrowing of the descending colon with nodular compression of the inner border.

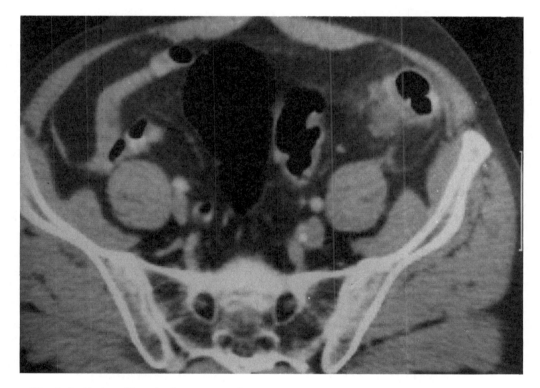

Fig. 8-4. Air insufflated CT scan reveals symmetric thickening of the wall of the descending colon. There is an associated area of increased density along the mesenteric border within the pericolic fat.

DIVERTICULITIS WITH INTRAMURAL MASS—cont'd

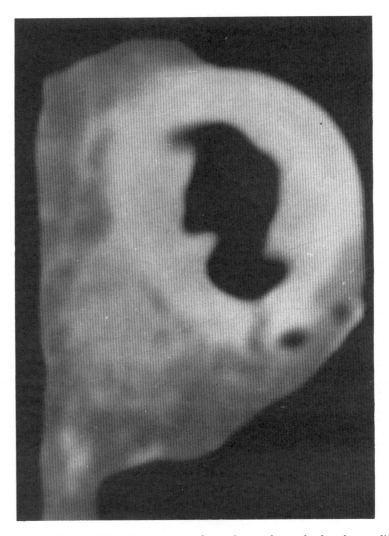

Fig. 8-5. Air insufflated CT of the resected specimen through the descending colon, corresponding to the level seen on the CT scan (Fig. 8-4). The inner border is smooth, and a few enlarged folds are noted. The wall is markedly thickened with a homogeneous appearance. The serosa is poorly marginated, and the mesentery is infiltrated. Notice the region of increased density along the mesenteric border.

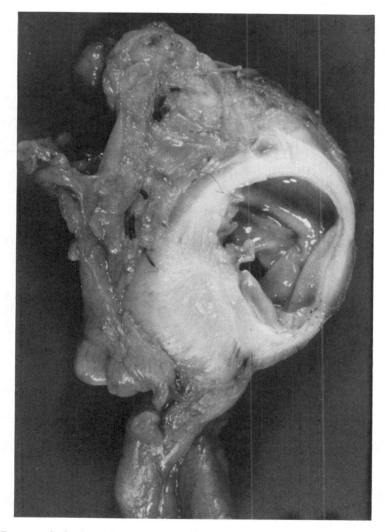

Fig. 8-6. Gross pathologic section corresponding to Figs. 8-4 and 8-5. There are thickened mucosal folds, a thickened wall, and dense mesenteric infiltration. Microscopically, a suppurative process is characterized by polymorphonuclear cells, and granulomas were present. Small microabscesses were also found. This combination suggests acute and chronic diverticulitis.

CROHN'S DISEASE—DOUBLE HALO
SIGN (Figs. 8-7 to 8-9)

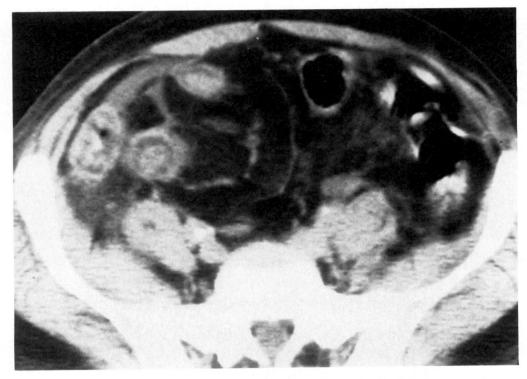

Fig. 8-7. CT of a patient with terminal ileitis. The ileal loops in the right lower quadrant reveal a double halo sign. There is fatty proliferation in the mesentery.

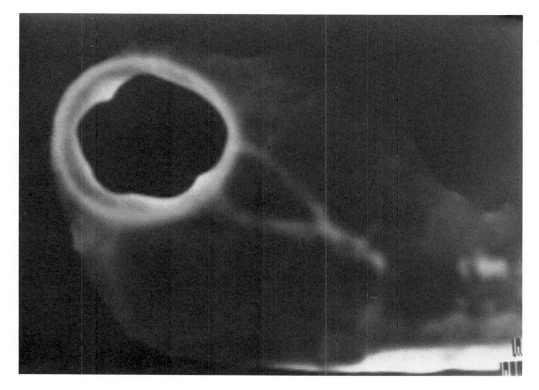

Fig. 8-8. CT of the resected ileum. Three layers are visualized in the bowel wall.

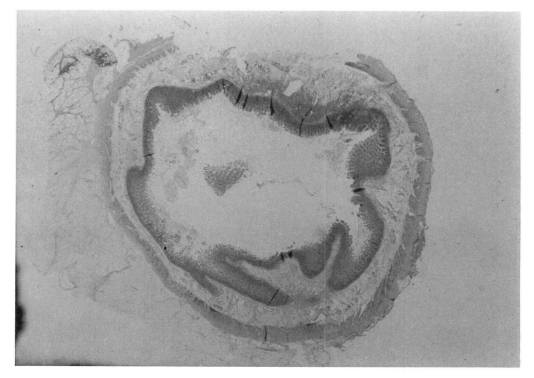

Fig. 8-9. Histologic section of specimen in Fig. 8-9. Three layers, the mucosa, submucosa, and muscularis, are visualized. Notice the widening of the submucosal layer as a result of marked edema.

CROHN'S DISEASE—COLITIS
(Figs. 8-10 to 8-13)

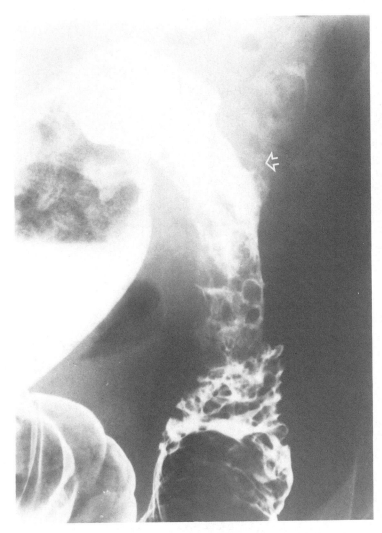

Fig. 8-10. Barium enema reveals a stenotic proximal descending colon. Apparent cobble-stoning is present in the distal aspect of the lesion. Extraluminal, barium filling sinus tracts are seen *(arrow)*.

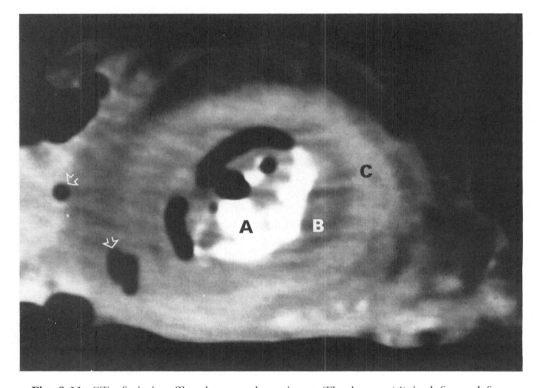

Fig. 8-11. CT of air insufflated resected specimen. The lumen (A) is deformed from multiple soft-tissue masses. There is relative lucency in the submucosa (B). The muscularis (C) is thickened. Notice the extraluminal gas in the bowel wall and mesenteric fat (*open arrow*).

CROHN'S DISEASE—COLITIS—cont'd

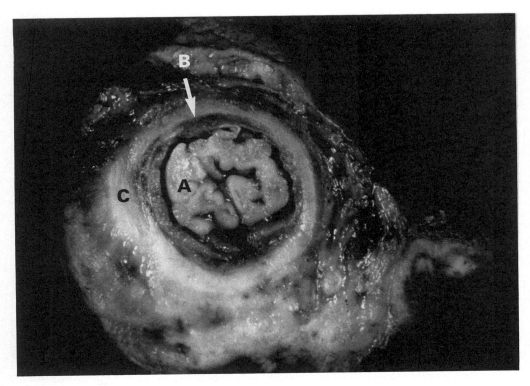

Fig. 8-12. Resected specimen reveals intraluminal pseudopolyps *(A)*, a lucent edematous zone *(B) (arrow)*, and a thickened muscularis *(C)*.

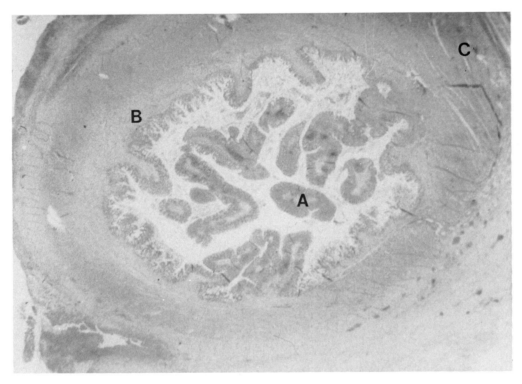

Fig. 8-13. Histologic section reveals the pseudopolyps *(A)*, edematous and fibrotic sub-mucosa *(B)*, and thickened muscularis *(C)*.

CROHN'S DISEASE—FISTULOUS
COMPLICATIONS (Figs. 8-14 to 8-17)

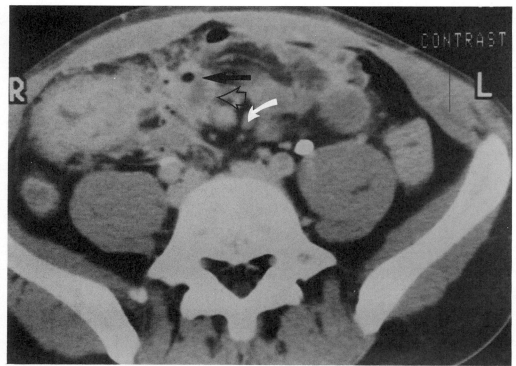

Fig. 8-14. CT scan from a 21-year-old male with Crohn's disease with signs and symptoms of acute abscess. There is marked thickening of the cecum. Mesenteric infiltration and air-filled fistulae are seen *(black arrow)*. An abscess cavity *(open arrow)* is seen below the fistulae. Enlarged regional mesenteric lymph nodes are present *(curved arrow)*.

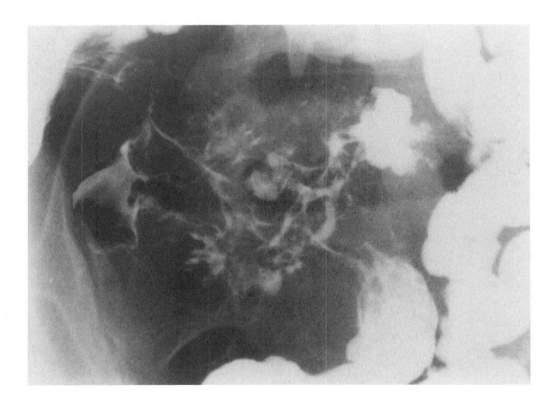

Fig. 8-15. Small bowel follow-through. The terminal ileum is narrowed, and multiple numerous sinus tracts and ileocolic fistulas are filled with barium. Barium also fills a large abscess cavity.

CROHN'S DISEASE—FISTULOUS
COMPLICATIONS—cont'd

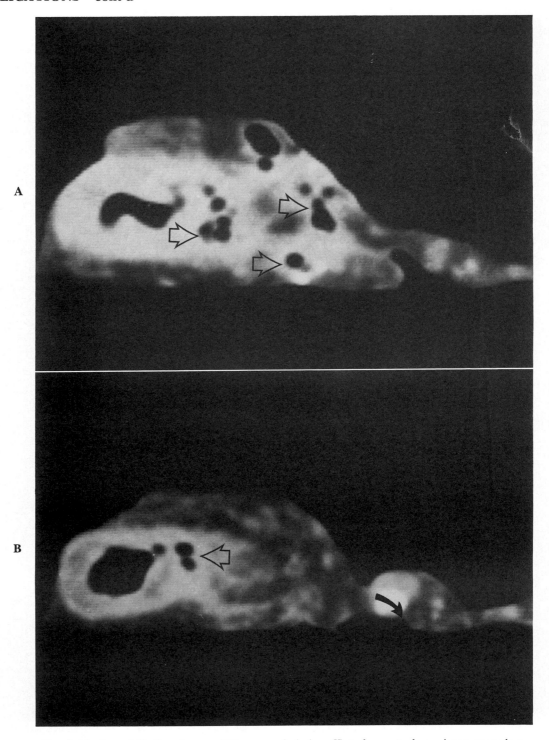

Fig. 8-16. A and **B,** Contiguous CT scans of air insufflated resected specimen reveals a thick-walled cecum. A double halo can be recognized. There is dense mesenteric infiltration. Extraluminal air is seen within the multiple fistulous tracts *(open arrows)*. The enlarged mesenteric lymph node is seen *(curved arrow)*. Fibrofatty sclerolipomatosis is seen in the mesenteric fat.

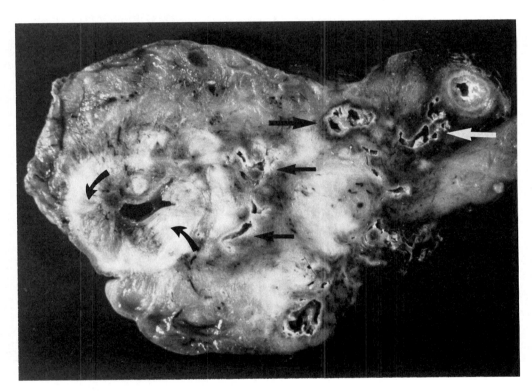

Fig. 8-17. Gross specimen reveals a thickened cecal wall with a double halo appearance *(curved arrow)*. There is dense sclerosis of the mesenteric fat, which appears white. Multiple cleftlike fistulae streak through the fibrofatty mesentery *(black arrows)*. They may be traced to an adjacent ileal loop *(white arrow)*.

COLONIC INVOLVEMENT BY ACUTE
PANCREATITIS (Figs. 8-18 to 8-21)

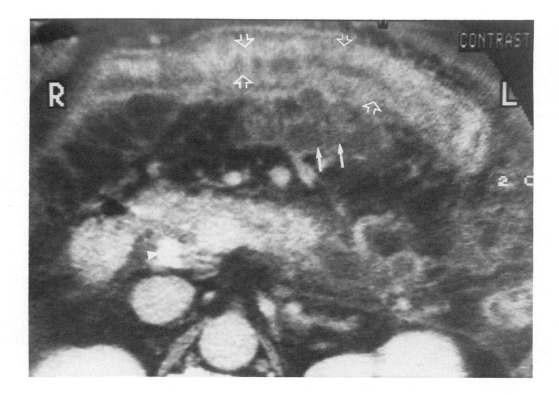

Fig. 8-18. CT section through the transverse mesocolon in a patient with acute pancreatitis reveals calcification in the pancreatic head *(arrowhead)* secondary to long-standing chronic pancreatitis. There is marked infiltration of the transverse mesocolon. Ill-defined fluid collections are seen along the inferior border of the transverse colon *(arrows)*. The colon shows a double halo appearance *(open arrows)*.

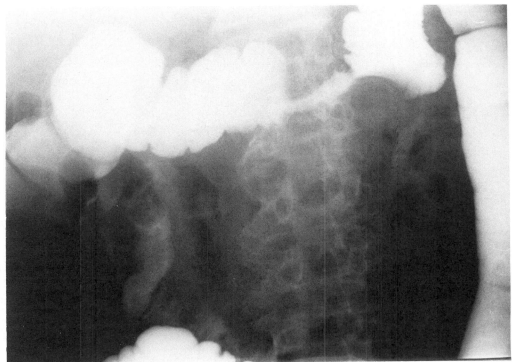

Fig. 8-19. Supine radiograph from barium enema demonstrates narrowing of the distal transverse colon with a smoothly marginated mass effect along the mesenteric border.

COLONIC INVOLVEMENT BY ACUTE PANCREATITIS—cont'd

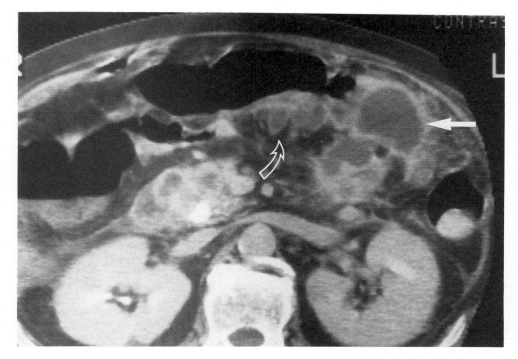

Fig. 8-20. CT scan performed 3 days following that in Fig. 8-18. Air insufflation of the colon reveals large cysts in the mesentery *(arrow)*. Multiple mesenteric fluid collections are seen. Notice the smooth narrowing of the air insufflated transverse colon with a thickened wall (revealing a double halo) along the mesenteric border *(curved arrow)*. The findings of acute and chronic pancreatitis are more evident. The asymmetry of the nephrograms is not apparent on other slices.

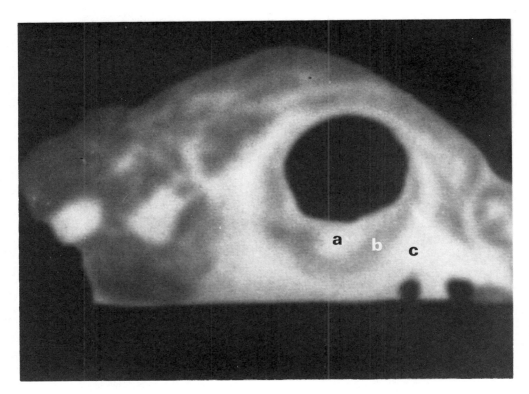

Fig. 8-21. CT of the resected colon reveals a smooth lumen and thickened mucosa *(a)*. An edematous submucosa *(b)* and dense infiltration of the mesentery *(c)* are seen. Notice the double halo effect, which is most pronounced adjacent to the mesenteric inflammatory infiltration and spares the anti mesenteric border.

ADENOCARCINOMA—RECTUM
(Figs. 8-22 to 8-24)

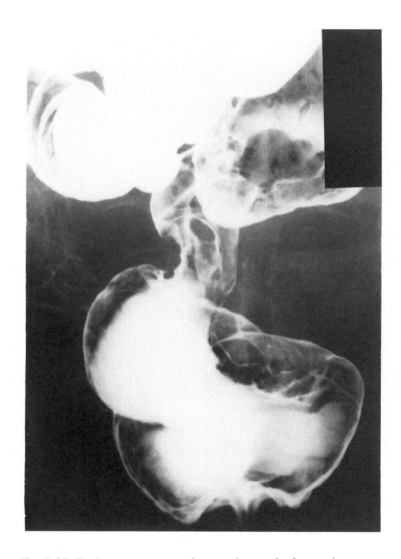

Fig. 8-22. Barium enema reveals stenotic rectal adencarcinoma.

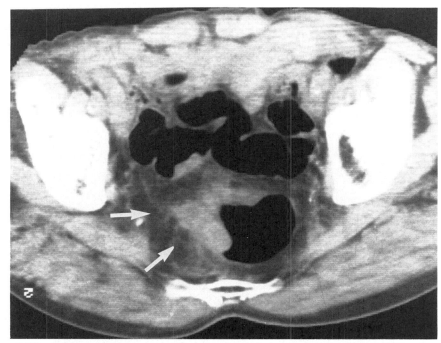

Fig. 8-23. Computed tomogram of the pelvis of the patient in Fig. 8-22 in the prone position. Air insufflation reveals a symmetric thickening of the right side of the rectum with well-defined soft-tissue extension *(arrows)*.

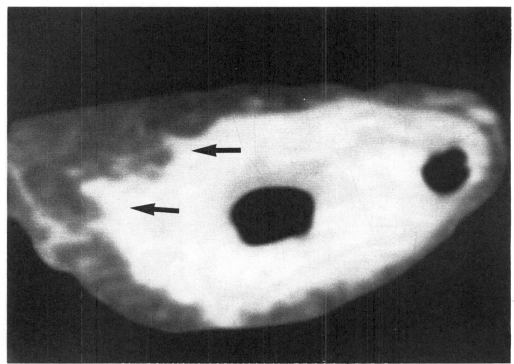

Fig. 8-24. Air insufflated CT section through the midportion of the tumor reveals a greatly thickened wall that is homogeneous. There are well-defined extensions of this process into the perirectal fat *(arrows)*. Compare the appearance of this well-defined neoplastic infiltration of perirectal fat with the less-defined mesenteric infiltration seen in inflammatory conditions. Whereas both processes involve the perivisceral fat and thicken the wall, the degree of thickening, homogeneity of the wall, and better definition seen more frequently in neoplastic disease influence the differential diagnosis.

INVASIVE ADENOCARCINOMA
(Figs. 8-25 to 8-28)

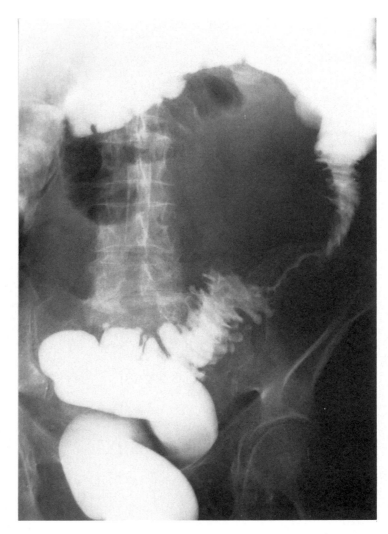

Fig. 8-25. Water-soluble contrast enema performed because of the patient's history of an elevated white count and abdominal tenderness reveals a neoplastic stenosis of the mid-portion of the descending colon.

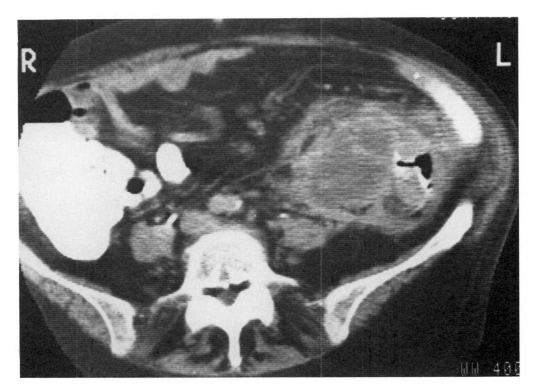

Fig. 8-26. Computed tomogram. The lumen of the air insufflated colon is irregular and ulcerated. There is a well-defined mass that produces irregular thickening of the bowel wall. Adjacent to the ulcerated mass is a larger mixed attenuation mass in the pericolic fat. There is no evidence of fistulization (i.e., no air or barium is seen) from the neoplasm into this mass.

INVASIVE ADENOCARCINOMA—cont'd

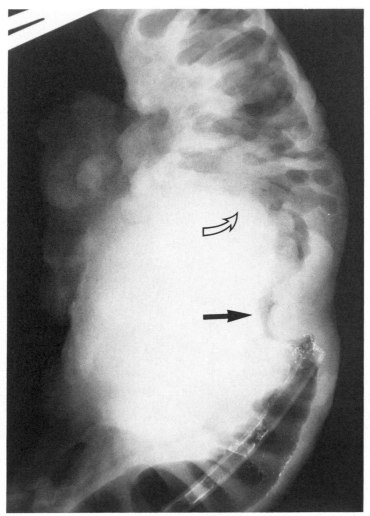

Fig. 8-27. Air insufflated resection specimen. The narrowed lumen is clearly seen *(straight arrow)*. Note the soft-tissue mass along the medial border of the lesion extending into the pericolic fat *(curved arrow)*.

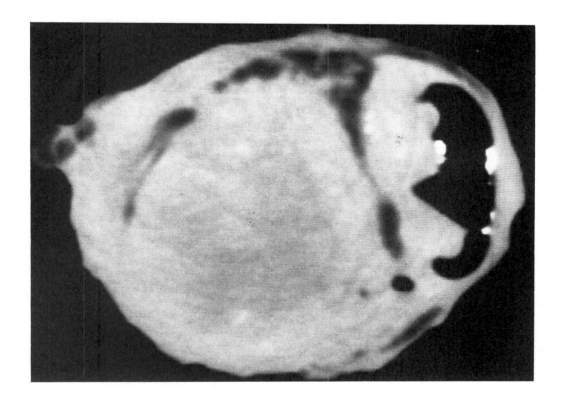

Fig. 8-28. Computed tomogram of the insufflated specimen reveals an irregular lumen with ulceration along the medial border. A well-defined mass thickens the bowel wall and displays a homogeneous attenuation. The larger mass can be identified separated by a cleft of pericolic fat. Serial sections confirmed the direct attachment to the primary tumor. Microscopically, the moderately differentiated adenocarcinoma accounted for all of the findings. The larger mass was predominantly necrotic, accounting for the mixed attenuation appearance on CT.

**ATYPICAL CT APPEARANCE IN
ENDOMETRIOSIS** (Figs. 8-29 and 8-30)

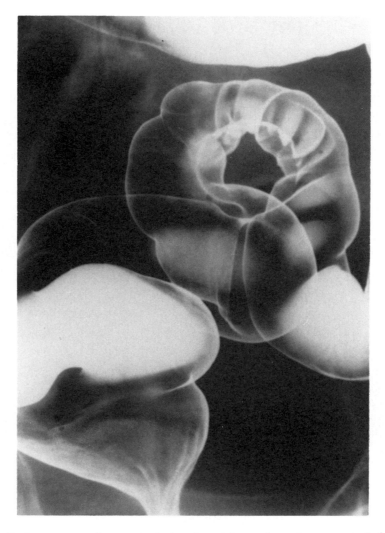

Fig. 8-29. Barium enema shows a typical endometrioma along the mesenteric border of
the sigmoid colon.

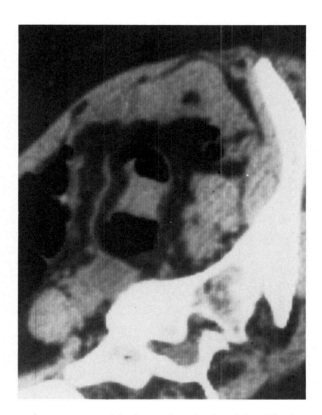

Fig. 8-30. Computed tomogram with the patient in the right-side-down decubitus position and following air insufflation has the appearance of a intraluminal mass with overhanging edges.

**ATYPICAL CT APPEARANCE IN
ENDOMETRIOSIS—cont'd** (Figs. 8-31 and 8-32)

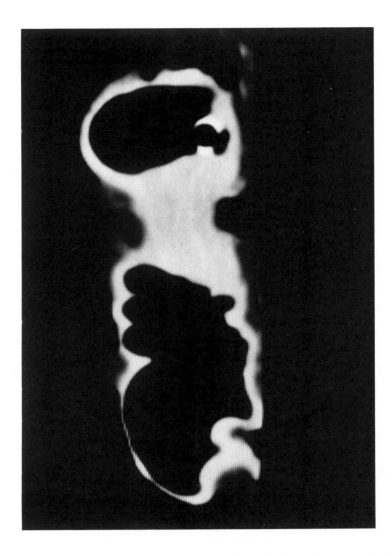

Fig. 8-31. CT of the air insufflated specimen oriented similarly to the CT scan in Fig. 8-32 reveals a dense mass with a retracted outer border.

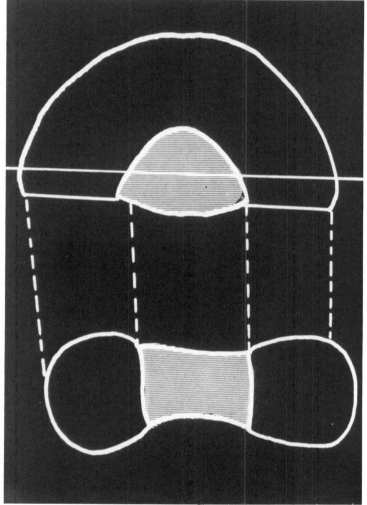

Fig. 8-32. Diagram explains how a predominantly intramural mass might be confused with a intraluminal mass if the inferior margin is included with adjacent normal bowel loops on a cross-sectional CT image.

INDEX

9